European Child Health Services and Systems:

Lessons without borders

The European Observatory on Health Systems and Policies supports and promotes evidence-based health policy-making through comprehensive and rigorous analysis of health systems in Europe. It brings together a wide range of policy-makers, academics and practitioners to analyse trends in health reform, drawing on experience from across Europe to illuminate policy issues.

The European Observatory on Health Systems and Policies is a partnership between the World Health Organization Regional Office for Europe, the Governments of Austria, Belgium, Finland, Ireland, the Netherlands, Norway, Slovenia, Spain, Sweden, the United Kingdom, and the Veneto Region of Italy, the European Commission, the European Investment Bank, the World Bank, UNCAM (French National Union of Health Insurance Funds), the London School of Economics and Political Science, and the London School of Hygiene & Tropical Medicine.

EUROPEAN PAEDIATRIC ASSOCIATION (EPA / UNEPSA)

European Observatory on Health Systems and Policies
a partnership hosted by WHO

European Child Health Services and Systems:

Lessons without borders

Edited by

Ingrid Wolfe and Martin McKee

Mc Graw Hill Education
Open University Press

Open University Press
McGraw-Hill Education
McGraw-Hill House
Shoppenhangers Road
Maidenhead
Berkshire
England
SL6 2QL

email: enquiries@openup.co.uk

world wide web: www.openup.co.uk

and Two Penn Plaza, New York, NY 10121-2289, USA

First published 2013

A catalogue record of this book is available from the British Library

ISBN-13: 978-0-33-526466-7 (pb)
ISBN-10: 0-33-526466-2

Library of Congress Cataloging-in-Publication Data
CIP data applied for

Typesetting by
RefineCatch Limited, Bungay, Suffolk

European Observatory on Health Systems and Policies Series

The European Observatory on Health Systems and Policies is a unique project that builds on the commitment of all its partners to improving health systems:

- World Health Organization Regional Office for Europe
- Government of Austria
- Government of Belgium
- Government of Finland
- Government of Ireland
- Government of the Netherlands
- Government of Norway
- Government of Slovenia
- Government of Spain
- Government of Sweden
- Government of the United Kingdom
- Veneto Region of Italy
- European Commission
- European Investment Bank
- World Bank
- UNCAM
- London School of Economics and Political Science
- London School of Hygiene & Tropical Medicine

The series

The volumes in this series focus on key issues for health policy-making in Europe. Each study explores the conceptual background, outcomes and lessons learned about the development of more equitable, more efficient and more effective health systems in Europe. With this focus, the series seeks to contribute to the evolution of a more evidence based approach to policy formulation in the health sector.

These studies will be important to all those involved in formulating or evaluating national health policies and, in particular, will be of use to health policy-makers and advisers, who are under increasing pressure to rationalize the structure and funding of their health system. Academics and students in the field of health policy will also find this series valuable in seeking to understand better the complex choices that confront the health systems of Europe.

The Observatory supports and promotes evidence-based health policy-making through comprehensive and rigorous analysis of the dynamics of health care systems in Europe.

Series Editors

Josep Figueras is the Director of the European Observatory on Health Systems and Policies, and Head of the European Centre for Health Policy, World Health Organization Regional Office for Europe.

Martin McKee is Director of Research Policy and Head of the London Hub of the European Observatory on Health Systems and Policies. He is Professor of European Public Health at the London School of Hygiene & Tropical Medicine as well as a co-director of the School's European Centre on Health of Societies in Transition.

Elias Mossialos is the Co-director of the European Observatory on Health Systems and Policies. He is Brian Abel-Smith Professor in Health Policy, Department of Social Policy, London School of Economics and Political Science and Director of LSE Health.

Richard B. Saltman is Associate Head of Research Policy and Head of the Atlanta Hub of the European Observatory on Health Systems and Policies. He is Professor of Health Policy and Management at the Rollins School of Public Health, Emory University in Atlanta, Georgia.

Reinhard Busse is Associate Head of Research Policy and Head of the Berlin Hub of the European Observatory on Health Systems and Policies. He is Professor of Health Care Management at the Berlin University of Technology.

European Observatory on Health Systems and Policies Series

Series Editors: Josep Figueras, Martin McKee, Elias Mossialos, Richard B. Saltman and Reinhard Busse

Published titles

Regulating entrepreneurial behaviour in European health care systems
Richard B. Saltman, Reinhard Busse and Elias Mossialos (eds)

Hospitals in a changing Europe
Martin McKee and Judith Healy (eds)

Health care in central Asia
Martin McKee, Judith Healy and Jane Falkingham (eds)

Funding health care: options for Europe
Elias Mossialos, Anna Dixon, Josep Figueras and Joe Kutzin (eds)

Health policy and European Union enlargement
Martin McKee, Laura MacLehose and Ellen Nolte (eds)

Regulating pharmaceuticals in Europe: striving for efficiency, equity and quality
Elias Mossialos, Monique Mrazek and Tom Walley (eds)

Social health insurance systems in western Europe
Richard B. Saltman, Reinhard Busse and Josep Figueras (eds)

Purchasing to improve health systems performance
Josep Figueras, Ray Robinson and Elke Jakubowski (eds)

Human resources for health in Europe
Carl-Ardy Dubois, Martin McKee and Ellen Nolte (eds)

Primary care in the driver's seat
Richard B. Saltman, Ana Rico and Wienke Boerma (eds)

Mental health policy and practice across Europe: the future direction of mental health care
Martin Knapp, David McDaid, Elias Mossialos and Graham Thornicroft (eds)

Decentralization in health care
Richard B. Saltman, Vaida Bankauskaite and Karsten Vrangbæk (eds)

Health systems and the challenge of communicable diseases: experiences from Europe and Latin America
Richard Coker, Rifat Atun and Martin McKee (eds)

Caring for people with chronic conditions: a health system perspective
Ellen Nolte and Martin McKee (eds)

Nordic health care systems: recent reforms and current policy challenges
Jon Magnussen, Karsten Vrangbæk and Richard B. Saltman (eds)

Diagnosis-related groups in Europe: moving towards transparency, efficiency and quality in hospitals
Reinhard Busse, Alexander Geissler, Wilm Quentin and Miriam Wiley (eds)

Migration and health in the European Union
Bernd Rechel, Philipa Mladovsky, Walter Devillé, Barbara Rijks, Roumyana Petrova-Benedict and Martin McKee (eds)

Success and failures of health policy in Europe: four decades of divergent trends and converging challenges

Johan P. Mackenbach and Martin McKee (eds)

Contents

List of contributors

Jasmine Armour-Marshall
Paediatrician, London, United Kingdom

Sven Bremberg
Senior Consultant at the Swedish National Institute of Public Health, Stockholm, Sweden

Ann van den Bruel
Clinical Lecturer, Department of Primary Care Health Sciences, University of Oxford, United Kingdom

Woody Caan
Professorial Fellow of the Royal Society for Public Health

Rose Crowley
Paediatrician, London. Honourary Research Fellow, London School of Hygiene and Tropical Medicine, United Kingdom

Peter Gill
Clinical Researcher, Department of Primary Care Health Sciences, University of Oxford. Honourary Fellow, Centre for Evidence-Based Medicine, United Kingdom

Rittakerttu Kaltia-Heino
Professor of Adolescent Psychiatry, Univeristy of Tampere, Finland

Marina Karanikolos
Research Fellow, European Observatory on Health Systems and Policies, London School of Hygiene and Tropical Medicine, United Kingdom

Sebastian Kraemer
Consultant Child and Adolescent Psychiatrist, Paediatric Department, Whittington Hospital, London, United Kingdom

Simon Lenton
Consultant Community Paediatrician; Chair British Association of Community Child Health, United Kingdom

Martin McKee
Professor of European Public Health, London School of Hygiene and Tropical Medicine, United Kingdom, and European Observatory on Health Systems and Policies

Arja Rimpelä
Professor of Public Health, School of Health Sciences, University of Tampere, Finland; Department of Adolescent Psychiatry, Tampere University Hospital, Finland

Giorgio Tamburlini
Scientific Director, European School for Maternal, Newborn, Child and Adolescent Health, Trieste, Italy; Honorary Consultant, Institute for Maternal and Child Health [IRCCS Burlo Garofolo], Trieste, Italy

June Thoburn
Emeritus Professor of Social Work, Centre for Research on Children and Families, University of East Anglia, Norwich, United Kingdom

Matthew Thompson
Reader in Primary Care, Department of Primary Care Health Sciences, University of Oxford, United Kingdom

Pieter Auke Wiegersma
University Medical Centre Groningen, Department of Health Sciences, Community and Occupational Health. European Public Health Assocation, President Section Child and Adolescent Health, the Netherlands

Ingrid Wolfe
Paediatric Public Health Consultant, Guy's and St Thomas' Hospital, London; Visiting Senior Lecturer, King's College London, Co-Chair British Assocation Child and Adolescent Public Health, United Kingdom

List of tables, figures and boxes

Tables

Figures

Boxes

Foreword

This book should serve as a wake-up call to all those concerned with the well-being of Europe's children, documenting some shocking variations in health outcomes, even among countries that, superficially, seem very similar. It also shows how, despite many opportunities for the exchange of ideas and knowledge, countries have adopted widely varying responses to the health needs of children, with no clear consensus on who should be responsible for their care, in what setting, and using which organizational models.

We in the European Paediatric Association (EPA-UNEPSA) warmly welcome this publication. We have long recognized the scope for Europe to act as a natural laboratory, but only if we have the necessary information on the diversity of models of care and health outcomes. Some of this diversity was already known, not least because of the work we have been doing over the past decade, but this is the first time it has been described so systematically and in so much detail.

This information is essential if we are to realize the aspirations set out by the Council of Europe in their programme for 'Child-Friendly Health Care in Europe', which calls for greater attention to meeting the needs of children in Europe, to maximize their chances of achieving the highest attainable level of mental and physical health and development.

This book makes a strong case for greater cooperation between all caregivers within Europe. This is important for child health, on many levels. First, there is a need for greater sharing of knowledge, on topics ranging all the way from basic sciences to health services organization and health systems policy. Second, there is much greater scope for cooperation among professionals in community, first-contact, and specialist care. Third, there is enormous scope for collaboration on research about children's health and well-being. EPA is contributing to this endeavour by embarking upon a major effort to understand the diversity of children's health care and its impact throughout our 39 Member States.

The European Paediatric Association especially commends this book to our colleagues working in paediatrics and child health across Europe, but we hope that it will also be read by many others, whether they be health professionals whose work brings them into contact with children or those responsible for developing health policy. Our children are our future and it is in our interests that they be enabled to grow into healthy adults who can make the world a better place for us all.

Professor Massimo Pettoello-Mantovani, Secretary General, European Paediatric Association, and Professor Jochen Ehrich, Treasurer, European Paediatric Association

Foreword

In the past few decades the health needs of children have changed beyond recognition. Large hospital wards that were once filled with children with infectious diseases requiring long periods of convalescence have been replaced with smaller units, typically managing short admissions of children with exacerbations of chronic disease. We have seen the creation of new care settings, such as highly specialized neonatal units caring for babies who, even a decade ago, would not have survived; oncology units that have transformed the management of many childhood cancers beyond recognition; specialist genetic teams who are exploiting an explosion of knowledge about the functions of cells; and mental health teams, supporting children struggling to cope in what can sometimes be an uncertain and confusing world.

Yet, despite the enormous magnitude of these changes, the delivery of care and the organizational structures within which services exist have not yet evolved sufficiently to meet the shifting burden of childhood disease and, especially, the growing importance of chronic conditions. The health care of children in many parts of Europe is still being delivered in systems that are based on patterns of illness and of care that prevailed in the early 20th century. As this book shows, this matters. Health outcomes for children vary markedly, as do models of care.

We value the opportunity to learn from the experiences of our European neighbours and for them, in turn, to learn from us where appropriate. We are grateful to the European Observatory, in which we are now partners, for the work that they do to make this possible.

The findings described in this book, and in other recent publications by the editors, have already informed our thinking on the way forward for children, most notably in the 'Report of the Children and Young People's Health Outcomes Forum', whose recommendations we are now taking forward. I am personally committed to this agenda and will be making the health of children a major focus of my next annual report. I commend this book to all those who seek to improve the care of children, wherever they are.

Professor Dame Sally C. Davies, Chief Medical Officer for England

Acknowledgements

The editors would like to thank the authors and all those who contributed their expertise to this volume.

Particular thanks go to: Dr Theo Bodin, for work on constructing the questionnaire survey for this work and for helping to design the project; Professor Michael Rigby, Nordic School of Public Health, Emeritus Professor of Health Information Strategy, Keele University, Adjunct Professor, School of Nursing, Dublin City University, for helpful discussions and constructive comments on the design of the project; Dr Mitch Blair, Consultant Community Paediatrician and Reader, Imperial College London, for informative and helpful discussions and comments; Nick Spencer, Professor Emeritus, Warwick School of Health and Social Studies, for inspiration and contributions to sections on social determinants; Neal Halfon, Director Professor, David Geffen School of Medicine UCLA, Department of Paediatrics, Professor, UCLA Fielding School of Public Health, Department of Health Services and Luskin School of Public Affairs, Department of Public Policy, for contributions, figures and comments; Sir Alasdair Breckenridge, Chairman, Medicines and Healthcare products Regulatory Agency, United Kingdom, for comments; Fliss Murtagh, Consultant and Clinical Senior Lecturer in Palliative Care, Cicely Saunders Institute, London, for contributions on palliative care; Harriet Yudkin, Public Health Practitioner, England, for contributions on public health interventions for young people; Ian Birrell, parent and journalist, London, for insightful contributions about difficult topics; Fiona Price-Kuehne, Staying Positive Programme, for her insights; Maria Ferris, David Wood and Cecily Betz, the International and Interdisciplinary Health Care Transition Research Consortium; Dr Simon Lenton for his contributions on child-friendly health care; Professor Staffan Janson, children's doctor and professor of Social Paediatrics at the Universities of Karlstad and Örebro, for education on child rights and social justice; country respondents to the questionnaire developed for this book; the European Paediatric Association; and the young people who wished to share their experiences of health care to enlighten us and motivate us to do better.

Finally, IW wishes to thank Richard and Isobel for patience, kindness and forbearance during the preparation of this book which was inspired by and is dedicated to them. MM similarly wishes to thank Dorothy, Rebecca and Charlotte.

Abbreviations

AAA	Alcohol Abuse among Adolescents (in Europe)
ADHD	attention-deficit hyperactivity disorder
ADP	Assistenza Domiciliare Pediatrica
ALD	affections de longue durée
ASD	autistic spectrum disorder
BMI	body mass index
BPCA	Best Pharmaceuticals for Children Act
CAMHEE	Child and Adolescent Mental Health in the Expanded European Union
CAMHS	child and adolescent mental health services
CASE	Child and Adolescent Self-harm in Europe
CBT	cognitive behavioural therapy
CCM	Chronic Care Model
CEHAPE	Children's Environment and Health Action Plan for Europe
CFS/ME	chronic fatigue syndrome/myalgic encephalomyelitis
CHE	comprehensive health examination
CHMP	Committee for Medicinal Products for Human Use
CI	confidence interval
DALY	disability adjusted life year
D.A.R.E.	Drug Abuse Resistance Education
DKA	diabetic ketoacidosis
DSM-IV	Diagnostic and Statistical Manual of Mental Disorders
DSS	Department of Social Services
DUP	duration of untreated psychosis

DWCB	disordered weight control behaviour
EAP	European Academy of Paediatrics
EARSS	European Antimicrobial Resistance Surveillance System
ECDC	European Centre for Disease Prevention and Control
ECHI	European Community health indicators
ECHO	European Collaboration for Healthcare Optimization
ECSA	European Child Safety Alliance
EEPP	European Early Promotion Project
ELIA	Emotional Literacy in Action
EMA	European Medicines Agency
Enpr-EMA	European Network of Paediatric Research
ENT	ear, nose and throat
EPA	European Paediatric Association
EU15	pre-2004 European Union countries
EU27	post-2007 European Union countries
EudraCT	European Clinical Trials database
EuTEACH	European Training in Effective Adolescent Care and Health
EWS	early warning system
FDA	Food and Drug Administration
FRESH	Focusing Resources on Effective School Health
GDP	gross domestic product
GP	general practitioner
HBSC	Health Behaviour in School-aged Children
HCPH	health care public health
HDL	high-density lipoprotein
HELENA	Healthy Lifestyle in Europe by Nutrition in Adolescence cross-sectional study
HFA	Health For All
HIV	human immunodeficiency virus
HPS	Health Promoting School
HPV	human papilloma virus
HRQoL	health-related quality of life
HSPR	health systems and policy research
ICD-10	International Classification of Diseases
ICF	International Classification of Functioning, Disability and Health
ISSOP	International Society for Social Pediatrics and Child Health
JSNA	joint strategic needs assessments
KOALA	Kinder Overweight Active Living Action plan
LBW	low birth weight
MEND	Mind, Exercise, Nutrition . . . Do it!
MICE	Medicines Investigation for the Children of Europe
MMR	measles, mumps, rubella
NCD	non-communicable disease
NEET	not in education, employment or training
NGO	non-governmental organization
NICE	National Institute for Health and Care Excellence
NSF	National Service Frameworks

OECD	Organisation for Economic Co-operation and Development
OR	odds ratio
PDCO	Paediatric Committee (of the EMA)
PIP	paediatric investigation plan
PPP	purchasing power parity
PREA	Pediatric Research Equity Act
PRISMA	Reflecting the **P**ositive Dive**R**sities of European Pr**I**orities for Re**S**earch and **M**easurement in End-of-Life C**a**re
PSHE	personal social health education
PUMA	Paediatric Use Marketing Authorisation
QALY	quality adjusted life year
RCPCH	Royal College of Paediatrics and Child Health
RCGP	Royal College of General Practitioners
RCT	randomized controlled trial
SBHC	school-based health centres
SDR	standardized death rate
SEAL	Social and Emotional Aspects of Learnings
SHS	School health services
SIDS	sudden infant death syndrome
SIGN	Scottish Intercollegiate Guidelines Network
SPZ	Social Paediatric Centres (Germany)
SROI	social return on investment
STI	sexually transmitted infection
TEDDY	Task-force in Europe for Drug Development for the Young
TESSy	The European Surveillance System
UNEPSA	Union of National European Paediatric Societies and Associations
WHO	World Health Organization
YHC	youth health care

chapter one

Child health in Europe: an overview

Ingrid Wolfe, Giorgio Tamburlini, Marina Karanikolos, Martin McKee

> The foundations for virtually every aspect of human development – physical, intellectual, and emotional – are laid in early childhood.
>
> *Sir Michael Marmot*

Introduction

Knowledge of how health care is delivered in different countries can test assumptions, offer insights into shared challenges and suggest ways in which services might be organized differently. Cross-country learning offers an opportunity to contribute to improvements needed in health systems to meet the demands of today and to ensure that they are able to respond to the challenges of tomorrow (WHO, 1999).

The boundaries of child health services, for the purposes of this book, encompass the activities, resources and institutions needed to deliver health care. However, since children's health and well-being are shaped by influences beyond health services, these factors will be considered where appropriate, as part of the wider health system. Thus, the World Health Organization (WHO) has defined a health system as comprising 'all organizations, people and actions whose *primary intent* is to promote, restore or maintain health' (Murray and Frenk, 2000). This includes efforts to influence determinants of health as well as more direct health-improving activities. A health system is therefore more than the pyramid of publicly owned facilities that deliver personal health services. It includes, for example, a parent caring for a sick child at home; private providers; behaviour change programmes; vector-control campaigns; health insurance organizations; and occupational health and safety legislation. It also includes intersectoral action by health staff, for example, encouraging the ministry of education to promote female education, a well-known determinant of better health (WHO, 2000). However, while such a definition of a health system is appropriately comprehensive, it is important that health advocates are aware that those from other sectors may not see the improvement of health as their primary intent.

Health systems across Europe are in the process of structural and organizational reform, struggling to meet the needs of their populations and to improve the quality of care they provide, while at the same time seeking to contain upward pressures on costs. Developments in several related areas underlie the drive for reform seen in many countries (Figueras and McKee, 2012). These are: demographic and technological change; the growth of evidence-based medicine; new approaches to quality improvement; recognition of the importance of integrating services; changing professional roles; a renewed focus on disease prevention and health improvement; developments in information technology; and, in some countries, an ideological belief in the role of market forces as an instrument for change. Health system responses to these pressures have been focused primarily on service delivery. Consequently, this book will focus on three key aspects of delivery: service integration and coordination; public health measures; and enhancing the quality of care for children. These aspects feature throughout the chapters, which are based around clinical scenarios.

Aims and methods of this book

Our aim is to increase understanding of child health and health services in Europe, and to present policy options underpinned by evidence from research and real-life experience. A move towards 'health for all', expressed in various terms, has been a widely accepted goal since the 1970s, but this requires health systems to respond to the challenges of changing health needs and social expectations. Many of the changes needed are summed up in the language of the primary care movement. However, health systems still focus disproportionately on hospital services and on short-term process-driven results, which can too easily fragment service delivery and diminish quality. Excessive specialization of health care can discourage a holistic child- and family-centred approach to health, with adverse consequences for continuity of care. Resources are disproportionately allocated for curative and acute services, rather than for primary disease prevention and health promotion, despite evidence that such a public health approach could prevent up to 70% of the disease burden (Fries et al., 1993).

This book deliberately takes a child-centric view on understanding how health services and systems work. Our aim is to contribute towards improving children's health through deepening the understanding of children's health services.

Gathering evidence about complex child health systems, making comparisons, and drawing conclusions is complex and fraught with difficulties. However, insights can be gained and lessons learned from a greater understanding of how other countries have attempted to solve similar problems. This book focuses mainly, although not exclusively, on the western European countries and relies on a combination of primary and secondary research on children's health services and wider child health systems. It draws extensively on a questionnaire distributed to child health leaders (paediatric society presidents and experts in relevant fields) in ten countries: Austria, the United Kingdom, Finland, France, Israel, Italy, Netherlands, Norway, Poland and Sweden. The questionnaire was constructed around clinical scenarios based on presenting complaints, clinical problems or established diagnoses, to gain understanding of how children with problems access and progress through health services in different countries. Each clinical scenario was based on the concept of tracer conditions, an established means of evaluating specific aspects of a health service organization or system (Kessner, Kalk and Singer, 1973; Nolte, McKee and Wait, 2005). Clinical vignettes can help to understand systematic differences in systems, cultures or language (Salomon, Tandon and Murray, 2004), and tracer conditions identify both condition-specific and generic health systems issues. Twelve tracer conditions were selected, each describing the various ways in which families and their children with these conditions negotiate health services. By this means it is possible to capture diverse aspects of each health system, enabling assessment of the ways health systems perform, the challenges involved, and their successes and failures. The tracer conditions formed one section of the questionnaire and three others asked specific questions on aspects of health systems such as the workforce. We obtained further primary data from the European Paediatric Association, WHO Regional Office for Europe databases, Organisation for Economic Co-operation and Development (OECD) and Eurostat. We conducted literature reviews, both systematic and purposive, and obtained further information from government websites and official reports. We also commissioned several case studies from experts.

This book cannot, unfortunately, provide a comprehensive account of European child health systems and services. Rather, we hope to identify common themes that are important contributors to child health, particularly where there are differences between countries that can offer policy-relevant learning points to others. Our selection of countries and examples is necessarily restrictive, and in many places focuses more on medical aspects of care than is fair given the invaluable contribution of nursing, other clinical and non-clinical workforce to children's health care. The choices made throughout this book partly reflect the availability of reliable material and therefore, by definition, include topics and countries that have been studied and written about. This also means that there will undoubtedly be numerous examples of good practice that are not included. By using a questionnaire based on clinical problems, we hoped to avoid confusion about terminology between countries. Health services and systems have unique lexicons in each country and the scope for confusion is great. 'Commissioning', for example, means the purchasing of health care in some countries, while a commissioner can be an ombudsman or advocate in others. 'Private paediatrician' can refer to the location of work (office) or funding model. The language around early years can be confusing too. There are babies, infants, children, adolescents and young people, as well as parents and carers. Inevitably we had to resort to shorthand and so, when we say children, we usually mean the entire spectrum of ages up to adulthood. When we say parents, we include carers.

How children's health needs differ from those of adults

Galen understood that patients explain their concerns, symptoms and pains best in their own words, rather than with a normative medical vocabulary. Indeed, he quoted his patients' words in his writings (Mattern, 2011). This is of course a truism, especially in paediatrics, but while it is a vital element of caring for children, it is often one of its most challenging aspects. Communication with children, including those who are pre-verbal, either directly or through their parents or carers, is one of the distinguishing characteristics of paediatric medicine, although an area that is still poorly understood (Niedel et al., 2012). Likewise, physical examination of children requires an opportunistic, sometimes creative, approach not usually necessary in general adult medicine.

Child health is influenced greatly by the environment and by familial, social and economic factors. Although this has long been recognized, medicine and public health through much of the 20th century focused heavily on technological advancements, with some remarkable successes. However, public health recognizes the diversity of influences on health. Social systems include health, education, political and economic activities that interact and contribute to individual and societal well-being (Figure 1.1). The relative contribution of each element, and the nature of their interactions, varies with age and the child's developmental stage.

Paediatric practice has become increasingly specialized, reflecting both an epidemiological shift in childhood illness, described in this chapter, and technological developments. Chronic diseases and other long-term conditions are increasingly important aspects of child health, while the prevalence and severity of acute illness has declined. At the same time there is insufficient attention paid to the psychosocial aspects of child health and the impact these have on the quality of outcomes of chronic disease care. Social functioning difficulties, behavioural problems and developmental disorders are everyday elements of paediatric practice. These 'new morbidities' of childhood are hardly new, but the term has come to represent a relearning of the importance of the psychosocial dimensions of child health.

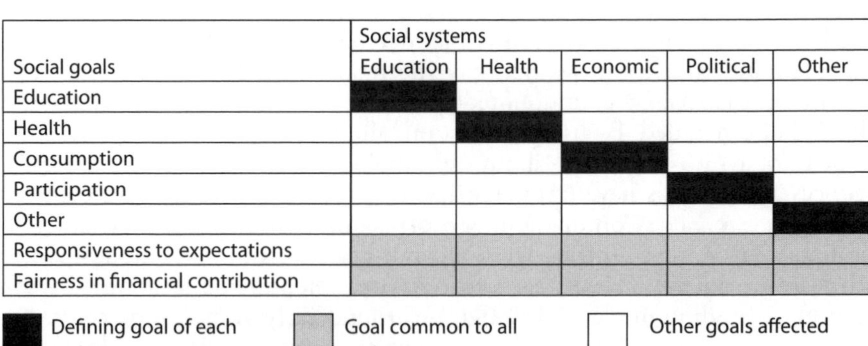

Figure 1.1 Influences on well-being

Source: Murray and Frenk, 2000

Although paediatrics came into its own during the latter half of the 20th century, children's medicine had traditionally been viewed as a subset of adult medicine, which may partly explain why progress lagged behind adult medicine in almost every regard. Children are not small adults. Thus, a representation of the infant Christ in a painting by Giotto from the 14th century is obviously a scaled-down version of an adult body, while one by Raphael, from two centuries later, accurately portrays a child's body proportions. In this example, medicine follows art.

Not only are children not small adults but each stage of early life has distinct concerns, maladies and developmental issues. Thus, we can differentiate preterm newborn infants, term newborn infants (0–28 days), infants and toddlers (>28 days to 23 months), children (2–11 years), and adolescents (12–18 years). Children's health needs change with their developmental stages from infancy to adolescence.

As well as there being many specific diseases of childhood, children can also manifest illnesses differently to adults, in terms of signs and symptoms, rapidity of decline and recovery, and behavioural response. Children also differ from most adults in their dependence on caregivers to seek health care, interpret their problems, administer interventions and communicate their views on the experience of care. Because of this dependence, child protection forms an important part of children's health care.

Finally, children are especially sensitive to the effects of social conditions. Child poverty rates vary between countries, but a very frequent finding among European countries is that the rates of children living in, or at risk of, poverty and social exclusion are greater than the rest of the population, as shown in Table 1.1.

Table 1.1 Population at risk of poverty or social exclusion, 2011

Country or region	*Total (%)*	*Children age 0–17 years (%)*	*Adults age 18–64 years (%)*	*Age 65 and over (%)*
EU27	24.2	27	24.3	20.5
Austria	16.9	19.2	16.2	17.1
Denmark	18.9	16	20.5	16.6
Finland	17.9	16.1	18	19.8
France	19.3	23	20.1	11.5
Germany	19.9	19.9	21.3	15.3
Italy	28.2	32.3	28.4	24.2
Netherlands	15.7	18	17	6.9
Spain	27	30.6	27.2	22.3
Sweden	16.1	15.9	15.4	18.6
United Kingdom	22.7	26.9	21.4	22.7

Source: Eurostat, 2013

Children are uniquely vulnerable, and the policy choices made by European countries have profound effects on their health, well-being and development.

Health policy begins with babies

The Rights of Man, Thomas Paine's call to action, was published in 1791 (Paine, 1985) and Mary Wollstonecraft's *A Vindication of the Rights of Women* in 1792 (Wollstonecraft, 1986). Notable public discourse on the rights of the child, however, was absent.

In nineteenth-century Victorian Britain, children worked in factories, few were educated, and they were not entitled to health care or meaningful legal protection. However, political revolution and economic upheaval in eighteenth-century Europe had laid the groundwork for social welfare movements. Literary illustrations of the poverty and hardship of children's lives, most notably by Charles Dickens (Dickens, 2012), pricked the consciences of powerful British philanthropists and law-makers. Early champions of social medicine, such as Edwin Chadwick (Golding, 2006), Louis-René Villermé (Julia and Valleron, 2011) and Rudolf Virchow (Virchow, 2006), began to describe and explain the importance of poverty and life circumstances to children's lives and health. A legal basis for the protection of children's health and lives began with employment law ensuring that child factory workers had protected rest periods, hygienic living conditions, and rudimentary education and health care. Politics and economics are vital forces that shape children's futures and it is now accepted that health and social welfare are inextricably linked.

Although the discourse on rights began in the 18th century, it was not until 200 years later that the United Nations issued their 'Convention on the Rights of the Child', stating that: 'the child, by reason of his physical and mental immaturity, needs special safeguards and care, including appropriate legal protection, before as well as after birth' (United Nations, 1989). Indeed, a remarkable transformation in European child health has occurred in the past two centuries, largely attributable to social reform and public health legislation rather than to paediatric medicine. The modern era of paediatric medicine began around the middle of the 20th century. Children's health care has advanced exponentially and so the marginal contribution of health care to health has become increasingly important. However, in contrast to children's life circumstances, the rights of the sick child have received little attention. Health services in many countries are largely designed according to adult models of care, and national and international health systems comparisons tend to focus on adult health. Reporting of health care quality concentrates on what is most easily measured, such as waiting times for hip replacements and cataracts. Incentive and remuneration systems focus on diseases of adults. Otherwise excellent national and regional strategies designed for the needs of children, such as 'Every Child Matters' in England and Wales (Department for Education, 2004), and the 'Child Friendly Healthcare' initiative (http://www.cfhiuk.org), are inadequately backed up by the policies and budgets necessary to realize their laudable aims (Chief Secretary to the Treasury, 2003). This is neglect of the rights of the sick child and is an issue of social justice, as poignant as the problems of child poverty in a wealthy world.

The rapid pace of growth and development that characterizes childhood has a profound impact on health and well-being throughout the life-course, so the early years of life represent a golden opportunity to improve the health of a population. Investment in the earliest years will pay the greatest dividends. The United Nations 'Convention on the Rights of the Child' reminds us of the moral imperative to improve children's lives and health. Marmot's work provides us with epidemiological evidence to justify the notion that societies focusing firmly on the early years is in the interests of everyone (Marmot, 2008).

A snapshot of child health in Europe

Child health in Europe has improved dramatically in recent decades, with child survival better than ever. However, there are profound socioeconomic and geographic inequalities in child health and life chances within and between countries. Social inequities in infant and child mortality are consistently reported in all countries (WHO Regional Office for Europe, 2005), and are greater in southern than in northern Europe (Mackenbach, 2006). Social gradients in pregnancy outcomes were described in many European countries up to the early 2000s, and more recent data from Finland, Germany, Italy, Netherlands, Spain, United Kingdom and the Nordic countries confirm these gradients (WHO Regional Office for Europe, 2009). The diseases, disabilities and problems children face are changing; non-communicable diseases (NCDs), long-term conditions and new morbidities have become increasingly important. The role of social determinants in shaping these trends is clearly shown by the unequal distribution of most of these indicators and conditions across social groups. Consequently, child health systems face several new and different challenges, which will require substantial changes. Strengthening child health systems will take years to accomplish and the benefits are likely to be realized well beyond the usual political cycle.

Mortality rates for children in the pre-2004 European Union countries (EU15) have dropped precipitously, and gaps between countries have narrowed for both children in (Figure 1.2) and after (Figure 1.3) the first year of life. However, considerable variation remains, so that many lives could still be saved if all countries achieved the death rates seen in Sweden, the best performing country (Table 1.2).

The reasons for these variations among countries are multiple but they include: national wealth (Figure 1.4) and levels of inequality (Figure 1.5); the proportion and type of social spending (Figures 1.6 and 1.7); and equitable accessibility of high-quality health care (Wolfe et al., 2013).

However, the effects of wealth and inequality can be influenced by political choices. Macroeconomic and fiscal policies deeply influence income distribution and, together with other social protection policies, represent the basis for

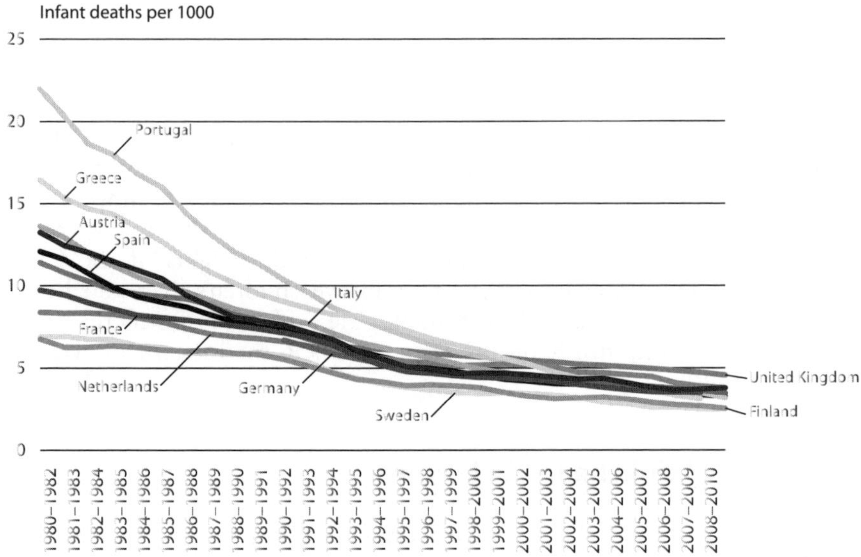

Figure 1.2 Trends in mortality rates, 0–1 year

Source: WHO Regional Office for Europe, 2012

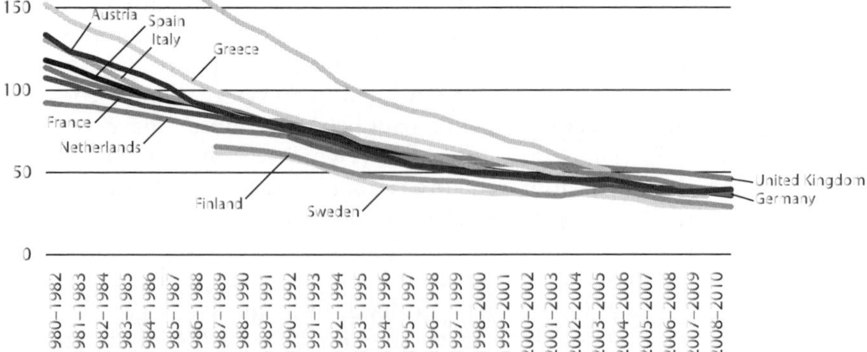

Figure 1.3 Age-standardized child death rates, all causes, per 100,000, 0–14 years (3-year moving averages) in selected EU15 countries

Source: Adapted from Wolfe et al., 2013

Table 1.2 Child mortality rates (0–14 years, all causes, 5-year average) and excess deaths per year (absolute number), compared with Sweden

Country	*Mortality rate (directly standardised) Deaths/100,000*	*Excess deaths compared with Sweden*
Sweden	29.27	0
Luxembourg	26.5	0
Finland	30.27	9
Slovenia	32.06	8
Cyprus	34.75	7
Czech Republic	35.1	89
Spain	37.4	545
Greece	37.86	135
Germany	37.88	815
Italy	38.07	683
France	38.25	962
Austria	39.09	106
Ireland	39.78	98
Netherlands	40.66	292
Portugal	40.73	176
Denmark	42.69	121
United Kingdom	47.73	1951
Belgium	47.77	304
Estonia	52.28	48
Malta	56.16	15
Poland	58.29	1614
Hungary	59.77	418
Lithuania	64.75	173
Slovakia	65.33	287
Latvia	80.92	160
Bulgaria	102.07	731
Romania	116.81	2666
total EU27		**12,412**

* Average for 2006–2010 for all except France, Greece, Hungary and Luxembourg (2005–2009); Denmark 2002–2006; Belgium 1998–1999 and 2004–2006; Italy 2003 and 2006–2009; Portugal 2003 and 2007–2010.

Source: WHO Regional Office for Europe, 2012

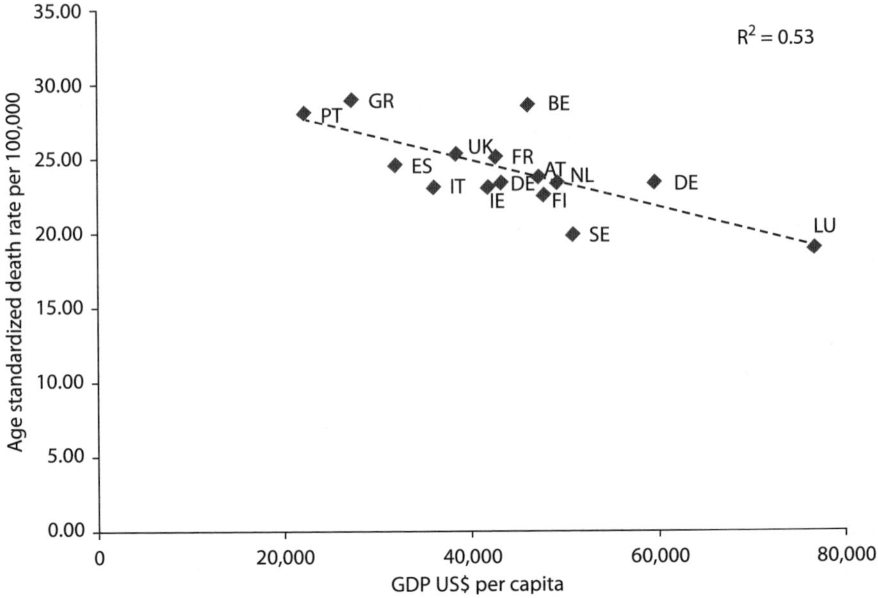

Figure 1.4 Mortality (1–14 years) and GDP

GDP: gross domestic product.

Source: WHO mortality files (updated July 2012); WHO European Health For All database (updated August 2012).
Key: AT Austria; BE Belgium; DE Germany; DK Denmark; ES Spain; FI Finland; FR France; GR Greece; IE Ireland; IT Italy; LU Luxembourg; NL Netherlands; PT Portugal; SE Sweden; UK United Kingdom.

ensuring equitable opportunities to all population groups and throughout all ages.

These associations are important because of the large numbers and high proportions (Table 1.1) of children in Europe living in poverty or material deprivation. However, this is not inevitable. Rates of childhood deprivation are determined substantially by political choices in relation to tax and benefit policies. Thus, as Table 1.3 shows, while both overall rates of deprivation vary considerably, there are also substantial differences within countries as to which groups suffer most. These differences reflect choices about not only the overall level of support for those at greatest risk but also how this is distributed – as direct expenditure on services or as benefits in kind. Denmark and Ireland are among the highest spenders on families and children, as a percentage of gross domestic product (GDP), but Ireland distributes more through cash transfers (benefits) while Denmark spends more on services, as shown in Figure 1.7, or by the priority in defining need that is given to education, employment, or migration status.

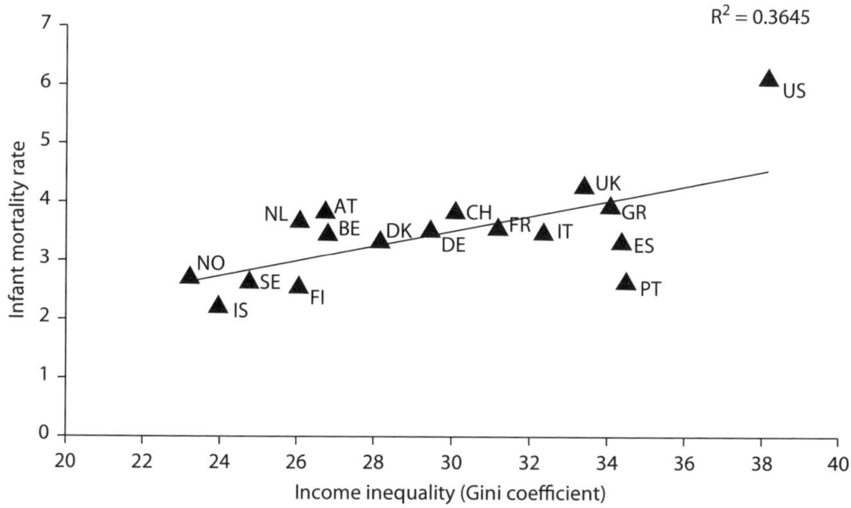

Figure 1.5 The association between infant mortality and income inequality in industrialized countries

Sources: Eurostat; OECD; WHO.
Key: AT Austria; BE Belgium; CH Switzerland, DE Germany; DK Denmark; ES Spain; FI Finland; FR France; GR Greece; IE Ireland; IS Iceland; IT Italy; LU Luxembourg; NL Netherlands; PT Portugal; SE Sweden; UK United Kingdom; US USA.

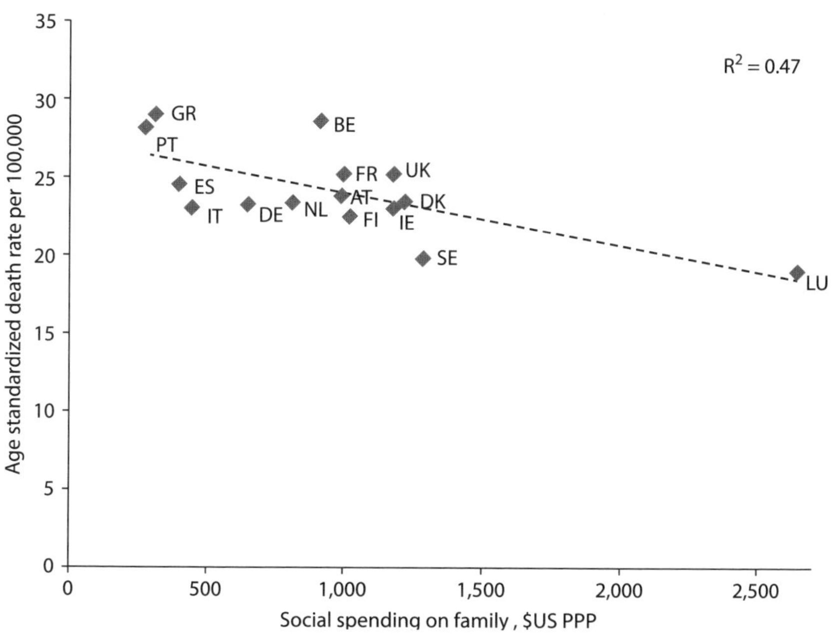

Figure 1.6 Mortality (1–14 years) and social protection spend

PPP: purchasing power parity
Source: WHO mortality files (updated July 2012); OECD.

Table 1.3 Child deprivation (lacking two or more household items) in at-risk groups

	Deprivation rate for children lacking two or more items	*Deprivation rate for children living in single-parent families*	*Deprivation rate for children living in families with low parental education (none, primary and lower secondary)*	*Deprivation rate for children living in households with no adult in paid employment*	*Deprivation rate for children living in migrant families*
Austria	8.7	16.9	19.2	40.7	17.9
Belgium	9.1	20	26.7	40.4	19.6
Bulgaria	56.6	76	89.6	85.2	
Cyprus	7	34.3	22.6	54.1	14.4
Czech Republic	8.8	29.7	59.5	50	18.8
Denmark	2.6	10.1	11.7	23.2	7.9
Estonia	12.4	22.3	29.4	55.5	16.6
Finland	2.5	6.8	2.5	26.2	11.8
France	10.1	21.5	34	45.6	20.5
Germany	8.8	23.8	35.6	42.2	16.7
Greece	17.2	24.3	50.8		42.2
Hungary	31.9	47.3	74.5	64.4	
Iceland	0.9	4.4	3.9	17.9	3.6
Ireland	4.9	13	12	19.4	3.1
Italy	13.3	17.6	27.9	34.3	23.7
Latvia	31.8	50.6	67.6	60.8	28.9
Lithuania	19.8	32.7	54.7	51	31.5
Luxembourg	4.4	23.4	9.9	29.3	5
Malta	8.9	31.2	15.8	38.1	10.1
Netherlands	2.7	14.9	13.8	20.1	7.8
Norway	1.9	4.1	5.9	14.6	3.4
Poland	20.9	42.6	61	46.8	
Portugal	27.4	46.5	37.9	73.6	33.6
Romania	72.6	85.4	92.4	95.8	
Slovakia	19.2	23.1	83.8	78.8	
Slovenia	8.3	17.3	32.9	43.6	15.5
Spain	8.1	15.3	19.2	33.5	19.4
Sweden	1.3	4.3	6.5	11.8	2.7
United Kingdom	5.5	12.2	19.3	13.3	7.4

Source: UNICEF, 2012

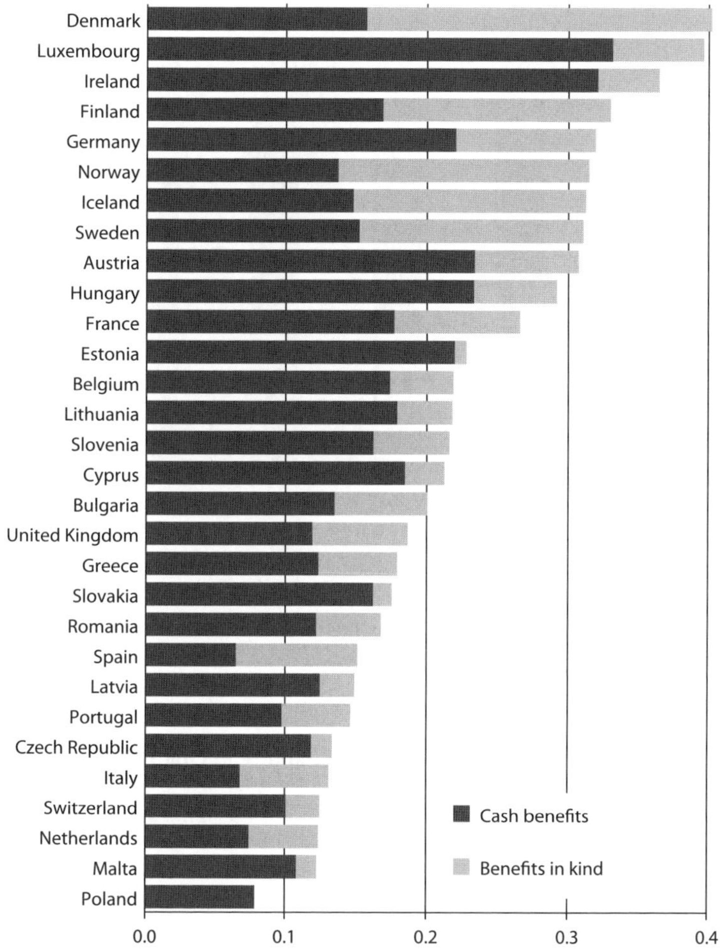

Figure 1.7 Spending on families and children as % of GDP, in the EU, Iceland, Norway and Switzerland, 2010

GDP: gross domestic product
Source: Eurostat data, 2010

The changing burden of disease

More children than ever are surviving, and the diseases and disabilities they suffer from are changing. Just as in the general population, NCDs or chronic conditions (often called long-term conditions in children) are increasingly dominant, while infectious diseases are decreasing in severity and incidence. Non-communicable conditions, such as congenital malformations, cancer and injuries, are responsible for an increasing proportion of childhood deaths (Figure 1.8).

The conditions affecting children's everyday lives are also dominated increasingly by chronic conditions (Table 1.4).

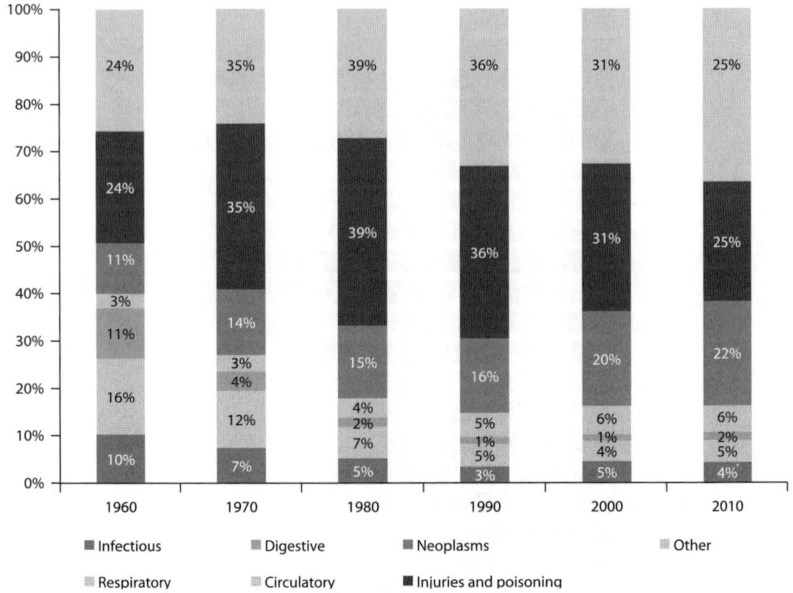

Figure 1.8 The changing causes of deaths (age 1–14 years) in the EU15, 1960–2010

Source: Adapted from Wolfe, 2013

Table 1.4 Overview of trends in disease and disability in children

Disease group	*Incidence (I) or prevalence (P)*	*Temporal trend*	*Comments*
Perinatal conditions, including low birth weight and prematurity	4–11% (<2500g) (I)	↑	Real increase in most countries
Communicable disease	Not applicable	↓	Real decrease in all countries
Congenital malformations	2 per 100 births (I)	↑↓	Increase or decrease depends on type of malformation
Overweight	33%	↑	Real increase over the last two decades
Neurological and developmental disorders	4–5% (P)	↑	Increase partially due to extended and improved diagnostic criteria
Mental health	12–16% (P)	↑	Increase partly due to extended and improved diagnostic criteria
Cancer	14 per 100,000 (0–14 years) (I)	↑	Real increase in all countries
Injuries	Not applicable	↓	Real decrease in all countries

Source: Cattaneo et al., 2012

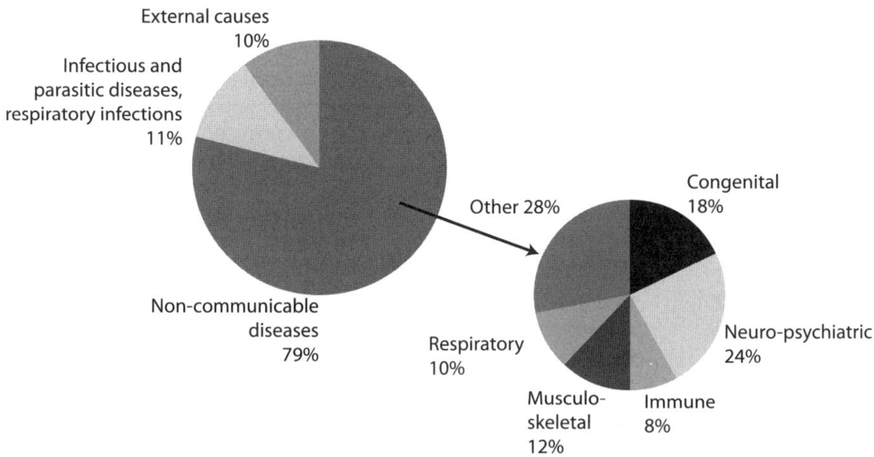

Figure 1.9 Childhood morbidity in western Europe (0–14 years)

Note: *Total DALYs excluding perinatal and maternal causes.
Source: Adapted from Wolfe et al., 2013

More than three-quarters of the total burden of disease, measured as disability adjusted life years (DALYs), for children under 15 years in western Europe is caused by NCDs. The most common causes are neuropsychiatric (largely depression), followed by congenital abnormalities, musculoskeletal disorders and respiratory disease (mostly asthma) (Figure 1.9).

The leading specific causes of DALYs in all age groups within childhood, as shown in Table 1.5 together with their risk factors (which include drug and alcohol use, smoking, and ambient particulate air pollution) are largely preventable.

Social determinants, daily life and demographics

This section complements information on risk factors and disease prevalence presented in other chapters, particularly Chapter 5 on child public health.

Market forces shape economic cycles, and therefore income distribution and employment, and have a profound influence on all health risks and health related behaviours. Socioeconomic status, women's condition, migration, ethnicity, market forces and the media are major distal determinants of child health in Europe. They influence child health and development through complex causal pathways and intermediate determinants, such as nutrition, physical and psychosocial environments, lifestyles and behaviours (Figure 5.2).

Table 1.5 Leading causes of death and DALYs among children in western Europe

Age	*Rank*	*Causes of death*	*Causes of DALYs*
0–6 days	1	preterm birth complications	preterm birth complications
	2	congenital anomalies	congenital anomalies
	3	neonatal encephalopathy	neonatal encephalopathy
	4	neonatal sepsis	neonatal sepsis
	5	lower respiratory tract infection	lower respiratory infections
7–27 days	1	preterm birth complications	preterm birth complications
	2	congenital anomalies	congenital anomalies
	3	neonatal encephalopathy	neonatal encephalopathy
	4	neonatal sepsis	neonatal sepsis
	5	SIDS	SIDS
28 days–1 year	1	congenital anomalies	congenital anomalies
	2	preterm birth complications	preterm birth complications
	3	SIDS	SIDS
	4	neonatal encephalopathy	neonatal encephalopathy
	5	lower respiratory tract infection	sickle cell
1–4 years	1	congenital anomalies	sickle cell
	2	road injury	diarrhoeal disease
	3	drowning	congenital anomalies
	4	leukaemia	eczema
	5	brain cancer	road injury
5–9 years	1	brain cancer	asthma
	2	road injury	major depressive disorder
	3	leukaemia	conduct disorder
	4	congenital anomalies	iron deficiency anaemia
	5	drowning	sickle cell
10–14 years	1	road injury	low back pain
	2	brain cancer	major depressive disorder
	3	leukaemia	asthma
	4	congenital anomalies	anxiety disorders
	5	self-harm	neck pain
15–19 years	1	road injury	low back pain
	2	self-harm	road injury
	3	leukaemia	major depressive disorder
	4	drug use disorders	anxiety disorders
	5	congenital anomalies	neck pain

SIDS: sudden infant death syndrome.
Source: Health Metrics and Evaluation, 2012

The early years of life are particulary vulnerable, in Europe, as elsewhere, so the socioeconomic, psychosocial and physical environments in which children are conceived, born and raised are important especially for their impact on child health outcomes, and for health later in life.

In Europe, poverty among children is 3% higher on average than among the population as a whole (TARKI Social Research Institute, 2010), with a few exceptions which include Denmark, Finland and Germany. This may be because few countries have instituted policies to reduce child poverty rates by income redistribution through tax exemption, child benefits and subsidized services (Bradshaw, 2006). In most EU countries, children living in lone-parent or otherwise vulnerable households and in large families are at an increased risk of living in poverty (UNICEF, 2005), as shown in Table 1.3. Some European countries provide significant financial support to families with children in order to combat child poverty and assist parents with child care responsibilities to help balance jobs and family life.

Socioeconomic gradients in pregnancy outcomes have been described in many European countries (WHO Regional Office for Europe, 2009). Preterm birth (22–32 weeks of gestational age) is 50% higher in the most deprived population quintile in England than in the least deprived (Smith, Allwright and O'Dowd, 2007). A Swedish study found a 49% higher risk of cerebral palsy among children in low-income households compared to those in high-income ones (Hjern and Thorngren-Jerneck, 2008).

Children, particularly those belonging to low-income and migrant households, are more vulnerable to the consequences of economic crises (UNICEF, 2007; UNICEF and Ankara University, 2009) (see Figure 5.3). Many families, particularly those with a lot of children or with disabled members, single-parent families (especially single-mother families) and migrant families, experience a decline in living standards and develop coping strategies, which typically include shifting to cheaper food and reducing expenditure on health and education (UNICEF and Ankara University, 2009). The stress of economic insecurity may add to pre-existing deprivation and psychosocial difficulties and produce a variety of adverse outcomes among children and adolescents, including worsening physical and mental health, intrafamilial violence, child abuse and neglect, all of which may have long-lasting consequences and lead to the reversal of previous gains. For example, the increase in mental health problems among children and young people in Europe, over the 20-year period starting in the early 1980s, has been linked to changes in the labour market for young people (Lager and Bremberg, 2009), a worrying observation since the rates of children living in unemployed households are likely to increase sharply in many European countries in the coming years.

Indirect effects of economic crises may also affect child health. Some countries are reducing public spending severely during the current economic crisis, with health and welfare systems representing prime targets for cuts. These effects combine to increase the risk for the most vulnerable (marginalized and minority groups, households depending on social support if working members become unemployed), by worsening their living conditions, and therefore their health, unless specific counteracting measures are taken to protect those most in need.

Adverse housing conditions, such as crowding, damp housing and living near a road with heavy traffic, have been associated with a lower socioeconomic position in several cross-sectional studies in school beginners (du Prel et al.,

2006; Bolte and Fromme, 2008). Resources like playgrounds and green areas are less common in disadvantaged areas, particularly in cities. Data from Germany indicate that poorer parents felt that they had less access to green spaces (Hornberg and Pauli, 2007).

Despite evidence that social spending in early childhood is likely to be most effective in promoting child development (Engle et al., 2011), very few EU countries (Finland, Hungary, Slovakia) spend a higher percentage of their financial support on families with children in the first years of life (OECD, 2009a) and spending on the middle and late years of childhood prevails in most countries. In all European countries, some form of child care and/or early childhood education is provided; enrolment rates, however, vary widely (OECD, 2009b). For newborn children and those up to the age of 3 years, enrolment exceeds 50% in Denmark but in many other countries, including Austria, the Czech Republic, Greece, Italy and Poland, rates are under 10%.

Maternity leave and maternity benefits play an important role in ensuring optimal pregnancy outcomes, and are offered to pregnant mothers in all European countries. Parental leave after the birth of an infant is offered in all countries but there is wide variation between countries in duration, financial support and flexibility (Pronzato, 2007). While many Nordic countries offer a high or moderate earnings replacement rate, other EU countries provide a more modest allowance or unpaid leave. In many European countries maternal health policies are adequate but there are pockets of underserved communities, essentially minority population groups.

Big differences exist in the status of migrant children depending on: country of origin; reason for and circumstances of migration; years spent in the host country; legal status; the legislation of the host country. Pregnancy outcomes differ between migrant women and native-born women in Europe. A review of 65 studies spanning nearly 40 years to 2004 found that migrant women have a 43% greater risk of having a baby with low birth weight, a 24% higher risk of a preterm delivery, a 50% higher risk of perinatal mortality and a 61% greater risk of congenital malformations (Bollini et al., 2009). Roma children are especially at risk, with higher rates of low birth weight and preterm birth (Hajioff and McKee, 2000). Migrant children are particularly dependent on their parents' ability to support them in adapting to their new environment. Unfortunately, migrant parents may suffer from poor mental health themselves, due to the many stressors and risks linked to the migration experience. Changing patterns of migration and a shift in attitude and policies in many EU countries are increasing the health risks of many migrating groups and particularly those of women and children. Depending on the host country's legislation and prevailing attitudes towards migrant people, migrant children may be subjected to discrimination based on nationality, origin, gender and religion. Those whose parents hold an illegal status are exposed to a combination of risks, including poverty, stress and lack of access to services. There are around 1000 children every year who enter the United Kingdom seeking asylum but are detained in immigration removal centres. Many of these children suffer mental health difficulties, including depression and suicidal behaviour; physical health problems such as weight loss; and inadequate pain relief for conditions such as sickle cell disease. Their care has been described as falling below the standards expected by the National Health Service, and as appalling failures in the duty of care to vulnerable children (UK Royal Medical Colleges, undated The Lancet, 2008).

The structure of family life has an important impact on children's health and well-being, as does parental educational achievement and employment (Bramlett and Blumberg, 2007). While women's education has improved over recent decades, their employment prospects, salaries and career opportunities lag behind those of men in most European countries. Women's status (education, role in society and within the family) has an important influence on child health and well-being, starting from reproductive behaviours and consequent reproductive outcomes, leading to long-term and even intergenerational effects (WHO Regional Office for Europe, 2005). Where women have a higher social status and more central role in decision-making, greater resources (at both public and household levels) tend to be directed towards child nutrition, welfare and education, ultimately contributing to child health outcomes (WHO Regional Office for Europe, 2005). Children from single-parent families may have a lower sense of well-being and worse educational outcomes, although of course there are many exceptions. For example, in the United States, the risk of developing behavioural problems, of having to repeat school years or leave school prematurely, are twice as high among single-parent families as in two-parent families, while the risk of teenage pregnancy is increased six-fold. However, approximately half of these differences can be attributed to the greater risk of poverty after family breakdown (McLanahan and Sandefur, 1994). Countries can protect children and families from some of these harmful outcomes. For example social protection policy can specifically help (or not) children from single-parent families. Thus, while there are more single-parent households in Sweden than in the United Kingdom, for example, there are many fewer Swedish children from otherwise vulnerable families live in poverty (See Table 1.3).

The quality of family and peer relationships is vital to child development, and the nature and structure of family life are changing. For example, it is much more common now for babies to be born to unmarried parents. In 1975, 8% of births were to single mothers, but by 2005, 35% of births were outside wedlock – although of course this does not always imply social instability or risk of poverty (European Commission, 2008). Divorce is also much more common; among children aged between 11 and 15 years, between 9% and 16% live in lone-parent households and so are at increased risk of poverty, while up to 14% live with step-parents (OECD, 2009a). Family cohesiveness, structure and functioning are important for many reasons (Sturge-Apple, Davies and Cummings, 2010), not least because maternal depression and paternal involvement affect child development (Sarkadi et al., 2008).

The Health Behaviour in School-aged Children (HBSC) study tracks progress throughout Europe, and some of its findings are causes for concern (Currie et al., 2012). For example, the survey measures the proportion of children who find it easy to talk to their mothers, since parental communication is an important protective factor for children and is associated with higher self-rated health, not smoking and higher life satisfaction (Pederson, 2004; Fenton et al., 2010). In almost all countries, the proportion of children who find it easy to talk to their mothers declines as they grow older, but the decline is faster in more deprived families and in northern Europe. Relationships with peers are also important for social development and are thought to protect against depression and isolation as friendship is associated with higher levels of well-being and happiness (Berndt, 1996; Zambon et al., 2010). Prevalence of close friendships reduces with age between 11 and 15 years, and again family wealth is important as it is associated with having more close friends. Electronic media use has become a common feature of childhood throughout Europe, and although there are benefits, there are also risks. Cyber-bullying is one, and excessive use of electronic media is associated with poorer self-reported health and engaging in risk-taking behaviour (Leena, Tomi and Arja, 2005; David-Ferdon and Hertz, 2007).

School is work for children. As such, the majority of children's daily lives are spent at school and with school friends; both are strong influences on development and well-being (Bradshaw, 2011), affecting health behaviour, such as the likelihood of taking up smoking (Williams et al., 2009). The HBSC survey looked at self-reported health among children and young people and found that, while most believe themselves to be in good health, there are some notable differences. Girls consistently report poorer health, lower life satisfaction and more dissatisfaction with body image. These are complex findings to interpret, since self-perceived health and well-being are, for example, closely associated with family and peer relationships. Risk-taking behaviours among children and young people are important, not least because they affect the likelihood of developing common chronic diseases that affect people later in life (such as diabetes, cardiovascular and respiratory disease) but also because, as discussed earlier, young people also increasingly suffer from chronic diseases.

The prevalence of obesity among children and young people in Europe is increasing, reflecting a complex interplay of factors culminating in an obesogenic environment in which it is easier to become overweight or obese than it is to maintain a healthy weight (Chow et al., 2009). Approximately 24% of schoolchildren between 6 to 9 years old are overweight or obese (Cattaneo et al., 2012) (see Chapter 5).

Tobacco use remains one of the main causes of disability and premature mortality worldwide (Lim et al., 2012), and is especially important in this discussion because for most people smoking begins in adolescence (Jarvis, 2004). Likelihood of smoking is associated with family breakdown, parental smoking and low family cohesion; conversely, strong family relationships and positive peer and friend relationships are protective. Boys are more likely to smoke than girls, generally. As with many risk behaviours there is an association with socioeconomic status. This also applies to exposure to environmental tobacco smoke. Social disadvantage is associated with more frequent prenatal and postnatal exposure (Bolte and Fromme, 2008), consistently across several countries. Tobacco use in pregnancy affects fetal development, and may also increase the risk of intrauterine growth retardation, low birth weight, and preterm birth (Tamburlini, von Ehrenstein and Bertollini, 2002).

Alcohol is responsible for 11% of deaths in men, and although a lower percentage of women die from alcohol (1.8%), there are other profound effects on women which either directly or indirectly affect children (WHO, 2009):

for example, drinking alcohol through pregnancy causing fetal alcohol syndrome; poverty; intimate partner violence; family breakdown (Cattaneo et al., 2012). The prevalence of alcohol use increases significantly through adolescence, in almost all countries, and in general boys drink more often and get drunk more often than girls, although the differences are narrowing rapidly in many countries. There is a less strong association with affluence, but family environment does affect the likelihood of alcohol use (Currie et al., 2012).

Early-onset sexual activity is associated with teenage pregnancy and sexually transmitted infection (STI). Age of beginning sexual activity is reducing throughout Europe and the prevalence of STIs is increasing accordingly. Over a quarter of 15-year-olds surveyed by HBSC have had sexual intercourse, with wide variation between countries – ranging from 2% (girls in Armenia) and 71% (girls in Greenland) (Currie et al., 2012). There is also significant variation in condom use. This variation, as in other risk areas, suggests scope for intervention.

Crucially, many of the problems discussed in this section, and in further detail in Chapter 5 on child public health, are amenable to intervention and policy, as will be discussed in subsequent chapters in this book.

Finally, the number of children in Europe is slowly decreasing (Figure 1.10), as is the proportion of young people in the population, with a corresponding increase in elderly people throughout Europe. Policy-makers often describe this as a demographic time-bomb. The resulting debate usually focuses on who will pay for pensions and who will care for the elderly. Yet there is a greater risk that, as the child population decreases in relative terms, the voices of children and young people will be even harder to hear among the clamour for steadily diminishing funds for health and social care.

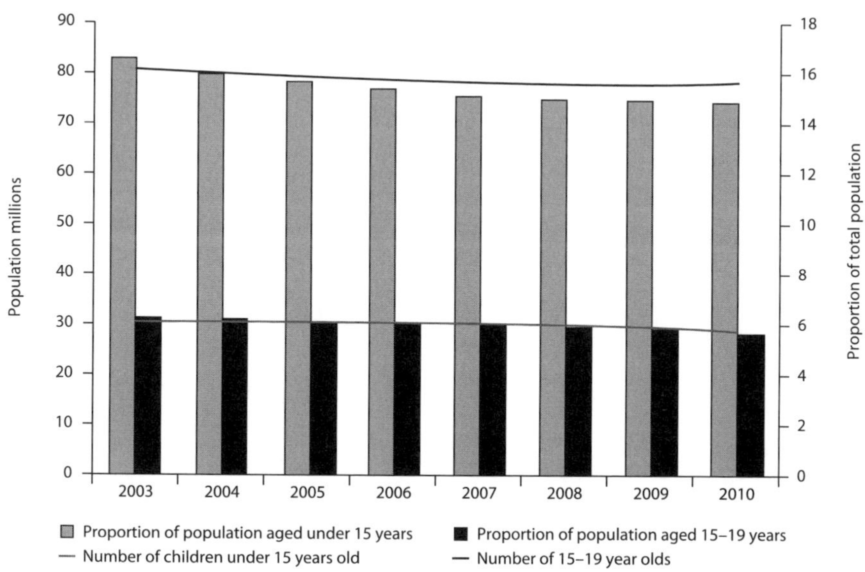

Figure 1.10 Child and adolescent population trends in the EU27

Source: Eurostat; WHO, 2013

Child health and health services policy in Europe

Child health systems in Europe need to meet the changing health needs that have been described in this chapter. Moreover, the pattern of demand for services is changing, with school and parental work demands, and also the 24/7 consumer culture that is increasingly promoted in some countries such as the United Kingdom. There is a strong policy imperative to improve effectiveness and efficiency of care, while competing for resources with other sectors. New solutions to health service problems are needed, which may require service redesign, innovative service models, technology and infrastructure. European countries need to find solutions to common pressures. Although there is a great deal of knowledge about health systems and services, what is less well understood is how (and how well) these deliver care for people. Even less is known about how health services and systems work for children. In most countries, children's services have developed as an 'add-on' to adult services. The same often applies to health policy responses to pressures and changing needs. It is becoming increasingly clear that this must change. Children's medicine was once a subset of adult health care, which was reasonable when medicine was rudimentary, but children's health needs are now recognized as being distinct from adults, with children's health care having become a sophisticated specialty with a discrete knowledge base. However, despite this progress and substantial changes in the burden of childhood disease, health services have failed to adapt adequately. Health systems still prioritize acute services for patients needing admission to hospital over care for long-term illness and disability, and health service planning and evaluation for children, which has distinct differences from that for adults, is still largely based on adult models of care (Forrest, Simpson and Clancy, 1997).

The 21st century should be the era when children's health care in Europe comes into its own and is fully recognized as distinctly different from health care for adults, requiring different methods for planning, training, delivery and evaluation. We hope that this book makes a small contribution towards that goal.

Acknowledgement

We are grateful to Professor Emeritus Nick Spencer (Warwick School of Health and Social Studies) for contributions to the sections on social determinants.

References

Berndt, T. (1996) Transitions in friendship and friends' influence. In: Graber, J. (ed.) *Transition through adolescence: Interpersonal domains and context*. Mahwah, NJ: Erlbaum.

Bollini, P. et al. (2009) Pregnancy outcome of migrant women and integration policy: a systematic review of the international literature, *Social Science and Medicine*, 68(3): 452–61.

Bolte, G. and Fromme, H. for the GME Study Group (2008) Umweltgerechtigkeit als Themenschwerpunkt der Gesundheits-Monitoring-Einheiten (GME) in Bayern [Environmental justice as a main topic of the health monitoring units in Bavaria, Germany], *UmweltMedizinischer InformationsDienst*, 2: 39–42.

Bradshaw, J. (2006) *A review of the comparative evidence on child poverty*. York: University of York.

Bradshaw, J. (2011) Trends in child subjective wellbeing in the UK, *Journal of Children's Services*, 6: 4–17.

Bramlett, M.D. and Blumberg, S.J. (2007) Family structure and children's physical and mental health. *Health Affairs (Millwood)*, 269(2): 549–58.

Cattaneo, A. et al. (2012) *Child health in the European Union*. Luxembourg: European Commission.

Chief Secretary to the Treasury (2003) *Every child matters*. Norwich: Her Majesty's Stationery Office.

Chow, C.K. et al. (2009) Environmental and societal influences acting on cardiovascular risk factors and disease at a population level: a review, *International Journal of Epidemiology*, 38(6): 1580–94.

Currie, C. et al. (eds) (2012) *Health Policy for Children and Adolescents, No 6. Social determinants of health and well-being among young people. Health Behaviour in School-aged Children (HBSC) study. International Report from the 2009–10 Survey*. Copenhagen: WHO Regional Office for Europe.

David-Ferdon, C. and Hertz, M.F. (2007) Electronic media, violence, and adolescents: an emerging public health problem, *Journal of Adolescent Health*, 41(6 Suppl 1): S1–5.

Department for Education (2004) *Every child matters: Change for children*. London: HM Government.

Dickens, C. (2012) *Oliver Twist*. London: Penguin English Library.

du Prel, X. et al. (2006) Preschool children's health and its association with parental education and individual living conditions in East and West Germany, *BMC Public Health*, 6: 312.

Engle, P.L. et al. (2011) Strategies for reducing inequalities and improving developmental outcomes for young children in low-income and middle-income countries, *The Lancet*, 378(9799): 1339–53.

European Commission (2008) *Demography Report 2008: Meeting social needs in an ageing society*. Brussels: European Commission.

Eurostat (2013) Children at risk of poverty or social exclusion. Statistics in Focus 4/2013. European Commission, Eurostat. http://epp.eurostat.ec.europa.eu/statistics_explained/index.php/Children_at_risk_of_poverty_or_social_exclusion and http://appsso.eurostat.ec.europa.eu/nui/show.do?dataset=ilc_peps01&lang=en

Fenton, C. et al. (2010) Sustaining a positive body image in adolescence: an assets-based analysis, *Health and Social Care in the Community*, 18(2): 189–98.

Figueras, J. and McKee, M. (2012) *Health systems, health, wealth and societal well-being: Assessing the case for investing in health systems*. Maidenhead: McGraw-Hill/Open University Press.

Forrest, C.B., Simpson, L. and Clancy, C. (1997) Child health services research. Challenges and opportunities, *JAMA*, 277(22): 1787–93.

Fries, J.F. et al. (1993) Reducing health care costs by reducing the need and demand for medical services. The Health Project Consortium, *New England Journal of Medicine*, 329(5): 321–5.

Golding, A.M. (2006) Sir Edwin Chadwick and inequalities, *Public Health*, 120(5): 474–6.

Hajioff, S. and McKee, M. (2000) The health of the Roma people: a review of the published literature, *Journal of Epidemiology and Community Health*, 54(11): 864–9.

Health Metrics and Evaluation (2012) *Global Burden of Disease 2010: leading causes and risks by region heat map.* http://www.healthmetricsandevaluation.org/gbd/visualizations/gbd-2010-leading-causes-and-risks-region-heat-map [accessed 22 June 2013].

Hjern, A. and Thorngren-Jerneck, K. (2008) Perinatal complications and socio-economic differences in cerebral palsy in Sweden – a national cohort study, *BMC Pediatrics*, 8: 49.

Hornberg, C. and Pauli, A. (2007) Child poverty and environmental justice, *International Journal of Hygiene and Environmental Health*, 210(5): 571–80.

Jarvis, M.J. (2004) Why people smoke, *BMJ*, 328(7434): 277–9.

Julia, C. and Valleron, A.J. (2011) Louis-Rene Villerme (1782–1863), a pioneer in social epidemiology: re-analysis of his data on comparative mortality in Paris in the early 19th century, *Journal of Epidemiology and Community Health*, 65(8): 666–70.

Kessner, D.M., Kalk, C.E. and Singer, J. (1973) Assessing health quality – the case for tracers, *New England Journal of Medicine*, 288(4): 189–94.

Lager, A.C. and Bremberg, S.G. (2009) Association between labour market trends and trends in young people's mental health in ten European countries 1983–2005, *BMC Public Health*, 9: 325.

Leena, K., Tomi, L. and Arja, R.R. (2005) Intensity of mobile phone use and health compromising behaviours – how is information and communication technology connected to health-related lifestyle in adolescence? *Journal of Adolescence*, 28(1): 35–47.

Lim, S.S. et al. (2012) A comparative risk assessment of burden of disease and injury attributable to 67 risk factors and risk factor clusters in 21 regions, 1990–2010: a systematic analysis for the Global Burden of Disease Study 2010, *The Lancet*, 380(9859): 2224–60.

Mackenbach, J.P. (2006) *Health Inequalities: Europe in profile. An independent, expert report commissioned by the UK Presidency of the EU.* Rotterdam: Erasmus MC, University Medical Center Rotterdam.

Marmot, M. (2008) *Closing the gap in a generation: Health equity through action on the social determinants of health.* Geneva: World Health Organization.

Mattern, S. (2011) Galen and his patients, *The Lancet*, 378(9790): 478–9.

McLanahan, S. and Sandefur, G.D. (1994) *Growing up with a single parent: What hurts, what helps.* Cambridge, MA: Harvard University Press.

Murray, C.J. and Frenk, J. (2000) A framework for assessing the performance of health systems, *Bulletin of the World Health Organization*, 78(6): 717–31.

Niedel, S. et al. (2013) Parallel vigilance: Parents' dual focus following diagnosis of Type 1 diabetes mellitus in their young child. *Health (London)*, 17(3): 246–65.

Nolte, E., McKee, M. and Wait, S. (2005) Describing and evaluating health systems. In: Bowling, A. and Ebrahim, S. (eds.) *Handbook of health research methods: Investigation, measurement and analysis.* Maidenhead: McGraw-Hill/Open University Press.

OECD (2009a) *Doing better for children.* Paris: Organisation for Economic Cooperation and Development.

OECD (2009b) *Education today: The OECD perspective.* Paris: Organisation for Economic Cooperation and Development.

Paine, T. (1985) *Rights of man.* New York: Penguin Books.

Pederson, M. (2004) Family and health. In: Currie, C. et al. (eds) *Health Policy for Children and Adolescents, No. 4: Young people's health in context. Health Behaviour in School-aged Children (HBSC) study: international report from the 2001/02 survey.* Copenhagen: WHO Regional Office for Europe.

Pronzato, C. (2007) *Return to work after childbirth: Does parental leave matter in Europe?* ISER Working Paper 2007–30. Colchester: Institute for Social and Economic Research, University of Essex.

Salomon, J.A., Tandon, A. and Murray, C.J. (2004) Comparability of self rated health: cross sectional multi-country survey using anchoring vignettes, *BMJ*, 328: 258.

Sarkadi, A. et al. (2008) Fathers' involvement and children's developmental outcomes: a systematic review of longitudinal studies, *Acta Paediatrica*, 97(2): 153–8.

Smith, S.M., Allwright, S. and O'Dowd, T. (2007) Effectiveness of shared care across the interface between primary and specialty care in chronic disease management, *Cochrane Database of Systematic Reviews*, CD004910.

Sturge-Apple, M.L., Davies, P.T. and Cummings, E.M. (2010) Typologies of family functioning and children's adjustment during the early school years, *Child Development*, 81(4): 1320–35.

Tamburlini, G., Von Ehrenstein, O.S. and Bertollini, R. (eds) (2002) *Children's health and the environment: A review of the evidence*. Copenhagen: European Environment Agency and WHO Regional Office for Europe.

TARKI Social Research Institute (2010) *Child poverty and child well-being in the European Union. Report for the European Commission DG Employment, Social Affairs and Equal Opportunities Unit E2*. Budapest: TARKI Social Research Institute.

The Lancet (2008) Health care for children in UK detention centres, *The Lancet*, 372(9652): 1783–9.

UK Royal Medical Colleges (undated) *Significant harm – the effects of administrative detention on the health of children, young people and their families*. Intercollegiate Briefing Paper. http://www.bacch.org.uk/publications/documents/Sgnificant_Harm_intercollegiate_statement_Dec09.pdf [accessed 23 June 13].

UNICEF (2005) *Child poverty in rich countries*. Florence: UNICEF Innocenti Research Centre.

UNICEF (2007) *Child poverty in perspective: An overview of child well-being in rich countries*. Florence: UNICEF Innocenti Research Centre.

UNICEF (2012) *Measuring child poverty: New league tables of child poverty in the world's rich countries*. Florence: UNICEF Innocenti Research Centre.

UNICEF and Ankara University (2009) *Report on review and analysis of poverty and child poverty*. Ankara: UNICEF.

United Nations (1989) *Convention on the rights of the child*. New York: United Nations.

Virchow, R.C. (2006) Report on the typhus epidemic in Upper Silesia, *American Journal of Public Health*, 96(12): 2102–5.

WHO (1999) *Making a difference*. Geneva: World Health Organization.

WHO (2000) *World Health Report 2000 – Health systems: Improving performance*. Geneva: World Health Organization.

WHO Regional Office for Europe (2005) *The European Health Report 2005: Public health action for healthier children and populations*. Copenhagen: WHO Regional Office for Europe.

WHO Regional Office for Europe (2009) *The European Health Report 2009: Health and health systems*. Copenhagen: WHO Regional Office for Europe.

WHO Regional Office for Europe (2012) *European Health for All Database (HFA-DB)*. http://www.euro.who.int/en/what-we-do/data-and-evidence/databases/european-health-for-all-database-hfa-db2 [accessed 23 June 2013].

Williams, G.C. et al. (2009) The importance of supporting autonomy and perceived competence in facilitating long-term tobacco abstinence, *Annals of Behavioral Medicine*, 37(3): 315–24.

Wolfe, I. et al. (2013) Health services for children in western Europe, *The Lancet*, 381(9873): 1224–34.

Wollstonecraft, M. (1986) *A vindication of the rights of woman*. London: Dent.

Zambon, A. et al. (2010) The contribution of club participation to adolescent health: evidence from six countries, *Journal of Epidemiology and Community Health*, 64: 89–95.

chapter two

Primary care for children

Matthew Thompson, Peter Gill, Ann van den Bruel, Ingrid Wolfe

> United by the common challenge of primary health care, the time is ripe, now more than ever, to foster joint learning and sharing across nations to chart the most direct course towards health for all.
>
> *Margaret Chan, WHO Director-General*

Introduction

The term 'primary care' is usually considered to have originated in 1920 in the Dawson report (Dawson, 1920), which described a hub and spoke model of health services in England that focused on the 'primary health care centre'. This was a milestone in the development of health services, noteworthy also because national approaches to health care diverged from this point. In many European countries, primary care and generalism developed to become the cornerstone of health services, in contrast to the United States, which became dominated by specialization (Starfield, Shi and Macinko, 2005).

Primary care further developed and matured as a concept in the 1970s. It is defined in many ways, each with particular implications and political consequences. The Institute of Medicine in the United States defines primary care as 'the provision of integrated, accessible health care services by clinicians who are accountable for addressing a large majority of personal health care needs, developing a sustained partnership with patients, and practicing in the context of family and community' (Institute of Medicine, 1978). This is similar to the 'Declaration of Alma-Ata' of 1978, which was the first major international statement on the importance of primary health care. In this definition, primary health care was defined as being the central focus of a country's health system, providing the first level of contact for individuals, family and community, providing universally accessible services as close as possible to where people live and work, and providing the first element of a life-long health care process (Chan, 2008). The Declaration of Alma-Ata signalled a major shift in thinking on health care and health systems as it emphasized the multifaceted nature of health and health care; that health inequities are unjust; and that primary health care is the key to attaining health for all as part of social justice. Poignantly, that aim was set in 1978 and was to be attained by 2000.

The Declaration specifies that primary health care should:

- reflect the economic, sociocultural and political characteristics of the country;
- be based on social, biomedical, health services and public health research;
- address the main health problems of the community; and
- include health promotion, disease prevention, curative and rehabilitative services.

Yet, 30 years after the Declaration of Alma-Ata, there is a sense of disappointment because health equity has not been achieved for all. Although considerable progress has been made in many areas of child health, with mortality decreasing substantially, progress has not been equally distributed worldwide and across populations, and stark inequalities remain (see Chapter 1).

In 2008, WHO reaffirmed the importance of primary health care in its report on the subject, identifying five key elements to achieving the goal of health for all (Chan, 2008):

- universal health coverage reforms
- service delivery reforms
- public policy reforms
- leadership reforms
- increasing stakeholder participation.

In essence, the modern primary health care movement aims to provide rational, evidence-based and anticipatory responses to health needs and social expectations (Saltman, Rico and Boerma, 2006).

There are more than 200 million children under 18 years of age living in Europe, with primary care being delivered to them in a variety of ways. This diversity provides opportunities to learn from each other. The focus of this chapter is mainly on medical aspects of primary care. This is because many of the key elements in the current debate around primary care reform centre on issues of the medical workforce. We recognize that this inevitably means an overly medical view of primary care may be conveyed; this is not intended to diminish the important role of nursing and other professionals in primary care, rather it is an attempt to address one important and topical issue in primary care. We open with a discussion of the role of primary care in children's health. We present: different models of organizing primary care and selected medical workforce issues; how services are used for urgent problems and care for children with long-term conditions; the role of primary care in disease prevention and health promotion. Finally, we will examine future challenges for children's primary care in Europe.

Primary care: the foundations of a health system

There is good evidence that countries with higher numbers of primary care physicians (e.g. family or general practitioners [GPs], general internists and general paediatricians) per population have better health outcomes, including lower rates of infant mortality and fewer babies born at low birth weight. These effects persist after controlling for important socioeconomic factors and income inequality (Shi et al., 2004) and occur at the individual level as well as the country level (Franks and Fiscella, 1998). A survey conducted in ten countries, including seven in Europe, found that those with a well-developed primary health care system provide better care and higher satisfaction in relation to the overall costs of the systems (Starfield, 1991).

There are many reasons why primary care provides greater health benefits at a lower cost than specialty-based systems:

- There are usually defined lists of patients, facilitating planning of population-based services such as screening.
- Primary care is ideally placed to provide continuity of care, helping to prevent repetition and duplication of services.
- Primary care is delivered in the context of changes in clinical, social, schooling and other factors (sometimes extending back to birth).
- It should facilitate coordination of care by acting as a hub between specialists, coordinating referrals and the results of diagnostic tests, and ensuring a comprehensive approach to treatment plans.
- It favours patient-centred care. For example, decisions regarding the need for referrals, diagnostics and hospital admission are made in collaboration with patients and parents, rather than either by patients independently or specialist clinicians who may have less expertise in caring for the 'whole' patient.

There is particularly strong evidence for the cost-effectiveness of continuity of care, or 'longitudinally' as Starfield (1998) puts it: 'a long-term personal relationship between practitioners and patients in their practice'. A study of 4134 patients in Belgium found that, even after accounting for many other factors known to influence health care costs (e.g. income and chronic disease), continuity of care with the same general practitioner was one of the strongest predictors of lower total health care costs (De Maeseneer et al., 2003). This echoes studies from the United States, which have shown that patients with continuity of care from the same health care provider had significantly fewer hospital admissions and lower health care costs (Flint, 1987; Gill and Mainous, 1998). However, although continuity of care may be highly valued by patients and be cost-effective, it is increasingly difficult to achieve with restrictions such as the European Working Time Directive and modern working practices such as large groups of primary care doctors working together and cooperative out-of-hours care models.

Primary health care has taken an increasingly central role in health systems throughout Europe over recent decades. Scope and responsibility for health care delivery, coordination of health with other sectors, and health system decision-making are changing the balance between generalism and specialism; localism and centralism; and access and expertise. The organizational changes happening in primary care are complex and difficult. They are profoundly important for children because, although primary care is the mainstay of care for children, primary care reforms often seem to be planned more for the needs and interests of adults than of children. By increasing its role relative to other levels of care, or extending the skill-mix of the team, primary care is often seen as the key to increasing the responsiveness of health care to patients' needs (Starfield and Shi, 2002). It is important that children's distinctive needs are accounted for adequately as primary care comes to the fore in health systems reform.

The major issues confronting children's primary care in Europe are: the different models of care; numbers and training of the professional workforce; and how services are used for urgent needs, children with long-term conditions, and preventive health care.

Primary care for children

In Europe, there are various definitions of paediatrics, general practice, primary care and types of health care providers (Table 2.1), as in the United States, where primary care includes family medicine, general internal medicine and office-based paediatrics. This reflects differences in types of doctor, whether their postgraduate (i.e. after medical school) clinical training involves children exclusively or includes a wide range of ages, and the clinical setting in which they provide care. In some cases, the same term can have a different meaning in different European countries.

Primary care for children in Europe is delivered using three main models based on the predominant type of doctor involved: GP-based, primary care paediatricians, and systems that combine GPs and paediatricians (Wolfe et al., 2011). Moreover, within a country there can be differences in how various aspects of primary care are provided in particular situations, such as out-of-hours care, adolescent care, school health or preventive care.

While it is true that most European countries have a stronger focus on primary care than the United States, there are important differences between countries in primary care provision for children; in particular the type of medical professional who is mainly responsible for delivery of care: GPs, primary care paediatricians, or a combination of these and the different training requirements and working relationships with other professionals in the primary care system (Wolfe et al., 2011). Table 2.2 describes important aspects of primary care systems for children that differ throughout Europe.

Models for delivering primary care for children

There is currently no Europe-wide database or high-level synthesis of evidence that allows comparisons of the effects of different models for delivering primary care for children on either process measures of care or health outcomes. In order to begin to understand the necessary conditions for high-quality primary care, researchers have started to describe the current system across Europe. Their findings point to significant variations.

Table 2.1 Definitions of providers and terms related to primary care for children

Primary care	'The provision of integrated, accessible health care services by clinicians who are accountable for addressing a large majority of personal health care needs, developing a sustained partnership with patients, and practicing in the context of family and community' (Institute of Medicine, 1978).
Clinical care	The type of clinician who will see a child first when they are acutely unwell; this may occur in primary care clinics staffed by general practitioners or paediatricians, urgent care, walk-in centres, out-of-hours care or emergency departments.
General practice/ general practitioner	Doctor trained for various lengths of postgraduate training to provide primary medical care for adults and children.
Family doctor	Doctor who provides primary care for both adults and children; the same meaning as GP in Europe, and family physician in the United States.
Paediatrician	Doctor trained (following medical school) to specialize in the care of children. Some may continue to work exclusively in hospital settings (hospital paediatricians), of whom some will be generalists (general paediatricians) while others will specialize in a medical or surgical specialty of paediatrics (e.g. paediatric surgeons, paediatric oncologists). In some countries, paediatricians work in primary care clinics and are called general paediatricians, primary care paediatricians or community paediatricians. In others, such as Germany, the term office paediatrician or private paediatrician describes a doctor who works in the community providing preventive, first-contact and planned care (the term 'private' does not refer to the mode of payment but to the setting).
General paediatrics	Refers to the care of children in either primary care clinics (primary care paediatricians) or in a hospital setting (e.g. paediatricians who provide care to children admitted to general paediatric inpatient wards).
Emergency care, urgent care and out-of-hours care	Children with acute health problems may seek care in: emergency departments (usually designed for more serious illness or trauma); urgent care settings (a form of 'walk-in' clinic where children with less severe problems are seen); or out-of-hours care which refers to clinics where children who would otherwise be taken to a GP can be seen out of normal working hours.

Two surveys approximately ten years apart reported somewhat different estimates of the proportion of primary care for children provided by different types of doctor (Table 2.3). In 1999, a survey of the national paediatric societies of 34 European countries noted that the most common model (47% of countries) was a combined system involving both GPs and paediatricians, followed by paediatricians alone (35%), and GPs/family doctors alone (18%)

Table 2.2 Key aspects of primary care for children

Systems	• **Choice available for parents in selecting type of primary care clinician:** In some countries there may be no choice, e.g. in the United Kingdom all children are registered with a GP, whereas in Germany parents may have choice about registering with a GP or primary care paediatrician (although there are financial incentives for parents to register with a GP). • **Extent of coordination of care between primary care and secondary care or specialists:** Integrated care, or the cooperation and coordination between general and specialized caregivers, can involve physical location (i.e. co-location) of services, shared clinical pathways and protocols or guidelines, information system/medical record-sharing, referral systems and pathways, urgent/acute management.
Services	• **Range of clinical services provided:** Acute and chronic conditions, preventive care, e.g. well-child checks, immunizations, mental health, sexual health clinics and adolescent health services. • **Acute care or after-hours care:** For acute health problems arising during or after normal working hours, including acute medical and surgical problems and acute trauma.
Workforce	• **Type of medical clinician responsible for providing the majority of care:** Predominantly GPs (e.g. Netherlands, United Kingdom) or paediatricians (e.g. Italy), or combinations. • **Doctor-to-population ratios:** Range widely across Europe, from as few as 112 children/primary care doctor (France) to 341/primary care doctor (Netherlands). This variation may arise from economic, geographical or historical factors. • **Primary care team working:** The extent to which primary care doctors work in isolation, or with various other members of a primary health care team involved in the care of children, including nurses, dieticians, community organizations, social workers, school nurses, etc.

(Katz et al., 2002). In contrast, the later survey reported that the majority of countries (41%) had a GP-based system, followed by combined systems (35%), and paediatrician-based systems (24%) (van Esso et al., 2010), although distinction is not made as to whether and how GPs are specifically trained in paediatrics. Developing a clear consistent taxonomy is essential for developing rigorous research in primary care for children.

Finally, a 2010 survey from 46 European countries provides greater detail about the types of clinicians involved in different aspects of primary care services for children. The survey questioned national leaders of child health organizations belonging to the EPA. The main question asked was which type of health professional is the main provider of care (defined as >50% care provided) (Figure 2.1).

Table 2.3 European surveys of main providers of primary care for children

	*Katz, 1999**	*Van Esso, 2007–09*
	National European Paediatric Societies (EU Members, Turkey, Switzerland, Israel, and countries in Scandinavia, East and Central Europe) *Responses from 34 countries (response rate 83%)*	European Academy of Paediatrics (EAP) of 31 countries (EU countries, Switzerland, Iceland, Norway and Israel) *Responses from 29 countries (response rate 94%)*
Paediatrician	12/34 (35%)	7/29 (24%)
GP or family doctor	6/34 (18%)	12/29 (41%)
Combined system involving both GP and paediatrician	16/34 (47%)	10/29 (35%)

* The main providers of health care for children, based on which kind of doctor provided care for >75% of child population in the public health care system for that country.

Source: Katz, 2002 and van Esso, 2010

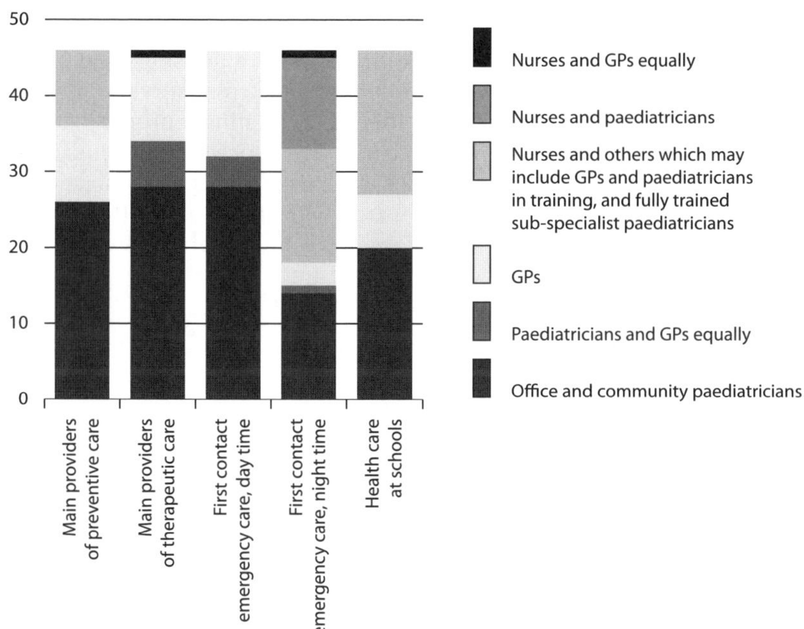

Figure 2.1 Diversity in primary care provision for children in Europe

Source: Adapted from Wolfe et al., 2013

However, these three surveys provide very limited evidence on the provision of primary care for children in Europe. The respondents to these surveys were typically individual paediatric leaders from each country, and they may lack comprehensive knowledge about the provision of primary care, especially by GPs. Another limitation is the extent to which routine primary care for children is provided by paediatric specialists (i.e. hospital outpatients, for example). The boundary between specialists and generalists is difficult to define at the best of times. In the United States, paediatricans can be considered both generalists and specialists; in Europe the terminology can be even more confusing. Caution is required when interpreting this research.

Primary care staff shortages, increasing demand, and pressure to reduce hospital use have increased interest in developing new models of care that transcend the boundaries between generalism and specialism, preserving the best features of primary care while strengthening the specialist expertise available and broadening the remit. The 'medical home' model for children in the United States aims to be accessible, comprehensive, compassionate, family-centred and continuous, as outlined in Box 2.1, and discussed further in Chapter 3.

Comparative merits of systems of paediatric primary care delivery

Understanding how and why services work, and relating structure and process to experience and outcomes, is essential in order to improve future services, particularly at a time of economic recession. There is a pressing need to collect such data, using more rigorous methodology than current surveys provide.

A survey of 15,996 adults visiting their GP in nine European countries (Belgium, Denmark, Germany, Netherlands, Norway, Slovenia, Spain, Switzerland, United Kingdom) provides evidence of overall satisfaction with different models of GP-based primary care (Wensing et al., 2002). Although based on adult patients (some of whom were presumably parents), overall evaluations were positive. The most consistent findings were that patients were

Box 2.1 The paediatric medical home model

1. Preventive care: immunizations, developmental assessments and surveillance, screening, counselling.
2. Ambulatory and inpatient care for acute illnesses at all times of day and night, every day of the year.
3. Continuity of care.
4. Referral to specialists and coordination of care.
5. Interaction with school and community agencies.
6. Centralized database with accessible, but confidential, shared medical records.

Source: American Academy of Pediatrics, 1992.

more satisfied with clinics that had fewer GPs, and those working longer hours rather than part time, apart from when seeking urgent care, when these factors were considered less important. A similar survey evaluated parents' perspectives of the quality and accessibility of paediatric primary care in Quebec, Canada (Lemoine, Lemoine and Cyr, 2006). In this setting, where 66% of care was provided by GPs and 19% by paediatricians, overall satisfaction with care was similar between both groups of providers.

Future issues facing primary care models

In the absence of sufficient evidence to demonstrate the relative merits of different types of primary care systems and different providers of care, debate about the optimal way(s) to deliver primary care for children will inevitably be strongly influenced by professional interests, often voiced through representative organizations. Nevertheless, several issues that are shared by all concerned are likely to dominate policy discussion on the reform of primary care for children in most European countries (Box 2.2).

Primary care medical workforce and training

Duration and types of training in primary care paediatrics

Paediatricians and GPs have different post-medical school training schemes in most European countries, and various professional bodies have recommended different components of training in children's health care for each. Proponents of different models (e.g. GP versus paediatrician) will claim that one type of

Box 2.2 Issues facing primary care for children in Europe

- **Integration:** avoiding fragmentation of delivery of services for children within the primary care team, between primary care and community services (e.g. social services), and between primary care and specialists.
- **Reducing costs**, or at least minimizing the rate of increase of health care costs for primary care for children; disinvesting in inefficient or outdated practices; and reducing inappropriate specialty referrals and admissions.
- **Workforce:** identifying the ideal balance of skill-mix, training and access, between paediatricians, GPs and other types of clinician.
- **Balancing choice** for types and location of providers, with workforce availability and costs of services, and increasing expectations of parents and children.
- **Supporting research** to evaluate current systems of care and new models for delivery.

provider is better trained to provide a high quality of care to children than others. Unfortunately, there is little evidence currently on the relative quality of care provided by different types of doctors.

GPs provide care for children in the context of their family and so should develop an in-depth appreciation of the wide-ranging influences on the health of the individual child. The European minimum standard for the length of training of GPs is three years, with minimum six-month requirements in both hospital care (though not necessarily paediatrics) and primary care (Stephenson, 2010). Training in general practice includes experience with primary care paediatrics, as well as learning opportunities with the wider primary health care team relevant to children's health, such as nurses, health visitors, school nurses, social workers and child protection services. In western Europe, the average length of training for GPs is four years, but there is considerable variability in the length, content, examination structure and regulation across countries (Stephenson, 2010; van Esso et al., 2010). Of the four years of training, only two are typically spent in general practice, with the other two years focused on clinical experience in other settings, mostly hospital-based (Stephenson, 2010). GP training in primary care for children emphasizes several key competencies (Table 2.4). Several professional organizations in Europe have published curricula relating to child health, such as the Royal College of General Practitioners (RCGP) in the United Kingdom (RCGP, 2010).

For paediatricians, the European Academy of Paediatrics (EAP) recommends five years of training, divided into core training for three years and specialized training for two years, in one of three branches: primary care, general paediatrics (hospital-based) and specialist paediatrics (such as paediatric nephrology) (van Esso et al., 2010; Wolfe et al., 2011). Table 2.5 outlines the training requirements of first-contact health care professionals in a selection of European countries.

Table 2.4 Key competencies for GP trainees

- Prevention
- Immunization
- Screening
- Child care
- Common minor illnesses
- Mental health
- Child protection
- Development
- Adolescent medicine
- Recognition of serious illness
- Basic resuscitation

Sources: Poole et al., 1982; Melville, Wall and Anderson, 2002; Stephenson, 2010; Duke, Curran and Hollett, 2011

Table 2.5 Training requirements for first-contact child health professionals

	UK	*Netherlands*	*Italy*	*France*	*Sweden*	*Germany*
First-contact model	GP	GP	Primary care paediatrics	Combined	Combined	Combined
Usual first-contact professional	GP or clinic nurse	GP or youth health worker	Primary care paediatrician	GP or paediatrician	GP or paediatrician	Family physician
Training of first-contact professional	40% of GPs have ≤6 months' training in hospital paediatrics; other child health training is in general practice	GPs not formally required to have postgraduate training in paediatrics	All professionals caring for children are specially trained in paediatrics	Postgraduate training for GPs includes either paediatrics or gynaecology	All GPs have postgraduate training in paediatrics	Most parents choose family physicians who are trained in paediatrics

Source: Adapted from Wolfe et al., 2011

Concerns with duration and content of training in primary care paediatrics

The content of training for both GPs and paediatricians may not adequately match children's primary care health needs. Paediatric training for GPs is largely based in hospital settings, sometimes emphasizing specialties with relatively little applicability and relevance to practice in the community (Melville, Wall and Anderson, 2002). Equally, for paediatricians, training provided by looking after hospitalized children, or in paediatric outpatient specialities, may not provide the skills or expertise for the range and scope of clinical and social problems encountered in community-based primary care practice (Melville, Wall and Anderson, 2002; Duke, Curran and Hollett, 2011).

Despite the recommendations for training in child health, the survey of members of the EAP found that the amount of formal training in paediatrics for GPs varied (median four months) but in some countries was not required or did not occur at all (van Esso et al., 2010). However respondents for the EAP survey were paediatric leaders, with no GP or family medicine representatives, so it is possible that a comprehensive view has not been obtained. In addition, the amount of training can vary within a given country; for example, in the United Kingdom, less than half of GP trainees have hospital paediatric training (RCPCH, 2007). The van Esso survey reported that the duration of training for paediatricians was five or more years in the majority of countries (20 of 29 surveyed), and less than five years in nine countries (van Esso et al., 2010).

It is extremely difficult to determine the effects of different lengths or types of training on process of care or clinical outcomes for children, not least because training is only one component in the quality of care provided to children. As noted in the section below, markers of quality of health care for children have only recently been proposed and few are used in Europe. However, data from the 'Confidential Enquiry into Maternal and Child Health' in the United Kingdom identified several deficiencies in the provision of care that contributed directly to child deaths, and identified avoidable factors in 26% of child deaths (Pearson et al., 2011). Where primary care was actively involved, the enquiry found avoidable factors in 20% of the deaths, with 'failure to recognise and manage severe infection' being the most common (Harnden et al., 2009; Pearson et al., 2011). Failures in each step in the clinical management of sick children (including patient history, physical examination, treatment and referral) were identified as avoidable factors (Harnden et al., 2009; Pearson et al., 2011).

In 2010, the United Kingdom's RCGP published a 'Child Health Strategy' emphasizing the importance of primary care professionals developing and maintaining competencies, for example, in the recognition of serious illness in children. The strategy calls for all GPs in training to have a 'sufficient amount of clinical exposure to sick children to ensure that they are competent in the assessment of the sick child' (RCGP, 2010). Further, GPs should be able to 'demonstrate the key skills and competencies required, maintain standards and regularly review their performance' (RCGP, 2010).

Improving training in primary care paediatrics

There is no clear data or European consensus on the appropriate length, structure or content of training in child health for GPs to be fully competent to care for children and encounter the challenges of primary care (Melville, Wall and Anderson, 2002; Stephenson, 2010). Some experts advocate that between 9 and 12 months will adequately prepare GPs to competently assess most paediatric primary care problems (van Esso et al., 2010), while others believe that the structure and content of training is more important (Duke, Curran and Hollett, 2011). For example, equivalent training programmes for family physicians in the United States require training in paediatrics, typically of five months' duration (Baldor and Luckmann, 1992).

In some countries there are opportunities for GPs to obtain more training and qualifications in particular clinical areas, based on personal interest or local health care needs, allowing them to provide expertise within a general practice, and sometimes within a region. For example, in the United Kingdom, GPs can undergo an additional examination in child health, following a period of hospital-based paediatric training. Indeed, there is some limited evidence from the United Kingdom that GPs' satisfaction with paediatric training increases with longer periods of training (Melville, Wall and Anderson, 2002).

The EAP's recommended training model of a common 'trunk' of training in child health for both GPs and primary care paediatricians is intended to offer an appropriate balance of training in both primary and secondary care, and to ensure that both types of doctor have appropriate clinical skills.

Service use in primary care: numbers, changes and trends

Common clinical problems in primary care paediatrics

Overall, children represent 25% of a typical practice population in general practice in the United Kingdom, yet are associated with 40% of the workload (Hippisley-Cox, Fenty and Heaps, 2007). Data from general practice settings in the Netherlands, United Kingdom and Germany show that the most common reasons for consultation in general practice are related to respiratory tract, skin, and ear, nose and throat (ENT) problems (Table 2.6). Within these systems the most frequently recorded diagnoses are related to acute infections, mostly of the respiratory tract and ENT. Chronic conditions are less frequent causes of consultation by children in primary care, but are dominated by eczema and asthma. However, recording of data is different between countries, depending on how care is provided. For example, in Germany, routine immunization is the third most frequent reason for consultation, whereas it does not appear in the most frequent lists in the Netherlands because this country has child health clinics that undertake routine vaccination. There are no data to compare the presentation patterns of children in general practice compared to paediatric practices across Europe, but it would be reasonable to assume these would be similar.

Table 2.6 Most frequent diagnoses and reasons for attendance in three countries

*Most frequent diagnoses in children under 17 years in Dutch general practice in 2001**		*Reasons for childhood consultations in United Kingdom general practice, 0–15 years, 2005–2007†*		*Most frequent reasons for encounter with GPs and its percentage in children 0–19 years in Saxony (Germany) 1999–2000***	
ICPC diagnosis	*incidence per 1000 years*	*Principal diagnosis category (ICD-9)*	*(%)*	*Reasons for encounter*	*(%)*
Acute respiratory tract infection	95.7	Respiratory conditions§	23.9	Cough	9.7
Acute otitis media	60.5	Ear conditions	9.1	Fever	9.0
Cough	51.0	Viral syndrome	8.3	Preventive immunization/injection	7.4
Warts	34.3	Eczema	7.6	Throat symptom/complaint	6.4
Acute bronchitis	26.3	Injury	6.8	Sneezing/nasal congestion	5.8
Dermatomycosis	25.4	Eye conditions	6.4	Respiratory: medical examination partial	3.4
Eczema	22.9	Asthma	3.3	Screening: medical examination complete	2.5
Gastrointestinal infection	21.0	Gastroenteritis	1.9	Diarrhoea	2.4
Impetigo	20.5	Bladder infection	0.8	Abdominal pain/cramps general	2.4
Infectious conjunctivitis	20.4	Well-child visit	—	Vomiting	2.4
Cut, laceration	20.3	All other	31.9	Respiratory symptom/complaint other	1.8
Acute tonsillitis	19.0			Headache	1.8
Fever	18.8			Ear pain/earache	1.7
Constitutional eczema	16.5			Nausea	1.5
Urinary tract infection	15.5			Dressing/compression/tamponade	1.4

General weakness	15.0	Weakness tiredness	1.4
Serous otitis media	14.3	Trauma/injury not other specified	1.2
Viral infection	13.9	Rash localized	1.2
Asthma	13.3	Ear: medical examination partial	1.1
Oral contraceptives	12.7	Tonsillar symptoms	1.1
		Pruritus	0.8
		Abdominal pain localized	0.5
		Rash generalized	0.3

Notes: United Kingdom data does not include well-child visits
[§] Excluding asthma

Sources: *Otters et al., 2005; [†]RCGP, 2008; **Frese et al., 2011; [†]Gill et al., 2011

Trends in child health attendances for first-contact care

The use of GP services by children has increased over recent decades in many European countries. Between 1984 and 1996, health care use of a sample of 15,000 children aged 2–17 years, in five Nordic countries (Denmark, Finland, Iceland, Norway and Sweden), showed a significant trend of increased attendance at GP services in four of the countries; Denmark was the only one in which there was no evidence of increased use (Virtanen et al., 2006). It is not clear whether these trends apply more generally across Europe, or to all aspects of primary care for children. However, it is clear that admission to hospital is common among children. In the United Kingdom, one in three children is admitted to hospital in the first year of life alone, of which two-thirds are short-stay admissions and nearly half for minor infections (Saxena et al., 2009). Two conclusions we can draw from this are:

1. Despite the decrease in incidence of serious illness in children (due to improved public health, nutrition and routine immunizations), levels of concern among parents, emergency department staff and hospital paediatricians regarding the possibility of serious illness continue to drive admissions.
2. A considerable proportion of short-stay admissions, i.e. those for minor infections, could potentially have been managed safely in the primary care setting.

Short emergency hospital admissions increased substantially in England over the decade from 1997 (Saxena et al., 2009); emergency hospital admissions in children under 10 years of age rose 22%, with a large increase of 41% in short less than 2 day admissions. In addition, there was a 42% increase in emergency department visits in the United Kingdom (Sands et al., 2012). There has also been a substantial increase in emergency admissions in England documented from the decade from 2003 onwards, particularly among children under 5 years old, admitted to hospital for short periods and for common infections. Notably, there has been a marked rise in admissions for conditions considered sensitive to primary care quality, including admissions for upper respiratory tract infections (increased by 22%), lower respiratory tract infection (up 40%), urinary tract infections (43% increase), and gastroenteritis (up 31%) (Gill et al., 2013). It is not known whether these hospitalization trends apply more widely to other European countries but this is widely held to be true.

It is also clear that the types of illness in children are changing. In western Europe, as elsewhere, NCDs and long-term conditions including mental health problems are increasingly common (see Chapter 1). Children with rare and congenital disorders are surviving ever longer, sometimes with residual complex problems. The pattern of children's needs for primary care is evolving.

Urgent access to primary care for children

A large proportion of the clinical problems in children seeking primary care still comprises acute illness. A critical element of first-contact care for children is distinguishing between minor and serious illnesses. This is one of the most difficult challenges in medicine, especially paediatrics, because children can deteriorate more suddenly than adults, and the clinical signs of acute serious illness may differ. This problem is illustrated by the failure to find simple solutions to resolving the tensions between generalism and specialism, and between access and expertise.

The most common presenting problems are: acute infections; difficulty breathing (including asthma exacerbations); and acute trauma. On average, a child under 1 year of age will have four consultations per year for infections; in older children aged 1–15 years, this falls to 1.3 consultations per year (Armon et al., 2001). Acute infections also represent a common cause for telephone consultations out of hours and up to a third of such calls to GP services are related to acute infections in children (Dale, Crouch and Lloyd, 1998).

Primary care services should be able to deal with the vast majority of acute medical illnesses and a significant proportion of minor traumas, without the need for hospital referral. One factor is parental perception of the severity of acute illness. In European settings, between 17% and 57% of patients presenting to hospital emergency departments have problems that could potentially have been managed in primary care (Dale et al., 1995; Murphy et al., 1996; Lee et al., 2000; van Uden et al., 2006; Department of Health, 2012). This potentially diverts attention away from children attending with more severe problems or from already hospitalized children, particularly as the same paediatric medical and nursing team may cover the entire hospital. Importantly, the emphasis of care is necessarily on children with urgent problems. Ensuring sufficient resources are available to provide preventive services and planned care for children with long-term conditions is essential, and many countries struggle with this problem.

Key attributes of urgent primary care systems

Primary care systems that provide safe and efficient medical care for children with acute health problems should have several core attributes (Table 2.7), while some may offer more advanced capabilities for diagnosis and management.

Different options for delivering urgent access primary care

Given the different systems of paediatric primary care, high demand for acute care and different attributes needed, it is not surprising that multiple systems for urgent care operate throughout Europe. Indeed, different systems exist not just between countries, but numerous systems may coexist within a single country. To some extent, the systems adopted may also be driven by other factors such as: changes in doctors' attitudes and expectations about lifestyle; increasing demand from parents accustomed to the 24-hour opening of supermarkets and shops; increasing work hours for both parents, limiting their ability to access care during daytime hours; and economic considerations such as the need to reduce 'inappropriate' or 'excessive use' of more costly

Table 2.7 Attributes of primary care systems providing acute or urgent care

Core attributes of urgent primary care systems:

- Easy access, with minimal financial or other barriers.
- Rapid access: in a short time period (usually the same day).
- Prioritization: use of triage (telephone or at presentation) to decide urgency of consultation.
- Availability of referral centre for onward hospital admission.
- Health care professionals with the ability to differentiate minor illness from more serious illness.
- Safety netting, i.e. follow-up systems in place to allow safe discharge home and reconsultation when and where necessary.
- Continuity between daytime and out-of-hours care, and between primary and secondary care.

Additional capabilities of more enhanced systems:

- Basic diagnostic tests are available on site, e.g. rapid antigen tests, point-of-care blood tests, imaging.
- Facilities and staff to allow short-term observation, e.g. for a few hours.
- Facilities and staff to provide immediate treatment, e.g. nebulizers for acute asthma.

after-hours services, for example, emergency departments and emergency paramedics.

Acute problems arise both during the daytime (normal working hours), and in the evenings or weekends (referred to as 'after-hours' or 'out-of-hours' care). The definition of daytime versus out-of-hours and the demarcation of workload between the two is important, and can vary between settings. For example, 'daytime hours' may extend late into the evening and include Saturdays.

Providing open access to primary care requires a carefully planned ratio of staff to patients to accommodate the inevitable peaks and troughs of attendance. In the United States, small primary care practices are evolving towards larger group practices (just as they are in many European countries) for economies of scale and due to a policy shift towards multidisciplinary teams that can provide coordinated care and economies of scope (Centers for Disease Control and Prevention, 2012). There is an inevitable tension between continuity and coordination: the former requires doctors to work full-time, long hours and to have relatively small patient list sizes, while the latter means teams of providers working together and depends on some role substitution. One study of a large number of (adult) patients found that continuity was not associated with better outcomes, while coordination and primary care team structure are significantly correlated with good outcomes (Parkerton, Smith and Straley, 2004). Many United States medical home models are developing teams of primary care providers with a physician (in the United States this means family doctor and/or paediatrician), nurse practitioners and physician assistants.

Nurse practitioners comprise nearly one-fifth of the primary care workforce in the United States, while physician assistants account for 7% (Ginsburg, Taylor and Barr, 2009; Dower and O'Neil, 2011). Nurse practitioners (according to a United States study) may be able to provide 60% of primary care of comparable quality to physicians (Mundinger et al., 2000; Ginsburg, Taylor and Barr, 2009). Primary care teams using electronic communication can also help meet demand in an open access primary care model (Green, Savin and Lu, 2013).

Access to urgent care during the daytime

Access to urgent care during the daytime is almost always part of routine primary care, but may involve a variety of methods of delivery. In most European countries, this means the provision of acute appointments in primary care clinics at which the patient or their family is registered. These arrangements can involve 'walk-in' systems, appointments provided on the same day, or triage at the individual practice level. In other systems, dedicated centres providing 'walk-in care' or 'urgent care' exclusively offer urgent primary care, which may be private or part of the statutory system.

Access to care out-of-hours

Access to primary care for children out-of-hours causes more difficulties than the delivery of daytime primary care services. To some extent this reflects a mismatch between the demands of parents and the realities of providing care. Parents increasingly want access to care outside normal working hours, but working at night is less attractive to clinicians (and thus more costly), and does not reflect initiatives to reduce working hours and increase the attraction of careers in primary care.

In general, the provision of out-of-hours care in many European countries has shifted from providing greater individual care (i.e. with the child's usual primary care doctor) to less individual care. Various models of providing this care have emerged. In some countries, the responsibility for offering access to urgent medical care remains that of individual primary care doctors; in others, this responsibility may lie with groups of primary care clinicians (usually in a defined locality). In other settings, the responsibility for out-of-hours may lie at a territorial level and may be subcontracted out to various providers to deliver the care.

Different ways of providing after-hours primary care include: practice-based services; cooperatives between GPs; primary care centres; telephone-based advice services; and hospital emergency departments (Table 2.8). Denmark, the Netherlands and the United Kingdom have made the most dramatic changes to the provision of out-of-hours care at a national level. A systematic review examined different types of after-hours care models and compared some of the advantages and disadvantages (Leibowitz, Day and Dunt, 2003). There are no data specific to the provision of after-hours care for children available, but it is likely that many of the findings are equally relevant for children.

Table 2.8 Different methods of providing after-hours primary care

		Country examples
Practice-based services	Provide access to a GP/ paediatrician, either individually or within a practice, looking after their own patients.	**Belgium:** Typical practice in many general practice settings, with care provided by the doctors from the practice, or from a small number of local practices.
Deputizing services	Commercial entities employ doctors to provide the service. This can reduce the need for practices and GPs/ paediatricians organizing the care.	**United Kingdom:** Changes in the general practice contract in 2004 led to provision of out-of-hours care being organized at the primary care trust level, with GPs employed either directly or via commercial subcontractors to provide care.
Co-operatives	Smaller or larger groups of GPs from local or regional practices form a shared organization to provide care.	**The Netherlands:** General practice cooperatives cover 90% of the population (Moll van Charante, van Steenwijk-Opdam and Bindels, 2007), and many of these are situated close or adjacent to hospitals (van Uden et al., 2006). • Telephone triage and advice is provided by nurses in most centres to decide on urgency and best place of care. • Improved general practice satisfaction. • Overall patient satisfaction is good, but patient satisfaction with telephone advice is lower than those receiving general practice contact at the primary care centre or home visit. • Greater proportion of telephone contacts and fewer home visits.
Primary care centres	Patients attend a dedicated centre without appointment. Some are provided by private organizations and some also offer alternatives to daytime care.	**United Kingdom:** Various types of walk-in centres are used, often in urban areas with less accessible general practice services.
Telephone triage and advice services	Regional or national systems of telephone consultations for parents seeking medical care or advice for children. The aim is to triage care and identify which children need immediate medical consultations and to help the medical workload.	**United Kingdom:** A trial comparing nurse telephone consultations with the usual practice of passing all calls to a general practice found nurses managed 49.8% of calls without referral to general practice, with 38% reduction in visits to a primary care centre and 23% fewer home visits, without increase in emergency department attendances or admissions (Lattimer et al., 1998).

		United Kingdom: National systems of telephone advice (NHS Direct; NHS 24) providing phone advice and on-referral to appropriate services. **Denmark:** Locally organized general practice after-hours services, replaced in 1992 with central telephone triage and advice service. It was found there has been a doubling in consultations dealt with by telephone (to 48%), and a reduction in home visits from 46% to 18%, but possibly accompanied by lower patient satisfaction (Christensen and Olesen, 1998; Hansen and Munck, 1998).
Emergency departments	Primary care patients seeking care in an emergency department. Can sometimes include GPs working in the emergency department.	**Ireland, United Kingdom:** Comparisons of GPs working in emergency departments in Ireland and United Kingdom found that GPs ordered fewer investigations and admitted 45% fewer patients than emergency department staff (all ages) (Dale et al., 1995; Murphy et al., 1996).

Future issues for urgent access primary care services

A comprehensive solution to the rising demand for immediate (same day) acute paediatric care is required. This system needs to enable coordination between primary care, hospital emergency and paediatric departments, and other sectors, while providing ready access to safe high-quality care that is affordable, sustainable and flexible enough to meet evolving health needs. Box 2.3 lists some of the future challenges in service provision.

Care for children with long-term conditions in primary care

Chronic diseases are defined by WHO as those that are of long duration and generally slow progression, and are associated with multiple contacts with a variety of different providers over long periods of time, even lifetime, often with a focus more on care than cure. As Chapter 1 illustrates, there has been a marked reduction in deaths overall, and a relative decrease in the proportion of deaths caused by communicable diseases in children. This includes improvements in overall survival of children with certain chronic diseases that previously had extremely poor outcomes, such as cystic fibrosis, prematurity and many malignancies. On the other hand, there is also good evidence that several chronic diseases are increasing in incidence, such as asthma (among some groups and in some ages) (Asher et al., 2006) and type 1 and type 2 diabetes mellitus (Patterson et al., 2009; Harron et al., 2011). Also, there is a growing recognition that some chronic diseases, which cause clinical sequelae

Box 2.3 Future challenges in urgent primary care services for children

Increasing expectations of parents and children for access to acute services, and balancing these pressures with providing services that meet their needs.

Coordination needs to improve between primary care, emergency departments, ambulance/paramedic services and social services.

Multiple points of access to urgent care may confuse parents and children, and hence it is important to signpost parents to access the right service at the right time.

Increasing availability of diagnostic resources at point of care for clinicians, or for home use.

Treatment services – facilities and staff to provide greater level of therapeutic services in primary care settings or in the home.

Cost minimization – increasing financial constraints on health funding necessitate tighter control of patient access or referral to the more costly facilities (e.g. emergency department; hospital), plus more cost-effective ways of providing acute care for minor illnesses are needed (e.g. pharmacy-based minor illness services, telephone advice lines).

in adults, have their origins at a very young age. For example, there is good evidence that several cardiovascular risk factors, such as hypertension and abnormal lipid profiles, in adolescents and young children can persist into adulthood. Moreover, many other chronic-disease risk factors also begin in childhood, such as obesity, smoking and alcohol abuse.

There are several possible ways to categorize chronic conditions in terms of the likely extent and complexity of primary care involvement:

- **Common conditions:** These include conditions that can be managed almost entirely within the primary care setting, such as asthma, eczema or chronic constipation. In some cases, this may involve additional members of the primary care team, for example, community nurses may be involved in providing parental support and education around the care of children with eczema. In other cases, a small number of children may need consultations with specialists, for example, those with poorly controlled asthma, causing repeated hospital admissions despite intensive primary care input.
- **Chronic diseases that are relatively rare:** A typical primary care doctor would usually only have a very small number of child patients with these conditions, for example, epilepsy, diabetes, juvenile rheumatoid arthritis. In these cases, the majority of the child's care for the condition is likely to be provided by specialists, who may be based in hospitals, but the ongoing care for the child may occur in primary care.
- **Complex chronic conditions and co-morbidities:** This could include children with severe cerebral palsy and with multiple problems such as feeding, breathing, mobility, congenital malformations, and learning disabilities. These children typically require a high intensity of care with multiple specialists, in addition to services such as respiratory specialists,

physiotherapy and occupational therapy. But these children will also have minor illnesses and require primary urgent and preventive care just as all other children.
- **Risk factors for chronic conditions** that may not occur until adulthood and are potentially modifiable, such as hypertension, obesity, smoking or lipid disorders. Because primary care doctors provide continuous long-term care to children and their families, they are in a unique position to opportunistically identify and manage such risk factors.

Recognizing these different aspects of chronic conditions is important in considering the roles of primary care in providing and improving care, and in strengthening the links between primary care, social care, specialty care and allied health professionals.

Problems with current primary care provision for children with chronic diseases and long-term conditions

Despite the epidemiological shift towards chronic and non-communicable diseases, services for children and young people with these types of condition are often poorly coordinated, inconvenient for families, and outcomes are frequently poor. As noted in Chapter 3, this includes suboptimal management of children with existing chronic disease and failure to adequately recognize and halt the progression of risk factors for chronic diseases that will track into adulthood (Friedemann et al., 2012).

The reasons underlying these problems are complex. Firstly, a large part of primary care for children is taken up with acute problems. This reflects the current demand for primary care for children, which, as noted above, is mainly driven by acute conditions, despite the reducing prevalence of many serious infectious diseases. This leaves fewer resources for the management of chronic care for children.

Secondly, the levels of skill and experience of primary care practitioners in chronic disease management are highly variable. This reflects the multiple paradigms of:

- disease incidence, ranging from common (e.g. eczema) to relatively rare (e.g. epilepsy, cystic fibrosis);
- disease longevity, including both chronic but time-limited conditions (e.g. infantile eczema) and lifelong (e.g. type 1 diabetes mellitus);
- potential consequences of management, ranging from possibly life-threatening consequences of poor management (e.g. type 1 diabetes mellitus causing diabetic ketoacidosis) to less serious but unpleasant consequences (e.g. exacerbations of eczema).

While it is sometimes possible for a primary care physician to become very familiar with some chronic diseases, the relative rarity of other conditions means that little experience can be gained, even over decades of clinical practice experience.

Thirdly, perhaps because of the heterogeneity in incidence, duration and consequences of chronic diseases, there have been relatively few attempts to design models of care for chronic disease in children.

Finally, available evidence suggests the lack of coordination of clinical services between primary and secondary care. In some countries, information is not exchanged optimally between primary and secondary care; shared information should not only contain all the essential details required to enable the provision of care a child needs, but should also be transferred in a timely fashion. Evidence also shows that primary care doctors do not always know whom to contact in secondary care when a patient with a chronic condition requires specialist advice (Torjesen, 2012). There are many other barriers to improved integration of health care systems, which can result from professional traditions, organization and funding (Smyth, 2009; Suter et al., 2009) (see Chapter 11).

Potential models for delivery of chronic disease care for children in primary care

Primary care for children offers many opportunities for better management of chronic disease, including prevention, early detection and ongoing management. Given the problems with current care provision, how can primary care services improve the management of children with chronic diseases?

The best evidence for how chronic care for children can be delivered comes from experience with a model of care in adults known as the 'chronic care model' (Coleman et al., 2009) which is starting to be adapted, in various ways, for children. This model and other aspects of developing chronic care for children will be discussed further in Chapters 3 and 11.

Screening for chronic diseases and risk factors: Primary care should also be able to play a major role in screening children for the presence of chronic diseases as well as risk factors for chronic diseases. This role is discussed further in Chapter 5.

Primary care and preventive services

Comparing models of surveillance versus well-child checks

There is substantial variability within Europe in terms of the frequency and content of preventive child health examinations (van Esso et al., 2010). In many European countries, the process for detecting health problems in children has undergone a shift from active surveillance, involving routine visits to a GP or paediatrician, to more passive systems that place more responsibility on the parent to detect abnormalities. In some countries, such as the United Kingdom, this has led to a reduction in the recommended number and content of surveillance visits. A recent survey among 29 European countries found the mean number of clinical visits for well-child checks was 14.7, with a huge range from 5 to 30 (van Esso et al., 2010).

Table 2.9 Differences between universal surveillance and voluntary well-child checks

Surveillance	*Well-child checks*
Clinician driven	Parent or caregiver driven
Occurs at regular or routine intervals	At the parent or caregiver's initiative
Expensive in health care provider time	Less costly
Early detection of disease or risk factors	Promoting a healthy lifestyle to prevent disease or risk factors
Universal for all children	May exclude the children most in need
May pick up too many false positives	May pick up fewer deviations from normal (false negatives)
Provides support for parents (including those with normal children)	Puts responsibility with parents and may widen inequalities

Other potential benefits of preventive health visits include parental support and reassurance. Indeed, attendance of routine health checks for preschool children is typically very high and parents welcome the opportunity to discuss their child's health and developmental progress (Hart, Bax and Jenkins, 1981). Some countries, such as France, offer financial incentives to mothers to attend the well-child clinic, but it is unclear how effective this is in improving child or parental health.

The dichotomy between active surveillance and passive well-child checks (Table 2.9) is increasingly outdated. For example, the United Kingdom has shifted from a strategy of 'seek and treat' to one of 'prevent and promote' (Blair and DeBell, 2011). Indeed, the new 'Healthy Child Programme' lists a number of aims, moving far beyond mere immunization against infectious diseases to a set of comprehensive goals encompassing the overall healthy growth and development of children, family interaction including comprehensive health promotion within schools, and the protection of children and young people from social, economic and environmental threats (see Chapter 5).

Moreover, the 'Healthy Child Programme' team is multidisciplinary and can include primary care, the school health team, community paediatricians, sexual health services, primary mental health workers, immunization teams, safeguarding professionals, youth workers, counsellors and a range of public health and health promotion specialists (e.g. for tobacco, drugs and dietetics). General practice has an important role through screening, surveillance and immunization, as well as opportunistically promoting health (Department of Health, 2009). Paediatricians and nurses play a role, along with members of the multidisciplinary team, in identifying and assessing neurodevelopmental and behavioural difficulties.

Assessment and measurement of quality of primary care for children

Defining the quality of primary care for children is a challenging task. Different groups have defined dimensions to evaluate quality of care for individuals and populations (Campbell, Roland and Buetow, 2000). The United States Institute of Medicine's quality framework includes safety, effectiveness, patient-centredness and timeliness (Beal et al., 2004), while other organizations evaluate the level of care provided, including diagnosis and treatment, access and patient experience (Center for Health Policy Studies, 1995; Lawthers, 1997). The widely used framework developed by Donabedian classifies markers as pertaining to the assessment of structures, processes or outcomes of care (Donabedian, 1966).

Quality indicators are 'specific and measurable elements of practice that can be used to assess the quality of care' (Marshall et al., 2001). Attributes of a good indicator include acceptability to those being measured, relevance to clinical practice, feasibility, and sensitivity to change, among others (Lester and Campbell, 2010; Gillam and Siriwardena, 2011). The nature of indicators reflects the particular health care settings where they will be used. For example, the National Institute for Health and Care Excellence (NICE) in the United Kingdom states that it will only develop indicators for common clinical conditions with a significant morbidity (Lester and Campbell, 2010). Although quality indicators should be based on scientific evidence, such evidence is often lacking for children in primary care and available evidence is often combined with expert opinion (Campbell et al., 2003). Extensive literature searches compile the evidence for each key indicator and this is then applied to consensus development techniques to ensure that those preparing indicators incorporate the best available evidence with their clinical expertise (Campbell et al., 2003).

Primary care health service performance indicators for children

Currently, there are few quality markers for children in primary care, reflecting the numerous challenges that apply to children's services. For example, children are rapidly progressing through developmental stages and are constantly changing physically, emotionally and cognitively (Beal et al., 2004). Quality measures in primary care will therefore likely differ based on age or developmental stage of the child assessed. In addition, most children are relatively healthy while special populations of children have complex needs (Beal et al., 2004). As a result, the application of adult quality indicators to children is inappropriate. While country-specific guidelines recommend measures based on best available evidence and consensus statements, such as the RCGP Toolkit for Safeguarding Children and Young People in General Practice, there is no clear set of quality measures for children in primary care (RCGP, 2010).

Internationally, a set of quality measures was developed by the OECD for the global assessment of primary care systems (Mattke et al., 2006). Its indicators include a few relevant to children (e.g. immunization for preventable diseases, provision of basic immunizations and asthma mortality rate) and these have been used to assess the performance of primary care systems in 23 primarily European countries. In 2004, the United Kingdom introduced a 'pay-for-performance' system in general practice, probably the largest such scheme ever introduced into primary care anywhere (Campbell et al., 2007).

Since it was implemented the quality of primary care has improved, especially in the most deprived areas, and there is less variation among practices (Doran et al., 2008). However, while children comprise 25% of a practice population, few markers relate to them and those that do are mainly focused on asthma management in older children and child developmental checks (NHS Confederation, 2011).

The Dutch College of General Practitioners used 61 national guidelines to develop 139 indicators for GPs, and many focused on child health (e.g. acute otitis media, asthma, acute diarrhoea, and fever) (Westert, Jabaaij and Schellevis, 2006). In Spain, researchers have developed a list of preventable emergency hospital admissions to be used by Spanish GPs to evaluate the effectiveness of primary care (Caminal et al., 2004). Several of the conditions are specific to children, including immunization, asthma and gastroenteritis. In the United States, government agencies and private foundations have developed systematic approaches to measuring and quantifying the quality of child health using various sets of indicators (Kavanagh, Adams and Wang, 2009). For example, the RAND Corporation developed over 400 indicators for paediatric primary care and have analysed the quality of care delivered to children (Mangione-Smith et al., 2007).

Quality measurement in Europe is in its infancy compared with the United States. Robust indicators of quality need to be developed, validated and implemented in order to measure and improve the quality of primary care for children in Europe.

The future

Primary care will remain the core system for delivering the vast majority of health care needs of children in Europe. Its key strengths are that it can provide continuity of care in the context of diverse clinical, social and school factors; can act as the coordinator of care within primary care, and between primary and secondary care; and its defined lists of patients facilitate the planning of population services such as screening. In addition, primary care is a more cost-effective way of providing health care for children than speciality-based models of health care.

What is equally clear is that multiple systems of primary care for children operate in Europe. These differ in terms of the range of clinical services offered, the extent to which care is provided for acute problems or after hours, the choice available for parents in selecting primary care clinicians, the extent of coordination between primary and secondary care, and the makeup of the primary care workforce, including the types and numbers of doctors (principally paediatricians or general or family practitioners) and other clinicians involved in the primary care team. Despite these differences, there is surprisingly little known about the relative merits of different models of primary care or the most important components of primary care that are associated with the best outcomes for children. Looking ahead, there are several issues that will dominate policy-making around primary care in most, if not all, European countries (Box 2.4).

Box 2.4 Future issues in models for delivering primary care for children in Europe

- **Integration:** avoiding fragmentation of delivery of services for children: within the primary care team; between primary care and community services (e.g. social services); and between primary care and specialists.
- **Reducing costs**, or at least minimizing the rate of increase of health care costs for primary care for children; disinvesting in inefficient or outdated practices; and reducing inappropriate specialty referrals and admissions.
- **Workforce:** identifying the ideal balance of skill-mix, training and access, between paediatricians, GPs , nurses, and other types of clinician.
- **Balancing choice** for types and location of providers, with workforce availability and costs of services, and increasing expectations of parents and children.
- **Supporting research** to evaluate current systems of care and new models for delivery.

Looking to the future, there are several priorities for improving the primary care of children in Europe.

Primary care should reflect the changing epidemiology of children's health

Currently, primary care for children is dominated by two main clinical areas: acute care for mostly respiratory and infectious diseases; and various types of health screening and preventive care. Acute care, in particular, dominates much of the day-to-day work of primary care for children, as well as much of the primary care provided in after-hours/out-of-hours and emergency department settings. At least in some European countries, there are increasing numbers of child admissions to hospital, mostly of very short duration and many potentially avoidable. However, significant epidemiological shifts in morbidity and mortality affecting children in Europe are occurring, with rises in chronic disease, NCDs and lifestyle-related illness (or risk factors). Changing how primary care is delivered is going to be critical in order to provide high-quality and cost-effective care for emerging priorities.

Improving chronic disease management in primary care

Managing children and young people with chronic diseases will require a shift in delivery (and resources) from acute care provision, plus the development of models of chronic care delivery, which are only now being explored in children. To some extent, primary care will be able to draw on many different chronic care models of care for adults, but few of these have been extensively trialled in children. A 'one size fits all' approach to chronic disease management will be particularly inappropriate for children, where chronic diseases in primary care encompass everything from common chronic conditions such as eczema or asthma (which are already largely managed in primary care) to less common diseases currently predominantly managed by paediatric subspecialists (for example, epilepsy and cystic fibrosis) and children with multiple co-morbidities resulting from complex multisystem illnesses (for example, severely disabled children with cerebral palsy). In addition, primary care is far behind adult practice in screening for and intervening on modifying risk factors for chronic conditions in children that will cause ill health later in adulthood (e.g. obesity, hypertension and lipid disorders).

The common features likely to be essential in improving the management of all chronic diseases in children will be:

1. More collaborative working across different parts of the primary and secondary care services.
2. Improved decision support for primary care paediatricians and GPs, including more effective ways of accessing speciality clinics and specialist advice.
3. More sophisticated information systems to facilitate sharing between primary and secondary care, as well as other parts of the health care system that may be involved in the care of children with chronic diseases (e.g. nursing, physiotherapy, occupational therapy), social services, as well as schools.
4. Supporting children/young people and their parents in managing more aspects of chronic diseases themselves.
5. Ensuring longitudinal care provision for children and their families with chronic diseases.
6. Developing effective methods to identify and modify risk factors of chronic disease.

Some European countries already have excellent models where this new type of working has occurred. This topic is discussed in further detail in Chapters 3 and 11.

Shifting resources from acute care

Shifting primary care resources from acute to chronic disease management will in itself be very challenging for many primary care systems in Europe. The paradoxical situation of rising demand for acute primary care (and indeed acute hospital admissions) at more convenient locations and times for parents, despite reductions in the incidence of many serious infections (due to vaccination and better health generally) is simply not going to be sustainable. It is not clear whether providing alternative methods for accessing acute care services, such as telephone advice lines or pharmacy-based minor illness services, reduces or increases demand for primary care medical services. Therefore, any disinvestments in acute primary care for children will simply not be possible (or acceptable to parents and policy-makers) if they are not accompanied by more effective and safe ways of coping with minor and mostly self-limiting illnesses.

Primary care medical workforce and training

In order to achieve many of these changes, it is also necessary to re-examine the primary care workforce for children. Both within individual countries as well as across different European countries, there is great variation in the types of doctor and training required in order to provide primary care for children. Whether primary care for children should be provided primarily by paediatricians, or by general or family practitioners, is unlikely to change within individual countries, as this largely reflects entrenched historic precedents among the professions. Perhaps a more realistic focus is therefore: a) finding more innovative ways for different health care professionals involved in primary care to work together and share best practices; and b) identifying the essential training needed by doctors in order to provide comprehensive, safe and effective primary care for children, given the changing epidemiology of child health and evolving demands in Europe.

Finally, it is important to recognize that the medical component of the primary care workforce is one part of a larger team and re-examining the primary care workforce must take into account this wider context.

Health care indicators of primary care quality for children

Developing indicators to measure and compare the quality of primary care for children is a major priority. Without robust quality measures it is difficult to compare the effectiveness of different models and systems of primary care within and between countries in Europe. This risks not only continuing ineffective (or even harmful) practices and policies, but also failing to adopt those that are most effective. Although there are several examples of indicators that have been developed for primary care, particularly for services designed for prevention and early detection of disease (immunization and screening), few have been developed especially to measure quality of curative primary care services for children (RICHE, 2012). Moreover, indicators are needed that can measure the quality of services when care is provided across many different elements of health and social care, particularly for children with complex problems, disabilities, mental health issues or who are at risk of maltreatment. See Chapters 5 and 11 for further discussion on child health indicators.

Filling the research gaps in primary care for children

Clinical practice and policy decisions relating to primary care for children are severely limited by a lack of research across multiple aspects of clinical practice and health services for children. This lack of primary research studies is reflected not only in the high proportion of off-label prescribing in children (see Chapter 10) but also the lack of systematic reviews on clinical topics relevant to child health (Gill et al., 2011). Identifying where specific research gaps exist in primary care has been haphazard, often driven by researcher interests rather than primary care needs. However, projects such as the EU's RICHE study providing an inventory of child health research in Europe will help to develop priorities for future EU research funding. Similar initiatives are needed at the national level to identify research gaps and set priorities for health research spending. In some European countries, the infrastructure to support primary care research is now well established, such as the United Kingdom, the Netherlands, Denmark, Sweden and Finland, with multiple linked data sources. Furthermore there are research networks of primary care practices such as the European Academy of Paediatrics Research in Ambulatory Setting network (EAPRASnet).

References

American Academy of Pediatrics (1992) Ad Hoc Task Force on Definition of the Medical Home: The medical home, *Pediatrics*, 90(5): 774.

Armon, K. et al. (2001) Determining the common medical presenting problems to an accident and emergency department, *Archives of Disease in Childhood*, 84(5): 390–2.

Asher, M.I. et al. (2006) Worldwide time trends in the prevalence of symptoms of asthma, allergic rhinoconjunctivitis, and eczema in childhood: ISAAC Phases One and Three repeat multicountry cross-sectional surveys, *The Lancet*, 368(9537): 733–43.

Baldor, R.A. and Luckmann, R. (1992) A survey of formal training in the care of children in family practice residency programs, *Family Medicine*, 24: 426–30.

Beal, A.C. et al. (2004) Quality measures for children's health care, *Pediatrics*, 113(1 Pt 2): 199–209.

Blair, M. and DeBell, D. (2011) Reconceptualising health services for school-age children in the 21st century, *Archives of Disease in Childhood*, 96(7): 616–18.

Caminal, J. et al. (2004) The role of primary care in preventing ambulatory care sensitive conditions, *European Journal of Public Health*, 14(3): 246–51.

Campbell, S. et al. (2007) Quality of primary care in England with the introduction of pay for performance, *New England Journal of Medicine*, 357(2): 181–90.

Campbell, S.M., Roland, M.O. and Buetow, S.A. (2000) Defining quality of care, *Social Science and Medicine*, 51(11): 1611–25.

Campbell, S.M. et al. (2003) Research methods used in developing and applying quality indicators in primary care, *BMJ*, 326(7393): 816–19.

Center for Health Policy Studies (1995) *Understanding and choosing clinical performance measures for quality improvement: development of a typology: Final report*. Rockville: Agency for Healthcare Research and Quality (AHRQ).

Centers for Disease Control and Prevention (2012) *National Ambulatory Medical Care Survey* (home page) [online]. National Center for Health Statistics. http://www.cdc.gov/nchs/data/databriefs/db105.htm [accessed 23 June 2013].

Chan, M. (2008) Return to Alma-Ata, *The Lancet*, 372(9642): 865–6.

Christensen, M.B. and Olesen, F. (1998) Out of hours service in Denmark: evaluation five years after reform, *BMJ*, 316: 1502–5.

Coleman, K. et al. (2009) Evidence on the Chronic Care Model in the new millennium, *Health Affairs (Millwood)*, 28(1): 75–85.

Dale, J., Crouch, R. and Lloyd, D. (1998) Primary care: nurse-led telephone triage and advice out-of-hours, *Nursing Standard*, 12(47): 41–5.

Dale, J. et al. (1995) Primary care in the accident and emergency department: II. Comparison of general practitioners and hospital doctors, *BMJ*, 311(7002): 427–30.

Dawson, B. (1920) *Interim report on the future provision of medical and allied services*. London: HMSO.

De Maeseneer, J.M. et al. (2003) Provider continuity in family medicine: does it make a difference for total health care costs? *Annals of Family Medicine*, 1(3): 144–8.

Department of Health (2009) *Healthy Child Programme: Pregnancy and the first five years of life*. London: Department of Health.

Department of Health (2012) *Report of the Children and Young People's Health Outcomes Forum*. London: Children and Young People's Health Outcomes Forum, Department of Health.

Donabedian, A, (1966) Evaluating the quality of medical care, *Milbank Memorial Fund Quarterly*, 44(Suppl): 166–206.

Doran, T. et al. (2008) Effect of financial incentives on inequalities in the delivery of primary clinical care in England: analysis of clinical activity indicators for the quality and outcomes framework, *The Lancet*, 372(9642): 728–36.

Dower, C. and O'Neil, E. (2011) *Primary care health workforce in the United States*. Princeton: Robert Wood Johnson Foundation.

Duke, P., Curran, V. and Hollett, A. (2011) Training family medicine residents to care for children: What is the best approach? *Canadian Family Physician*, 57(2): e46–50.

Flint, S. (1987) *The impact of continuity of care on the utilization and cost of pediatric care in a Medicaid population* [dissertation]. Chicago: University of Chicago.

Franks, P. and Fiscella, K. (1998) Primary care physicians and specialists as personal physicians. Health care expenditures and mortality experience, *Journal of Family Practice*, 47(2): 105–9.

Frese, T. et al. (2011) Children and adolescents as patients in general practice – the reasons for encounter, *Journal of Clinical Medicine Research*, 3(4): 177–82.

Friedemann, C. et al. (2012) Cardiovascular disease risk in healthy children and its association with body mass index: systematic review and meta-analysis, *BMJ*, 345: e4759.

Gill, J.M. and Mainous, A.G., 3rd (1998) The role of provider continuity in preventing hospitalizations, *Archives of Family Medicine*, 7(4): 352–7.

Gill, P.J. et al. (2011) The evidence base for interventions delivered to children in primary care: an overview of cochrane systematic reviews, *PLOS One*, 6(8): e23051.

Gill, P.J. et al. (2013) Increase in emergency admissions to hospital for children aged under 15 in England, 1999–2010: national database analysis, *Archives of Disease in Childhood*, 98(5): 328–34.

Gillam, S. and Siriwardena, A.N. (eds) (2011) *The Quality and Outcomes Framework*. Abingdon: Radcliffe Publishing Ltd.

Ginsburg, J., Taylor, T. and Barr, M.S. (2009) *Nurse practitioners in primary care. A Policy Monograph of the American College of Physicians*. Philadelphia: American College of Physicians.

Green, L.V., Savin, S. and Lu, Y. (2013) Primary care physician shortages could be eliminated through use of teams, nonphysicians, and electronic communication, *Health Affairs (Millwood)*, 32(1): 11–19.

Hansen, B.L. and Munck, A. (1998) Out-of-hours service in Denmark: the effect of a structural change, *British Journal of General Practice*, 48(433): 1497–9.

Harnden, A. et al. (2009) Child deaths: confidential enquiry into the role and quality of UK primary care, *British Journal of General Practice*, 59(568): 819–24.
Harron, K.L. et al. (2011) Rising rates of all types of diabetes in south Asian and non-south Asian children and young people aged 0–29 years in West Yorkshire, U.K., 1991–2006, *Diabetes Care*, 34(3): 652–4.
Hart, H., Bax, M. and Jenkins, S. (1981) Use of the child health clinic, *Archives of Disease in Childhood*, 56: 440–5.
Hippisley-Cox, J., Fenty, J. and Heaps, M. (2007) *Trends in consultation rates in general practice 1995 to 2006: Analysis of the QRESEARCH database*. QRESEARCH. http://www.qresearch.org/Public_Documents/Trends%20in%20consultation%20rates%20in%20general%20practice%201995%20to%202006.pdf [accessed 23 June 2013].
Institute of Medicine (1978) *A Manpower Policy for Primary Health Care*. Washington, DC: National Academy of Sciences.
Katz, M. et al. (2002) Demography of pediatric primary care in Europe: delivery of care and training, *Pediatrics*, 109(5): 788–96.
Kavanagh, P.L., Adams, W.G. and Wang, C.J. (2009) Quality indicators and quality assessment in child health, *Archives of Disease in Childhood*, 94(6): 458–63.
Lattimer, V. et al. (1998) Safety and effectiveness of nurse telephone consultation in out of hours primary care: randomised controlled trial, *BMJ*, 317(7165): 1054–9.
Lawthers, A.W. and Palmer, H. (1997) In search of a few good performance measures. In: Seltzer, J. and Nash, D. (eds) *Models for Measuring Quality in Managed Care: Analysis and impact*. New York: Faulkner and Gray's Healthcare Information Center.
Lee, A. et al. (2000) Factors associated with non-urgent utilization of Accident and Emergency services: a case-control study in Hong Kong, *Social Science and Medicine*, 51(7): 1075–85.
Leibowitz, R., Day, S. and Dunt, D. (2003) A systematic review of the effect of different models of after-hours primary medical care services on clinical outcome, medical workload, and patient and GP satisfaction, *Family Practice*, 20(3): 311–17.
Lemoine, M.H., Lemoine, C. and Cyr, C. (2006) Paediatric primary care quality and accessibility: Parents' perspective, *Paediatrics and Child Health*, 11(1): 25–8.
Lester, H. and Campbell, S. (2010) Developing Quality and Outcomes Framework (QOF) indicators and the concept of 'QOFability', *Quality in Primary Care*, 18(2): 103–9.
Mangione-Smith, R. et al. (2007) The quality of ambulatory care delivered to children in the United States, *New England Journal of Medicine*, 357(15): 1515–23.
Marshall, M. et al. (2001) *Quality Indicators for General Practice: A practical guide for primary health care professionals and managers*. London: RSM Books.
Mattke, S. et al. (2006) *Health Care Quality Indicators Project Initial Indicators Report*. OECD Health Working Papers, No. 22. Paris: Organisation for Economic Co-operation and Development.
Melville, C., Wall, D. and Anderson, J. (2002) Paediatric training for family doctors: principals and practice, *Medical Education*, 36(5): 449–55.
Moll van Charante, E.P., van Steenwijk-Opdam, P.C. and Bindels, P.J. (2007) Out-of-hours demand for GP care and emergency services: patients' choices and referrals by general practitioners and ambulance services, *BMC Family Practice*, 8: 46.
Mundinger, M.O. et al. (2000) Primary care outcomes in patients treated by nurse practitioners or physicians: a randomized trial, *JAMA*, 283: 59–68.
Murphy, A.W. et al. (1996) Randomised controlled trial of general practitioner versus usual medical care in an urban accident and emergency department: process, outcome, and comparative cost, *BMJ*, 312(7039): 1135–42.

NHS Confederation (2011) *Quality and Outcomes Framework guidance for GMS contract 2011/12: Delivering investment in general practice*. http://www.nhsemployers.org/Aboutus/Publications/Documents/QOF_guidance_GMS_contract_2011_12.pdf [accessed 23 June 2013].

Otters, H.B. et al. (2005) Changing morbidity patterns in children in Dutch general practice: 1987–2001, *European Journal of General Practice*, 11(1): 17–22.

Parkerton, P.H., Smith, D.G. and Straley, H.L. (2004) Primary care practice coordination versus physician continuity, *Family Medicine*, 36(1): 15–21.

Patterson, C.C. et al. (2009) Incidence trends for childhood type 1 diabetes in Europe during 1989–2003 and predicted new cases 2005–20: a multicentre prospective registration study, *The Lancet*, 373(9680): 2027–33.

Pearson, G.A. et al. (2011) Why children die: avoidable factors associated with child deaths, *Archives of Disease in Childhood*, 96(10): 927–31.

Poole, S.R. et al. (1982) Pediatric training in family practice: a core curriculum, *Journal of Family Practice*, 15(6): 1145–56.

RCGP (2008) *Weekly Returns Service Annual Prevalence Report 2007*. Birmingham: Birmingham Research Unit, Royal College of General Practitioners.

RCGP (2010) *RCGP Child Health Strategy 2010–2015*. London: Royal College of General Practitioners.

RCPCH (2007) *Response to "Our NHS, Our Future"*. London: Royal College of Paediatrics and Child Health.

RICHE (2012) Quality of child health service indicators. Final Report, RICHE Work Package 2. *Research Inventory for Child Health in Europe*. http://www.childhealthresearch.eu [accessed 23 June 2013].

Saltman, R.B., Rico, A. and Boerma, W. (2006) *Primary care in the driver's seat? Organisational reform in European primary care*. Maidenhead: Open University Press.

Sands, R. et al. (2012) Medical problems presenting to paediatric emergency departments: 10 years on, *Emergency Medicine Journal*, 29(5): 379–82.

Saxena, S. et al. (2009) Increasing short-stay unplanned hospital admissions among children in England; time trends analysis '97–'06, *PLOS One*, 4(10): e7484.

Shi, L. et al. (2004) Primary care, infant mortality, and low birth weight in the states of the USA, *Journal of Epidemiology and Community Health*, 58(5): 374–80.

Smyth, L. (2009) Making integration work requires more than goodwill, *Healthcare Quarterly*, 13 Spec No: 43–8.

Starfield, B. (1991) Primary care and health. A cross-national comparison, *JAMA*, 266(16): 2268–71.

Starfield, B. (1998) *Primary Care: Balancing Health Needs, Services, and Technology*. New York: Oxford University Press.

Starfield, B. and Shi, L. (2002) Policy relevant determinants of health: an international perspective, *Health Policy*, 60(3): 201–18.

Starfield, B., Shi, L. and Macinko, J. (2005) Contribution of primary care to health systems and health, *The Milbank Quarterly*, 83(3): 457–502.

Stephenson, T. (2010) Paediatric primary care in Europe: variation between countries, *Archives of Disease in Childhood*, 95(10): 767–8.

Suter, E. et al. (2009) Ten key principles for successful health systems integration, *Healthcare Quarterly*, 13 Spec No, 16–23.

Torjesen, I. (2012) Care of IBD patients compromised by poor communication between primary and secondary care, *BMJ*, 344: e2675.

van Esso, D. et al. (2010) Paediatric primary care in Europe: variation between countries, *Archives of Disease in Childhood*, 95(10): 791–5.

van Uden, C.J. et al. (2006) Development of out-of-hours primary care by general practitioners (GPs) in The Netherlands: from small-call rotations to large-scale GP cooperatives, *Family Medicine*, 38(8): 565–9.

Virtanen, J.I. et al. (2006) Children's use of general practitioner services in the five Nordic countries, *Journal of Epidemiology and Community Health*, 60(2): 162–7.

Wensing, M. et al. (2002) Patient satisfaction with availability of general practice: an international comparison, *International Journal for Quality in Health Care*, 14(2): 111–18.

Westert, G.P., Jabaaij, L. and Schellevis, F.G. (2006) *Morbidity, Performance and Quality in Primary Care: Dutch General Practice on Stage*. Abingdon: Radcliffe Publishing Ltd.

Wolfe, I. et al. (2011) Improving child health services in the UK: insights from Europe and their implications for the NHS reforms, *BMJ*, 342: d1277.

Wolfe, I. et al. (2013) Health services for children in western Europe, *The Lancet*, 381(9873): 1224–34.

chapter three

Health services for children with long-term conditions and non-communicable disease

Ingrid Wolfe

"very sore nights and days" a child's experience of chronic illness

Newton (2011)

Introduction

Non-communicable diseases (NCDs) have become the leading cause of morbidity and mortality in Europe. Children have not been spared from this trend, with an epidemiological shift away from acute infectious diseases. This has important implications for children, leading to diminished quality, and sometimes duration, of life. Furthermore, children with long-term conditions are often unable to attend and participate fully in school, which may compromise their future development and potential. There are indirect effects on parents through depressed labour market productivity, with subsequent macroeconomic and wider social consequences.

The growing importance of NCDs poses challenges for health services and systems. Health care systems in European countries were designed as an episodic care model, in which acute infectious illnesses predominated and the expected outcomes of contact with the health service were usually cure or death (Allotey et al., 2011). Children with NCDs need a different model of care, tailored specifically to their needs and not fitted in around the demands of acute illness. They need long-term, often complex, packages of care, provided by different health professionals, often working in different organizations, and they may also require input from social services, such as special educational support. New service models will be needed, and providers will have to work in different ways from the past.

The term NCDs, as used in this chapter, includes long-term and ongoing conditions and chronic diseases. There is a dual purpose in using this term: partly for brevity, but also to support the idea that children and young people should be included in the wider discourse on NCDs in adults, which is at last attracting high-level political attention.

This chapter begins with an overview of the challenges facing policy-makers and service-providers that look after children with NCDs. The second section examines strategies for the prevention and management of chronic disease in childhood. The chapter concludes with recommendations for improving chronic care systems for children and young people.

Assessing the challenges

Children and young people with NCDs: a neglected priority

NCDs rose rapidly up the political agenda in 2011, when they were the subject of a United Nations High-Level Meeting for heads of governments. However, thus far, efforts to tackle them have focused largely on adults, with a few notable exceptions (NCDCHILD, 2013). Yet, children are directly affected by NCDs and, as future adults, measures to improve their health can play an important role in stemming the future epidemic of NCDs in the whole population. Finally, the lack of attention to children with NCDs is unjust. The United Nations Convention on the Rights of the Child, Article 24 asserts that children have a right to the highest attainable standard of health, with the provision of health care and disease prevention based on primary care (United Nations, 1989). The contribution of conditions in early life to NCDs in adulthood is now well recognized (Kuh et al., 2003), as discussed in Chapter 1, leading to acceptance of the need for a life-course approach to NCD prevention. Children are affected by the four major NCDs that also afflict adults: cardiovascular disease, respiratory disease, cancer and diabetes; and by the common risk factors: tobacco use, alcohol abuse, unhealthy diet and physical inactivity. The health (and financial) gains that can be accrued by preventing and treating NCDs in early life are substantial (Marmot et al., 2012).

Trends in childhood NCDs

The terms 'chronic disease', 'long-term condition', 'ongoing condition' and 'non-communicable disease' are sometimes used interchangeably. However, there are many definitional problems; for example, many children with cerebral palsy might not consider themselves to have a disease at all. Some infections are chronic; for example, children may live for decades with human immunodeficiency virus (HIV), requiring services planned and delivered in much the same way as for children with NCDs. A definition that considers the impact on children's lives, and that takes into account their health service needs, is more useful than one restricted to aetiology or disease category.

The substantial decline in childhood mortality in the past 50 years has involved both communicable and non-communicable diseases, but the reduction in NCDs has been much less marked. As a consequence, the relative importance of NCDs has markedly increased (Viner et al., 2011). NCDs cause approximately 77,000 deaths among children 0–14 years old per year in western Europe (Wang et al., 2012) and the burden of disability caused by NCDs now represents the largest category among children (see Chapter 1).

Asthma is one of the most common chronic diseases in childhood, responsible for 1.0 million DALYs in 2010 (Murray et al., 2012). Its epidemiology is complex. Standardized international comparisons report wide variation in the prevalence of asthma symptoms (up to 20-fold differences) (Beasley, 1998) and in trends, with evidence of decreases in prevalence in some countries, particularly among older children and adolescents, while in other countries and particularly among younger children it is increasing (Asher et al., 2006). While there has been little change in the overall prevalence of wheeze symptoms, there is an increase globally in the percentage of children with a diagnosis of asthma (Pearce et al., 2007), perhaps reflecting improved awareness and diagnosis. In the United States, the prevalence of asthma has been estimated by measuring the use of medicines for asthma. This indicates a near 50% increase (in medicine use) between 2002 and 2005 (Cox et al., 2008).

In contrast, trends in diabetes mellitus (type 1) are clearer: it is becoming increasingly common in young children and appears to be presenting earlier in childhood. The incidence of type 1 diabetes mellitus among children younger than 5 years is projected to double, causing the prevalence for children under 15 years in Europe to increase by 70% between 2005 and 2020 (Patterson et al., 2009). This rapidly rising incidence of diabetes mellitus will place considerable demands upon health services. Yet, while children with diabetes place a significant demand on health services, diabetes is only responsible for a small proportion (less than 1%) of DALYs in children under 14 years (135,000 DALYs in 2010 in western Europe) (Murray et al., 2012). Similar trends are evident for type 2 diabetes, once seen almost exclusively in adults but now being detected at much younger ages (Dabelea, Bell and D'Agostino, 2007). In the United States, the prevalence of type 2 diabetes in 5–19-year-old children, estimated by the use of medications, has doubled between 2002 and 2005 (Cox et al., 2008). Indeed, it is now the major form of diabetes in adolescence in certain populations such as Native Americans, Asian and Pacific islanders. If obesity trends continue as predicted, it is likely to become an increasingly significant part of childhood disease.

Childhood cancer is responsible for over 13,000 deaths and 1 million DALYs per year (approximately 5% of NCD-related DALYs) in 0–14-year-olds in 2010 in western Europe (Murray et al., 2012; Wang et al., 2012). More effective treatments have achieved remarkable improvements in recovery rates. However, with longer survival, increasing complications and long-term problems are becoming apparent. Late treatment-related problems include secondary cancers, organ dysfunction, and cognitive and psychological problems. The likelihood of long-term complications varies according to the cancer site and treatment, but approximately 75% of children who have survived childhood cancer will develop at least one adverse event, and around a quarter will develop five or more (Geenen et al., 2007).

The complications of premature birth are the leading cause of disability (DALYs) among children under 5 years in western Europe (IHME, 2012); for example, children born prematurely are at increased risk of cerebral palsy, a long-term condition that can lead to a variety of difficulties and dependent states. It is thought to affect around 2 in every 1000 live births. There have been small increases over time among normal birth-weight babies, declines among premature and low birth-weight babies, and stable or decreasing rates among babies born before 27 weeks' gestation and whose birth weight was between 500g and 1249g (Pharoah et al., 1990; Stanley and Watson, 1992; Pharoah, Platt andCooke, 1996; Robertson, Svenson and Joffres, 1998; Hagberg et al., 2001; Winter et al., 2002; Surman, Newdick and Johnson, 2003; Himmelmann et al., 2005).

Cardiovascular disease accounted for 500,000 DALYs among children aged 0–14 years in 2010 in western Europe, representing 2% of all DALYs related to NCD (Murray et al., 2012). The incidence of stroke is increasing in young people, reflecting the rise in risk factors such as hypertension, diabetes and obesity (Bigi et al., 2011). Cerebrovascular disease accounted for 120,000 DALYs or 1 in 5 of all cardiovascular DALYs among children aged 0–14 years in 2010 in western Europe (Murray et al., 2012).

Inequities and NCDs

Poorer children are at greater risk of NCDs than their wealthier peers (Marmot, 2010). Their disadvantage begins *in-utero* and, as discussed in Chapter 1, there are socioeconomic effects on pregnancy outcomes that can affect the entire life-course.

Modifiable risk factors for NCDs: a public health approach

From a public health perspective, the first step in any response to NCDs is to prevent them from occurring. Many NCD risks are modifiable by public policy, for example, intermediate risk factors (such as overweight and obesity) or upstream determinants (such as nutrition, physical activity, tobacco, alcohol and air quality). Chapter 1 outlines some of the more important risk factors and Chapter 5 examines in detail the policy implications of addressing these issues and interventions to promote and protect health. Finally, Chapter 11 describes a comprehensive approach to preventing and treating NCDs as part of the wider health system.

Life circumstances of children with NCDs

Living with NCDs can present distinct challenges in a child's life: at home, at school and in the health care system. For example, children with chronic health conditions are at increased risk of abuse and neglect (Jaudes and Mackey-Bilaver, 2008). A nationwide study in Sweden documented an increased risk of physical abuse for children with chronic conditions (odds ratio [OR] 1.67), substantially further increased if there is also intimate partner violence (OR 2.54), and that these risks are even higher among families living in poor areas, who have migrated to Sweden, and where the child is not living with both biological parents (OR 4.14) (Svensson, Bornehag and Janson, 2011).

Life at school poses practical difficulties for children with NCDs, ranging from the need to take medicines during the school day, to requiring special support in a mainstream school or attending a dedicated school for children with special or additional needs. The experience of illness can diminish school attendance, participation and performance, and reduce potential employability as an adult (Maslow et al., 2011). Children with NCDs can also be indirectly affected by the impact of their parents' or carers' reduced ability to work and earn due to reduced workforce participation and wages, increased job turnover or early retirement.

Worryingly, the quality of care that children with NCDs receive may vary according to ethnic origin; for example, in the Netherlands, there is evidence to suggest that children with asthma who have migrated to Holland may receive suboptimal care compared with ethnic Dutch children (Urbanus-van Laar et al., 2008). Qualitative research in the United Kingdom suggests that many families with children who have severe and enduring health needs and disabilities see the need for a key worker to coordinate services (such as organizing hospital discharges so that community or home-based services are in place) and to coordinate the range of services needed for a coherent package of care. Many complain that:

- there are few or no regular reviews of their care needs;
- there is a lack of appropriate services for acute problems in the context of an ongoing chronic illness;
- there are insufficient services in place to meet their needs at times of transition to adult services;
- professionals involved in their care fail to treat children and young people with chronic conditions with dignity and respect.

Mismatch between health services and children's needs

Children with NCDs need an ongoing relationship with health professionals that focuses on more than simply managing their condition. It should be about ensuring maximum capability and minimum complications for both child and family, with 'care more than cure' often being the expected outcome. Although children with long-term conditions will experience acute episodes requiring discrete health care interactions, continuity of care is a key goal. This presents challenges to most European health systems, which were configured largely to cope with the acute infectious illnesses that dominated health care in the early to mid-part of the 20th century. This 'tyranny of the urgent' (Bodenheimer, Wagner and Grumbach, 2002a) increases the difficulties in shifting health systems towards services for children with long-term conditions.

The story of a child with asthma (Box 3.1) illustrates some of the complex needs of a child with a common chronic illness, and demonstrates many of the challenges in obtaining the services he deserves.

The mismatch between children's health needs and the provision of services causes many problems. First, health outcomes for children with NCDs are suboptimal in many countries. Asthma, a common childhood NCD managed predominantly in primary care, exemplifies the problems that can arise when there is insufficient focus on prevention and effective first-contact care. Around

Box 3.1 Asthma: a case study of a common chronic illness

Thomas is a 5-year-old boy who wheezes with every cold he gets. He has been ill at least eight times in the past year and has been admitted to hospital as an emergency with difficulty breathing three times this winter. He has eczema. His immunization history is unclear, but he may not have had all his routine immunizations. He is the third child of his parents who are long-term unemployed. His mother has depression. Both his parents have allergies to pets and his mother has hay fever. Both parents smoke, but not indoors. The family live in a one-bedroom apartment, on the fourth floor of a building with no elevator. They have moved three times in two years. Thomas has been given two inhalers to use when he gets a cold, but his parents don't think they help him very much. The family regularly use multiple different hospitals, emergency departments and primary care providers.

What does a child like Thomas need?

- Thomas will need care, advice and support for the multiple risk factors, upstream determinants and manifest clinical problems he has.
- He needs access to a health system that will deliver high-quality multidisciplinary care; be sensitive to the risks he is exposed to; anticipate his needs; and respond to his development and evolving health needs.
- Thomas's family may need housing support and smoking cessation advice.
- The health team should follow evidence-based clinical guidelines.
- Support and follow-up at home should be available if necessary.
- There should be ready access to advice at night and during weekends.
- Clinical information systems should underpin the whole system: allowing data to be collated appropriately to track progress and plan services; ensuring that medical follow-up appointments are planned and reminders sent; and enabling multidisciplinary discussions beyond the health sector.

No single professional or organization can provide all the care and advice Thomas needs.

Table 3.1 Comparison of diabetes control in children and young people in England and Wales, and Germany and Austria

NICE HbA1c target, 2004	*England and Wales, 2010/2011*	*Germany and Austria, 2011*
HbA1c <58mmol/mol	15.1% females 16.4% males	50–55%
HbA1c considered to be at risk levels	Over 30% (>80mmol/mol, 9.5%)	10% (>75mmol/mol, 9.0%)

NICE: (UK) National Institute for Health and Care Excellence
Source: de Beaufort et al., 2007; Gerstl et al., 2008; Cinek et al., 2012

60% of hospital admissions for asthma could be avoided with more effective prevention, such as written care plans to prevent and manage exacerbations, better health education, and support for parental smoking cessation (Reindal and Oymar, 2006; Fuhrman et al., 2011). However, first-contact services are not the only sector failing to deliver high-quality care for children with NCDs. Hospital-based or specialist paediatricians usually provide care for children with diabetes, and outcomes are poor in many cases. For example, fewer than 6% of children with diabetes in England receive care consistent with the guidelines, and preventable diabetic emergencies and deaths still occur (RCPCH, 2012b). England's performance as measured by HbA1c, an important indicator of diabetic control is comparatively poor, as shown in Table 3.1.

Second, services are used in inefficient ways, so that urgent services may become overwhelmed, leaving insufficient capacity for planned services for children with NCDs. This means that: health services are inevitably reactive; opportunities for prevention are missed; services become fragmented and inconvenient for families; and preventable emergency admissions are a frequent result. Most importantly, the chasm between needs and services causes unnecessary suffering for children and families. A parent's description of trying to fit his child's care (for a rare and complex condition) within the constraints of a system clearly ill-suited to her needs vividly portrays the consequences for the child and her family (Box 3.2). Their experiences are crystallized into specific recommendations for how to improve services from the child and family's perspectives.

The ever-increasing demand for urgent care is one of the factors contributing to poor outcomes for children with NCDs, as hospital services are overwhelmed (Gill et al., 2013). The immediacy of acute illness and risk of adverse serious outcomes inevitably mean that urgent services take precedence over planned care, and if first-contact care is inefficient, services for children with NCDs will fall behind. 'Failure demand' is what happens when a child and their family get to a health care setting and fail to find the right care for their concern or condition, leading to repeated attempts to access the care they need. This is an inefficient and costly use of health services and resources. Poorly planned and inefficiently delivered first-contact care produces a bottleneck problem,

Box 3.2 Struggling against the system: caring for a child with a complex chronic condition

My daughter has a rare complex condition that most people haven't heard of; it is known by the genetic mutation that causes it – CDKL5. It causes my daughter to suffer terrible seizures and she is blind, cannot walk, talk or eat unaided. She has reached adult age now, but my wife and I continue to look after her, just as we have done every day since she was born. But all these years in contact with the National Health Service have brought a harsh dose of reality to our lives. We have battled bureaucracy, fought lethargy, observed inefficiency, and had to guard against outbreaks of incompetence.

To take one small example: we needed larger nappies for her after an adolescent growth spurt. It took five weeks, several phone calls and visits from community nurses, and a great deal of paperwork before we succeeded. Our daughter was distressed, we were frustrated, and the pile of laundry was immense.

The problems were apparent from the earliest days. While waiting to see a specialist in a famous children's hospital we met an anxious young couple who had travelled across the country for their newborn sick baby's first appointment there. 'Didn't anyone tell you?' asked the receptionist breezily, 'Your appointment's been cancelled.'

When our daughter was 7 years old, she had a major neurological review, spending three days and nights with sensors connected to brain-scanning devices glued to her head, under constant video surveillance, while my exhausted wife comforted her and tried to keep her from ripping off the sensors: a huge strain but worthwhile, we thought, in our hope for answers and help. A few weeks later, after the usual waiting-room delays, the neurologist summoned us and asked us why we were there. She opened our daughter's notes and asked what was wrong with her. Then she couldn't find the results. We stormed out, me in fury and my wife in tears.

Or there was the nurse (despite having been told our daughter was blind) who asked if she would like to watch a video. The blood samples taken (badly) from our child . . . and then lost. Results delayed. Needless tense weeks of waiting.

A celebrated neurologist measured our heads and blithely asserted that our daughter, then suffering up to 30 seizures a day, would have a just slightly lower than average IQ.

Blasé receptionists. Unanswered emails. Overcrowded clinics.

So what do I think children with complex chronic illnesses need?

- All services should be run for the needs of the child and family rather than for the producers and managers. This simple statement means that appointments are kept, doctors bother to read clinical notes rather than endlessly repeat questions, consultations are held in pleasant friendly environments, with staff who are compassionate, open-minded, supportive and professional.

- There should be expert points of contact available, who know the details of a child's condition and are available out-of-hours, rather than relying on often junior staff at A and E who have no knowledge of a highly complex condition.
- There needs to be someone who knows our child and ourselves, our personal circumstances and her medical history; who can help us find our way through the health service and negotiate with social services, schools, transport and other local authority services; and who will be with us for the long-term – someone to share the pressures of being full-time carers. We have found this with a palliative care team, but only after many years and in the most extreme circumstances.
- The ability to choose what sort of services are used, within set budgets, and the freedom to seek better care elsewhere with ease when experiencing poor-quality care.
- There needs to be as much transparency as possible, for everything from spending to health outcomes. Relying on hospital reputation is not enough. We need information to make intelligent choices.
- Health service workers should remember they are there to serve the public: there should be as much emphasis on personal skills in health services as on academic achievement. It is meant to be health *care*, after all.

Source: Ian Birrell, personal account.

preventing chronic care services from receiving the attention they require, and explains why a whole-systems approach is necessary.

Integrated care, where services transcend boundaries between providers and organizations are an attempt towards such a comprehensive approach, and has become a widespread policy objective. However at least for children, little progress has been made (Wolfe et al., 2011).

The reasons for the failure to make sufficient progress in adapting systems are complex and include barriers arising from organizations, management, governance, finance and the workforce. The reluctance to cooperate often begins with different, sometimes competing, approaches to care, and professional rivalries and perceived threats to medical monopolies may ensue (Baerlocher and Detsky, 2009). Other structural, organizational and financial barriers include: providers with separate management structures, often competing for resources, and sometimes with explicit disincentives to cooperate; and a lack of clarity and accountability about professional roles. Professionals, services and sectors may adopt dichotomous opposing perspectives, for example, primary care versus hospital; generalist versus specialist; health versus social care. The increasing specialization of child health professionals – especially doctors – that has accompanied advances in medical practice may, ironically, have prevented health systems being sufficiently responsive to the changing needs and demands of the population. Professional health education and training have not kept up with changing health needs because of fragmented and outdated curricula that produce doctors ill-prepared to address the needs of the population they will serve. Efforts to address these problems have largely failed, partly because of professional tribalism, for example, between GPs and paediatricians in the case of child health. Indeed, human resources are central to the ability of any country's health system to deliver care effectively, and it is widely recognized that there is a need to transform the education of health professionals as part of strategies to strengthen health systems (Frenk et al., 2010). These issues are discussed further in Chapter 11.

The ways in which health services are planned further explain the lack of progress in developing new models of care and the limited ability to adapt to the needs and demands of children and families. Historical patterns of service use, rather than contemporary estimations of need, usually determine service configuration. Staff numbers and distribution are planned on the same basis. This situation of supply determining demand is inherently flawed and perpetuates systems that are not designed around the needs of children and families.

As the prevalence of chronic disease continues to rise, the pressure on health services and systems will undoubtedly grow. Furthermore, financial constraints on health service budgets throughout Europe add to the pressures to increase efficient service use, prevent disease and reduce future use of health services. Developing new models of care and closing hospital beds feature widely in the policy discourse of many countries.

NCD strategies for children and young people: a review of the evidence and European experience

Concepts in chronic and integrated care

While most approaches to chronic disease care share the aims of improving outcomes and efficiency of care for patients with complex needs, usually by linking elements of cure and care, there is a spectrum of complexity. A comprehensive definition of integrated care is provided by Kodner and Spreeuwenberg (2002), writing that:

> Integration is a coherent set of methods and models on the funding, administrative, organisational, service delivery and clinical levels designed to create connectivity, alignment and collaboration within and between the cure and care sectors. The goal of these methods and models is to enhance quality of care and quality of life, consumer satisfaction and system efficiency for patients with complex, long term problems cutting across multiple service, providers and settings. The result of such multi-pronged efforts to promote integration for the benefit of these special patient groups is called "integrated care" (Kodner and Spreeuwenberg, 2002).

Although their definition specifies collaboration within and between cure and care, much of the discourse on integration focuses on closer working between health and social services, so integration within the health sector may be considered to be of secondary concern. In reality, there is often a significant gap between primary and secondary health care for children (Wolfe et al., 2011).

WHO's definition is helpful as it addresses the problem of fragmented care familiar to many patients with chronic conditions, describing integrated care as:

> bringing together inputs, delivery, management and organization of services related to diagnosis, treatment, care, rehabilitation and health promotion . . . as a means to improve services in relation to access, quality, user satisfaction and efficiency (Grone and Garcia-Barbero, 2001).

Thus integrated care (perhaps the most popular current concept in health care), promises to deliver more efficient and higher quality care in keeping with what children and families want: smooth, seamless care regardless of the boundaries between professions, organizations and sectors. A recent review suggests that clinical coordination, especially when combined with other measures such as admission avoidance management, can improve quality of care and reduce costs (Øvretveit, 2011). Integration of clinical services is important, but it is one part of many aspects of coordination required to improve services for children with NCDs. Children need care that is not only integrated between primary and secondary care providers (vertical integration) and across providers such as physical health and mental health services (horizontal integration), but also integrated across time (longitudinally) (Halfon, Du Plessis and Inkelas, 2007). Integration over time is necessary to ensure that services are coordinated and appropriately adapted to fit the changing developmental context of the child and family. This requires joined-up anticipatory care and a data system that allows monitoring of individual and population children's health and developmental trajectories.

Bridging the boundaries between providers, organizations and sectors is important for providing high-quality, responsive services for children with long-term conditions across the continuum of care (Ouwens et al., 2005). Such complex models of care, relying on professionals from different specialties and organizations, as well as clinical and non-clinical backgrounds, necessitate collaboration and cooperation between organizations and individuals who may usually work separately. A system is needed that is flexible enough to configure care according to the long-term needs of the child and family, while also providing care through episodes of acute illness and for the duration of childhood, finally managing a smooth and effective transition to adult chronic care services or, if the illness is progressive, to palliative care services. Finally, to be wholly successful, a chronic care system must include disease prevention and early detection.

Integration is comprehensive when it links public health, population-based and patient-centred approaches to health care, focusing on the diverse needs of whole populations, not just care groups or diseases. Systemic integration of this kind requires alignment of functions and activities, such that there is a coherence of policy at all levels of organization, producing an integrated delivery system; it is characterized by common values, or a shared philosophy of care, between providers, a normative process whereby shared commitment underpins the delivery of care (Nolte and McKee, 2008; Curry and Ham, 2010). Whole-systems thinking underpins this approach to improving care (de Savigny and Adam, 2009).

Chronic care and integrated service models

The Chronic Care Model (CCM) (Figure 3.1) was developed in the United States and has been very influential (Coleman et al., 2009). It was not designed specifically for children but its aims (to overcome the barriers to effective, coordinated and efficient care for people with chronic disease, inherent in hospital-centric health care systems that were built to cater for acute episodes of illness) apply equally to all age groups (Bodenheimer, Wagner and Grumbach, 2002a, 2002b). The CCM encompasses assessment, treatment and follow-up. The model is built on four interacting components: supported self-management; service delivery system redesign to support collaboration; decision support; and clinical information systems to facilitate integrative working. To function optimally, these elements should be within a health system that links the model appropriately with resources and policies in the wider context. The CCM seeks informed active patients (and families) working with prepared and proactive teams of professionals to deliver interactive care and, ultimately, improved outcomes of chronic conditions. The CCM combines various interacting system components that are considered to be effective individually.

To date, most evidence of the effectiveness of the CCM is limited to individual components rather than to the model as a whole, and relates to conditions such as diabetes in adult populations. A meta-analysis of trials including patients with diabetes, asthma, congestive heart failure and depression, showed that interventions comprising at least one element of

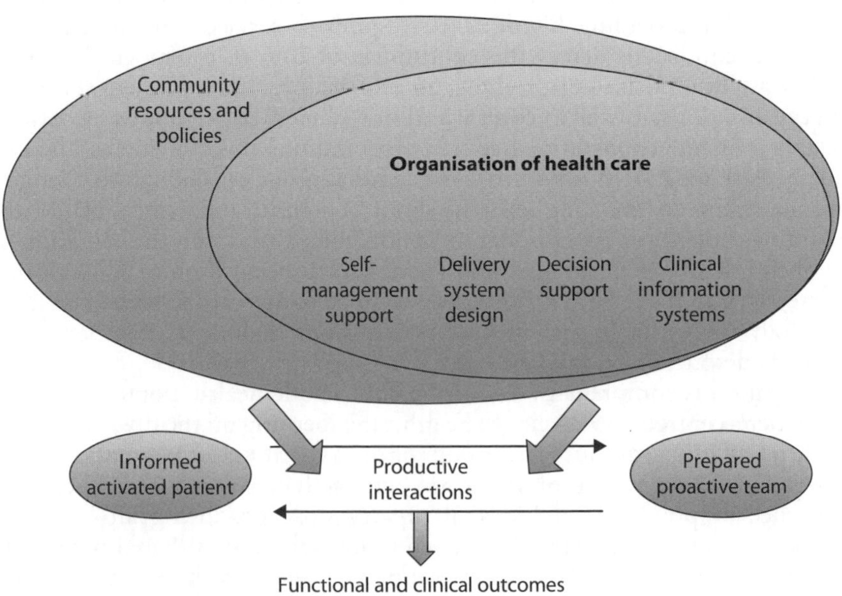

Figure 3.1 The Chronic Care Model

Source: Epping-Jordan et al., 2004

the CCM could improve both clinical outcomes and processes of care (Tsai et al., 2005). Delivery system design and self-management support are the modules most consistently found to be effective, however most studies have been in adults with diabetes (Zwar et al., 2006). Many early studies were weak methodologically, or had findings unlikely to be generalizable to the whole population (let alone children). Most were unable to demonstrate a relationship between specific aspects of intervention and outcome (Nolte and McKee, 2008). Although the CCM has intuitive appeal, and individual components are accepted as being effective in some settings, there is little evidence, to date, that the model as a whole is effective. However, because of methodological challenges in evaluating the CCM, and the relative novelty of the concept, absence of evidence may not constitute evidence of ineffectiveness.

The CCM has been most comprehensively adapted for children within the United States, where the system is known as the 'medical home' (also called the 'patient-centred medical home'). See Chapter 2 for discussion of the CCM regarding primary care aspects. This aims to deliver coordinated, personalized and high-quality care for patients with long-term conditions (Cooley et al., 2009). The key features are that each child has a personal physician (key worker), who provides first-contact, continuous and comprehensive care. Care is coordinated with comprehensive teams across all elements of the health system, working closely together in 'flat management' structures without hierarchies. Teams include primary care and specialist doctors, nurses, other professionals, and patients as active participants. Systems supporting such integrated care include patient registries and information technology designed for the purpose. A study of medical home services for children with chronic conditions, including asthma, diabetes, attention-deficit hyperactivity disorder (ADHD), cerebral palsy and epilepsy, reported a significant association between a strong medical home model (as measured by an index of implementation) and reduced hospital admissions, and a non-significant association with reduced emergency department visits (Cooley et al., 2009). A review of the evidence for its effectiveness provides some, albeit weak, evidence that medical homes may achieve improved health outcomes, timeliness of care, family-centredness and family functioning for children with special health care needs and their families (Cooley, 2004; Homer et al., 2008).

Integration has wide appeal and offers logical solutions to some of the problems experienced by children with long-term conditions and their families. There is some evidence of improved processes, but evidence of improved health outcomes is limited. A review of 20 studies of services (not specifically for children) that provide integrated primary and secondary care (defined as joint planning and delivery of care, and enhanced information exchange), which included randomized controlled trials (RCTs), controlled before-and-after studies and interrupted time series analyses, found no consistent evidence of improved outcomes in physical and mental health, psychosocial well-being, hospital admissions or satisfaction with treatment, but did demonstrate improved prescribing. Most of the studies examined complex interventions and were of short duration, so it is possible that beneficial results had not yet been realized (Smith, Allwright and O'Dowd, 2007). However, a review of interagency collaboration to improve health at the level of the individual found no evidence of health gain (Hayes et al., 2012).

One explanation for the limited evidence of successful health outcomes from the CCM as a whole may be due to the difficulties of evaluating complex health service interventions. Moreover, there is comparatively little work to develop models of integrated services for children with chronic illnesses and evaluation inevitably lags further behind. There are some individual studies that suggest promising results for the child population; for example, a pre- and post-intervention comparison of patients participating in integrated services for children with asthma, with matched controls at non-participating sites, found that clinically important processes of care, health-related quality of life and asthma-specific quality of life, all improved significantly in the intervention group (Mangione-Smith et al., 2005). An RCT of a clinical pathway for asthma in general practice achieved reduced numbers of hospital admissions and emergency department attendances, but as there was improvement in both intervention and control groups there may have been an alternative explanation, such as 'contamination' between the arms of the trial (Mitchell et al., 2005). Another study comparing quality of care between specialists and generalists for children with asthma found significantly more compliance with national guidelines for children looked after by specialists; they were 6.7 times more likely to use controller medications (95% confidence interval [CI] 1.5–30.4), 6.5 times more likely to have had lung function tests (95% CI 2.4–18.1) and 5.9 times more likely to have been given advice about asthma triggers and avoidance (CI 1.3–26.2). These are important, if indicative, results since under-treatment is an important element in poor outcomes for children with asthma (Asthma UK, 2007). An RCT investigating the effects of an integrated care model (Hospital at Home) for children with acute asthma found that home care was as effective as hospital care and more acceptable to parents and children (Sartain et al., 2002). Finally, specific multiprofessional intervention packages, which would form a component of an integrated care model, have been shown to improve outcomes in diabetes. Children and young people who receive intensive medical management together with psychosocial support, and whose families receive tailored education, have improved glycaemic control and diabetes outcomes (Diabetes Control and Complications Trial Research Group, 1994; White et al., 2001).

The international experience

Many European countries deliver some elements of care through multiprofessional teams. At the micro level of the CCM framework, most countries have made good progress in recognizing the need for partnerships between the children and their family and the professionals, and many countries have developed some aspect of CCM for children (Table 3.2).

Table 3.2 Models of care for children with chronic conditions in Europe

Sweden and Finland: *Chains of care; supplemented in Sweden by multiprofessional primary care centres, where GPs, paediatricians and children's nurses work closely together.*	Chains of care are designed to improve integration between services for children with specific chronic conditions and therefore quality of care. The system was developed as a response to the fragmentation of care resulting from excessive decentralization of services, with professionals working in separate organizations, which resulted in a lack of coordination. Together with increasing professional specialization, this contributed to a lack of general oversight of patient care. Early evaluation revealed problems with weak incentives for collaboration, perceived challenges to existing power structures, and conflicting values among participants, especially physicians. Implementation was facilitated by: involving patients as active participants; allowing sufficient time for change; developing supportive policy and financing instruments; and maintaining motivation by focusing strongly on quality improvement (Ahgren, 2003). A further element of integration in Sweden comprises community-based children's health centres, staffed by GPs, paediatricians and children's nurses working closely together. When a child needs more specialist care, a referral is made to a hospital-based paediatrician. A named physician coordinates the individual child's care. By contrast, Finnish paediatricians are responsible for groups of patients with a particular condition. Specialist nurses provide a point of contact for urgent problems in both countries, and there are education programmes for families to encourage supported self-management.
France: *Coordinated care for patients with a specified list of conditions (affections de longue durée [ALD]) and national standards.*	France has extensive health networks designed to improve care across the primary–secondary care boundary for patients with chronic disease. In addition, it has a system of financial incentives for using evidence-based guidelines for the management of chronic conditions. Recently, France introduced mandatory registration of patients with GPs, as part of a gatekeeping strategy, and to enhance patients' abilities to navigate through the health care system (Nolte and McKee, 2008). The system of coordinating care for children with certain specified chronic conditions, or ALD, is intended to ensure that children receive personal treatment plans with lists of investigations and interventions covered by health insurance and according to prescribed national standards of care. Children receive routine care from a specialist service, such as paediatric pneumology. However, for an acute illness parents are entitled to choose any doctor. Coordinated planned care is achieved through multidisciplinary appointments in specialist centres. This system, with its focus on only one specialist aspect of the child's health and development, is considered expensive, and does little to bridge gaps between generalists and specialists.

(*Continued*)

Table 3.2 Models of care for children with chronic conditions in Europe (continued)

The Netherlands: *Transmural care, a collaborative integrated system of care delivered by professionals working together within and outside hospitals, in mutual agreement and according to patients' needs, supplemented by a system of youth health care (YHC) services.*	The Netherlands has a complex health system of multiple insurers and providers that risks fragmentation of care. The 'transmural' system approximates the CCM, and was developed specifically to bridge the gap between primary and secondary care. Health professionals have explicit individual and shared responsibilities. For example, specialist nurses manage hospital admissions and discharge planning. The Dutch experience early on in the process of establishing transmural services provides an example of organizational integration occurring without sufficient clinical and service integration. Stronger legal frameworks and financial incentives were put in place to strengthen these aspects. The problem of integrated structures failing to create actual integration of delivery of patient care is well recognized (Burns and Pauly, 2002). A further distinct feature of the Dutch approach to integrated services is that YHC physicians provide some primary and preventive care alongside GPs. GPs and nurses provide care for simple chronic illnesses, such as uncomplicated asthma, while hospital-based paediatricians provide the mainstay of care for children with severe or complex illnesses. Either a GP or paediatrician assumes the coordinating role and offers urgent advice, depending on the nature and severity of the child's illness and care needs. There are shared professional guidelines, which further strengthen links between primary and secondary care (van der Linden, Spreeuwenberg and Schrijvers, 2001; Zwar et al., 2006). Evaluations of transmural care have been mixed, with persisting evidence of discontinuity between primary and secondary care, while organizational integration has not always led to clinical and service integration (van der Linden, 2001).
United Kingdom: *Clinical networks and Team around the Child.*	Although components of a CCM have been widely implemented in the United Kingdom, there is some evidence that the relevance to children's services is not clear (Campbell et al., 2005). Children with chronic illnesses may not have a specific professional who coordinates their care. This function may be provided by a GP or paediatrician but, anecdotally, is often the responsibility of parents, for whom it may represent a considerable commitment of time and energy. A variety of formal and informal networks have been set up, but with limited evaluation to date. Difficulties encountered include: resistance to change; lack of evidence to demonstrate benefits; financial disincentives to cooperation (promoting competition instead of collaboration); and organizational boundaries preventing cooperation between providers (RCPCH, 2012a). A child-specific integrated service 'Team around the Child' focuses on children with complex social and educational needs, and has a relative lack of health sector input. It has been criticized for being overly bureaucratic (Jones, 2006).

Italy: *Health and Social Care Networks, Assistenza Domiciliare Pediatrica (ADP).*	Italy's child health care is delivered almost exclusively by paediatricians, who assume responsibility for monitoring and managing children with long-term conditions, and act as the first point of access for urgent advice and consultations; for example, when drug doses need adjustment during intercurrent acute illness. Children with very severe or complex conditions who require specialist paediatric management are often followed up in hospitals rather than by primary care paediatricians in community settings. ADP is a bridge between specialist centres, community services provided by health districts and family paediatricians, ensuring that as much care as possible is delivered at home. ADP is being increasingly widely implemented and focuses on chronic conditions requiring, for example, parenteral nutrition, oxygen therapy, physiotherapy or frequent blood sampling (Tamburlini, 2012).
Germany: *Specialist multidisciplinary teams, Social Paediatric Centres (SPZ), and ModuS.*	GPs with an interest in a particular chronic disease, such as asthma or allergies, provide care in offices or hospitals. Specialized paediatricians, who coordinate care for children with complex or rare chronic illnesses, work in teams with other professionals, such as nurses, dieticians and physiotherapists. Pathways are organized on an individual patient basis, and it is rare for children to have multiple appointments in different places or on different days. Children with developmental disorders, epilepsy, behavioural disorders, learning difficulties and all forms of chronic disease with additional psychosocial problems, receive their care through SPZ, which are multidisciplinary teams of paediatricians (mostly specializing in neuropaediatrics), psychologists, physiotherapists, occupational therapists, speech therapists and social workers. SPZs are usually co-located with hospitals to facilitate the transfer of acutely ill children. Coordinated multidisciplinary care in Germany is facilitated by funding packages of care with a single provider organization rather than the usual fee-for-service model (Strassburg, 2011). ModuS is a teaching programme for patients and families that aims to integrate the management of chronic conditions into everyday lives (Szczepanski, 2010).
Norway	Norway's health system is strongly centred on primary care. Children with chronic illnesses have individualized written plans, setting out roles and responsibilities for all providers involved in their care, with a local health worker taking the coordinating role, while hospital-based paediatricians provide most of the specialist medical care. Urgent questions or problems are dealt with by paediatricians working on call in local hospitals. Parents are able to telephone directly for advice when needed. All hospitals have learning or mastering centres that provide information and training for families after a child has been diagnosed with a chronic disorder. Other families with similar problems are available for advice and support. Children with ongoing conditions almost always attend mainstream schools, with support from teachers and local health workers liaising closely with the school.

Source: Adapted from Wolfe et al., 2013

Risk reduction and disease prevention: a public health approach

Many chronic diseases have social, political and economic causes and consequences. An unhealthy diet, physical inactivity, tobacco and excessive alcohol use are major risk factors for NCDs. The globalization of many aspects of lifestyles throughout Europe has contributed significantly to the rising prevalence of these risk behaviours. Although chronic care models of health services are designed to manage people with chronic diseases, a more strategic approach is required to address disease determinants and prevent disease.

Despite the limited evidence of effectiveness, the CCM has been widely influential in the United States and, more recently, some aspects have been adopted in some European countries, such as England and Germany (Gensichen et al., 2006; Department of Health, 2010). The CCM has also been adapted by WHO into an 'Innovative Care for Chronic Conditions Framework' designed to be more flexible and useful in diverse settings (WHO, 2002; Epping-Jordan et al., 2004). This framework describes macro, meso and micro levels of operation for integrating services into a CCM, and builds on the 'Ottawa Charter for Health Promotion', which emphasizes the importance of social change for improving health (WHO, 1986). Key features include: partnership between children and their families and health care and other professional teams; continuity and coordination of the health care organization and community within which it operates; and a supportive macro-level policy environment to enable compassionate, effective and efficient care. An expanded model (Glasgow, Orleans and Wagner, 2001; Barr et al., 2003) sets the CCM within the context of the wider social and economic policy action that is needed to ensure a comprehensive approach to NCD prevention and management.

Strategies for risk reduction and disease prevention range from those targeted at individual children and families who are at increased risk, to population-based approaches for all people, irrespective of risk, with the intention of shifting the population risk profile. Furthermore, fiscal policy and legislation offer effective means of producing population-level behaviour change in favour of healthier lifestyles, as discussed in detail in Chapter 5, and informing the comprehensive strategy set out in the final chapter of this book.

WHO has produced a series of recommendations for population-based interventions to reduce NCD risk factors (Table 3.3), many specifically targeted at the child population (WHO, 2011). Individual interventions for prevention or early detection of NCDs among high-risk groups include vaccination and screening.

While these population-level approaches are usually most effective, there can also be a role for individual-level interventions. However, there are many barriers, including lack of awareness of risk and the solutions; practical constraints, such as lack of time or money; varying perceptions of risk; lack of accessibility; affordability; and acceptability of healthy lifestyle options. For example, social perceptions of 'overweight' have changed so that recognition and acknowledgement of the problem have become even more challenging. A United States study found that few parents of overweight children recognized that their child was overweight or were worried about the weight of their child (Eckstein et al., 2006).

Table 3.3 Selected population-wide interventions for reducing risk factors for NCDs

WHO recommended policies for immediate implementation to prevent disease, save lives and reduce costs	*Additional cost-effective and low-cost interventions to reduce risk factors*	*Interventions with strong evidence for effectiveness but lacking cost-effectiveness research*
Protect people from tobacco smoke and ban smoke in public places	Nicotine dependence treatments	Healthy nutrition environments in schools
Warnings about dangers of tobacco use	Promote adequate breastfeeding and complementary feeding	Nutrition information and counselling in health care settings
Enforce bans on tobacco advertising, promotion and sponsorship	Enforce drink–driving laws	National physical activity guidelines
Raise taxes on tobacco	Restriction on marketing of foods and beverages high in salt, sugar and fats, especially to children	Physical activity programmes for children in schools
Restrict access to alcohol sale	Food taxes and subsidies to promote healthy eating	Physical activity and healthy diet programmes in workplaces
Enforce bans on alcohol advertising		Community programmes for healthy eating and physical activity
Raise taxes on alcohol		Improving the design of the built environment to promote healthy lifestyles
Reduce salt intake and content of food		
Replace trans-fat with polyunsaturated fat		
Promote public awareness about diet and physical activity		

Source: WHO, 2011

There are, however, examples of individualized programmes that may prevent or reduce obesity, although evidence is limited. One is the 'Kinder Overweight Active Living Action' (KOALA) programme. Qualitative evidence suggests that parents, children and teachers value interventions that link home with community and school programmes. Long-term weight loss has not, however, been documented (Smibert et al., 2010). MEND (Mind, Exercise, Nutrition . . . Do it!) is the largest obesity treatment programme in England. It comprises

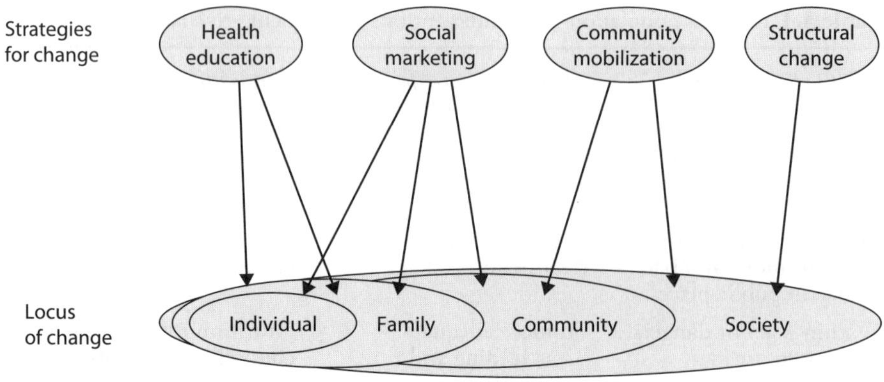

Figure 3.2 Strategies for achieving changes in knowledge, attitudes and behaviours to prevent chronic disease in children and young people

Source: Adapted from O'Connor Duffany et al., 2011

behavioural change techniques to help parents and children improve diet and activity, an exercise programme and nutrition guidelines. MEND has been evaluated in a randomised controlled trial (RCT), showing significantly reduced waist circumference and body mass index (BMI), with benefits in cardiovascular fitness, physical activity levels and self-esteem. Moreover, this intervention was perceived as acceptable by many families and some results were sustained for at least 6–12 months after the intervention (Sacher et al., 2010).

A child's knowledge, attitude and behaviour are influenced by their family, friends and wider community. Consequently, there is scope for policy-makers to influence environments in ways that enable healthier lifestyles. Tackling upstream determinants of many chronic diseases requires a variety of approaches including, for example, structural interventions, community mobilization, health education and social marketing (O'Connor Duffany et al., 2011) (Figure 3.2).

Furthermore, the long-term nature of NCDs means that prevention and treatment require a comprehensive and sustained response. A Europe-wide review of social determinants of health recommends specific actions in prevention, treatment and strategy (Marmot et al., 2012), as summarized in Table 3.4.

Paediatric palliative and end-of-life care

In some cases, a child's illness may be such that it progresses towards an inevitable death. Palliative care services for children are developing slowly, but have a long way to go. There are no reliable data on the number of children who require palliative care each year in Europe, but 16 children per 10,000, or 15 children per 10,000 if neonates are excluded, die from causes likely to have required such care (Cochrane, Liyange and Nantambi, 2007) (Table 3.5).

Table 3.4 A comprehensive response to preventing and treating long-term conditions in childhood

Prevention	• Reduce harmful alcohol consumption • Reduce consumption of fats, especially trans-fats • Reduce smoking • Encourage active living
Early detection	• Design screening programmes that ensure access for the most vulnerable children
Treatment	• Ensure equitable access to health care • Remove barriers to effective planning and delivery of integrated care for NCDs
Strategies	• Strengthen health promotion, protection and disease prevention programmes, ensuring that social determinants of health are addressed • Improve quality of and access to health services • All strategies should focus efforts towards addressing inequities
Evaluation	• Monitor and assess the effects of a comprehensive response to childhood NCDs by measuring population health and equity, using indicators specific to important developmental stages and key socioeconomic determinants

Source: Adapted from Marmot et al., 2012

Paediatric palliative care aims to improve the quality of life for children living with life-limiting conditions, and provides care and support for the child's family. A comprehensive paediatric palliative care service includes physical, emotional, social and spiritual care, based on early and continuous assessment, and ensuring adequate symptom and pain management (Sepulveda et al., 2002).

PRISMA is a multinational European project that aims to inform practice, policy and research around end-of-life care for cancer patients but it is restricted to adults; to our knowledge, no similar project exists for children.

Making it happen

A comprehensive chronic care system for children and young people that encompasses all aspects of prevention and care is needed to offer a solution to the rising tide of chronic conditions in childhood. However, there is no strong evidence, nor consensus, about how best to adapt health systems to meet the needs of increasing numbers of children with NCDs. Integrating services and developing chronic care models have intuitive appeal and are logical responses to some of the known deficits in care. Although evidence is weak or lacking as to whether these are the best responses, there is evidence about what makes

Table 3.5 The Association of Children's Hospices' four major categories of conditions that may require palliative care

Category 1	Life-threatening conditions for which curative treatment may be feasible but can fail. Access to palliative care services may be necessary when treatment fails or during an acute crisis, irrespective of the duration of that threat to life. On reaching long-term remission, or following successful curative treatment, there is no longer a need for palliative care services.
	Examples: cancer, irreversible organ failures of heart, liver, kidney.
Category 2	Conditions where premature death is inevitable, where there may be long periods of intensive treatment aimed at prolonging life and allowing participation in normal activities.
	Examples: cystic fibrosis, Duchenne muscular dystrophy.
Category 3	Progressive conditions without curative treatment options, where treatment is exclusively palliative and may commonly extend over many years.
	Examples: Batten disease, mucopolysaccharidoses.
Category 4	Irreversible but non-progressive conditions causing severe disability leading to susceptibility to health complications and likelihood of premature death.
	Examples: severe cerebral palsy, multiple disabilities e.g. following brain or spinal cord injuries, complex health care needs and a high risk of an unpredictable life-threatening event or episode.

Source: Cochrane, Liyange and Nantambi, 2007

health systems work more generally. This includes a clear vision of what needs to be achieved; good communication with those who have to implement the changes; reforms appropriate to context; an ability to take advantage of events; and maintaining the stability of institutions (Balabanova, McKee and Mills, 2011). That said, there is a clear policy imperative in many countries to develop integrated services. So with these caveats in mind, the following sections describe barriers, possible solutions and necessary preconditions for developing chronic care models for children (see also Chapter 11).

Integrating services and developing chronic care models

Evidence from a variety of countries suggests that integrated care services do not develop or evolve spontaneously as a response to health needs. This is irrespective of the health system, and applies just as much in countries with a nationalized tax-funded health system (such as the United Kingdom) as it does in countries with a social insurance system (for example, the Netherlands) or the United States, where private insurance dominates the health care market. Systemic structural barriers to integration include resistance among professionals; separate organizational processes (such as information management and clinical guidelines); payment systems that provide perverse incentives; policies that hinder collaboration between organizations; regulation that focuses on single episodes of health care use or single organizations; insufficient reliable data on health needs and service use; lack of skills in planning, organizing and purchasing services; and lack of political will (Curry and Ham, 2010; Ham, 2010; Rosen et al., 2011).

Information needs and research

In order to plan services to match health needs, policy-makers and health service managers need reliable data on chronic disease prevalence and trends. However, a common unifying definition of chronic disease in childhood is lacking and this lack of clarity may partly explain widely differing prevalence estimates ranging from 0.22% to 44% (van der Lee et al., 2007). The picture is further complicated by the difficulties inherent in interpreting data on co-morbidity. Although no international consensus on definitions of NCDs in childhood exists, a conceptual framework has been described (van der Lee et al., 2007), which starts with two broad categories. The first comprises children with chronic diseases, diagnosed according to professional standards, where the condition is expected to last 3 months at least (for example, a child with diabetes). The other category includes children with special health care needs: these are children who have, or are at risk of having, chronic physical, developmental, behavioural or emotional conditions that mean they are more likely to use health and related services than other children of the same age (for example, a child with Trisomy 21, or Downs' Syndrome).

In practice, there are few data as yet on actual prevalence. Most available data relate to service utilization, being largely based on inpatient episodes and outpatient visits. Although understanding how many children have a particular disease or problem is important *per se*, it becomes more meaningful information if there is also an indication of the impact of the illness on the child and family. For example, we need to be able to capture data about children's functional ability, and how children with chronic illness or complex needs experience health services. (Lollar et al., 2012). The WHO International Classification of Functioning, Disability and Health (ICF) is an aid to understanding the functional dimensions of chronic disease. It has categories for: body functions and structures; activity and participation; and environmental factors (Madden, Sykes and Ustun, 2007).

Information is also important for measuring the effects of health services. Comprehensive indicators for the quality of chronic disease management for children are lacking, as are means of tracking children's health and development across sectors and over time. These tools are urgently needed as part of a child health information system that could support efforts to improve child health across Europe. See Chapter 11 for further discussion on indicators and monitoring systems.

Child health services research is lagging behind other areas of child health research, and the same applies to research on children's chronic disease prevention and policy analysis (Modi et al., 2013). There are some signs of change though: a project funded by the European Union has compiled an inventory of child health research, identifying priorities for future funding (RICHE, 2012).

A renewed focus on primary care and transformative medical education

The community setting, family focus and holistic approach of primary care mean that it is best placed to become the focus of chronic disease care for children. This will necessitate finding a better balance between access and expertise than is currently the case in many countries.

Teams of professionals from different backgrounds and organizations will be required to deliver optimal care for children with chronic and complex conditions. Historically, the health care workforce has been developed to deal with acute infectious illness, but children with complex, sometimes lifelong, health care needs, such as those with cancer, chronic respiratory disease and neurological impairment, need ongoing support outside hospital settings. Training programmes have varied in the extent to which they have kept pace with the changing nature of illness. A transformative programme of medical education is called for – one which keeps pace with the changing needs of children and families (Frenk et al., 2010).

A whole-systems approach

An effective and efficient health system response to the rising burden of chronic disease across the whole population must include mechanisms to address determinants from the earliest years of childhood through to adolescence and beyond. Intervening as early as possible in life to prevent NCDs will pay the greatest dividends. Renewed efforts are needed, underpinned by the principles of the 'Convention on the Rights of the Child', to raise the profile of children in the global NCD discourse (NCD Alliance, 2011). Health services and systems must adapt to deliver coordinated compassionate care for increasing numbers of children with chronic diseases and complex long-term conditions.

Acknowledgement

We are grateful to Dr Fliss Murtagh (Consultant and Clinical Senior Lecturer in Palliative Care, Cicely Saunders Institute) for contributions to the section on palliative care, to Professor Neal Halfon (Director Professor, David Geffen School of Medicine UCLA, Department of Paediatrics, Professor, UCLA Fielding School of Public Health, Department of Health Services and Luskin School of Public Affairs, Department of Public Policy) for comment and advice, and to Ian Birrell for his personal account and insightful recommendations.

References

Ahgren, B. (2003) Chain of care development in Sweden: results of a national study, *International Journal of Integrated Care*, 3: e01.
Allotey, P. et al. (2011) Rethinking health-care systems: a focus on chronicity, *The Lancet*, 377(9764): 450–1.
Asher, M.I. et al. (2006) Worldwide time trends in the prevalence of symptoms of asthma, allergic rhinoconjunctivitis, and eczema in childhood: ISAAC Phases One and Three repeat multicountry cross-sectional surveys, *The Lancet*, 368(9537): 733–43.
Asthma UK (2007) *The asthma divide: inequalities in emergency care for people with asthma in England*. London: Asthma UK.
Baerlocher, M.O. and Detsky, A.S. (2009) Professional monopolies in medicine, *JAMA*, 301(8): 858–60.
Balabanova, D., McKee, M. and Mills, A. (2011) *Good health at low cost 25 years on: what makes a good health system*. London: London School of Hygiene and Tropical Medicine.
Barr, V.J. et al. (2003) The expanded Chronic Care Model: an integration of concepts and strategies from population health promotion and the Chronic Care Model, *Hospital Quarterly*, 7(1): 73–82.
Beasley, R. (1998) Worldwide variation in prevalence of symptoms of asthma, allergic rhinoconjunctivitis, and atopic eczema: ISAAC, *The Lancet*, 351(9111): 1225–32.
Bigi, S. et al. (2011) Acute ischemic stroke in children versus young adults, *Annals of Neurology*, 70(2): 245–54.
Bodenheimer, T., Wagner, E.H. and Grumbach, K. (2002a) Improving primary care for patients with chronic illness, *JAMA*, 288(14): 1775–9.
Bodenheimer, T., Wagner, E.H. and Grumbach, K. (2002b) Improving primary care for patients with chronic illness: the chronic care model, Part 2, *JAMA*, 288(15): 1909–14.
Burns, L.R. and Pauly, M.V. (2002) Integrated delivery networks: a detour on the road to integrated health care? *Health Affairs (Millwood)*, 21(4): 128–43.
Campbell, S.M. et al. (2005) Improvements in quality of clinical care in English general practice 1998–2003: longitudinal observational study, *BMJ*, 331(7525): 1121.
Cinek, O. et al. (2012) Heterogeneity in the systems of pediatric diabetes care across the European Union, *Pediatric Diabetes*, 13(Suppl 16): 5–14.
Cochrane, H., Liyange, S. and Nantambi, R. (2007) *Palliative care statistics for children and young adults*. London: Department of Health.
Coleman, K. et al. (2009) Evidence on the Chronic Care Model in the new millennium, *Health Affairs (Millwood)*, 28(1): 75–85.
Cooley, W.C. (2004) Redefining primary pediatric care for children with special health care needs: the primary care medical home, *Current Opinion in Pediatrics*, 16(6): 689–92.
Cooley, W.C. et al. (2009) Improved outcomes associated with medical home implementation in pediatric primary care, *Pediatrics*, 124(1): 358–64.
Cox, E.R. et al. (2008) Trends in the prevalence of chronic medication use in children: 2002–2005, *Pediatrics*, 122(5): e1053–61.
Curry, N. and Ham, C. (2010) *Clinical and service integration: the route to improved outcomes*. London: King's Fund.
Dabelea, D., Bell, R.A. and D'Agostino, R.B.J. (2007) Incidence of diabetes in youth in the United States, *JAMA*, 297(24): 2716–24.

de Beaufort, C.E. et al. (2007) Continuing stability of center differences in pediatric diabetes care: do advances in diabetes treatment improve outcome? The Hvidoere Study Group on Childhood Diabetes, *Diabetes Care*, 30(9): 2245–50.
de Savigny, D. and Adam, T. (eds) (2009) *Systems thinking for health systems strengthening*. Geneva: Alliance for Health Policy and Systems Research.
Department of Health (2010) *From the ground up. A report on integrated care design and delivery*. London: Department of Health.
Diabetes Control and Complications Trial Research Group (1994) Effect of intensive diabetes treatment on the development and progression of long-term complications in adolescents with insulin-dependent diabetes mellitus: Diabetes Control and Complications Trial, *Journal of Pediatrics*, 125(2): 177–88.
Eckstein, K.C. et al. (2006) Parents' perceptions of their child's weight and health, *Pediatrics*, 117(3): 681–90.
Epping-Jordan, J.E. et al. (2004) Improving the quality of health care for chronic conditions, *Quality and Safety in Health Care*, 13(4): 299–305.
Frenk, J. et al. (2010) Health professionals for a new century: transforming education to strengthen health systems in an interdependent world, *The Lancet*, 376(9756): 1923–58.
Fuhrman, C. et al. (2011) Hospitalizations for asthma in children are linked to undertreatment and insufficient asthma education, *Journal of Asthma*, 48(6): 565–71.
Geenen, M.M. et al. (2007) Medical assessment of adverse health outcomes in long-term survivors of childhood cancer, *JAMA*, 297(24): 2705–15.
Gensichen, J. et al. (2006) Case management to improve major depression in primary health care: a systematic review, *Psychological Medicine*, 36(1): 7–14.
Gerstl, E.M. et al. (2008) Metabolic control as reflected by HbA1c in children, adolescents and young adults with type-1 diabetes mellitus: combined longitudinal analysis including 27,035 patients from 207 centers in Germany and Austria during the last decade, *European Journal of Pediatrics*, 167(4): 447–53.
Gill, P.J. et al. (2013) Increase in emergency admissions to hospital for children aged under 15 in England, 1999–2010: national database analysis, *Archives of Disease in Childhood*, 98(5): 328–34.
Glasgow, R.E., Orleans, C.T. and Wagner, E.H. (2001) Does the chronic care model serve also as a template for improving prevention? *Milbank Quarterly*, 79(4): 579–612, iv–v.
Grone, O. and Garcia-Barbero, M. (2001) Integrated care: a position paper of the WHO European Office for Integrated Health Care Services, *International Journal of Integrated Care*, 1: e21.
Hagberg, B. et al. (2001) Changing panorama of cerebral palsy in Sweden. VIII. Prevalence and origin in the birth year period 1991–94, *Acta Paediatrica*, 90(3): 271–7.
Halfon, N., Du Plessis, H. and Inkelas, M. (2007) Transforming the U.S. child health system, *Health Affairs (Millwood)*, 26(2): 315–30.
Ham, C. (2010) The ten characteristics of the high-performing chronic care system, *Health Economics, Policy and Law*, 5(Pt 1): 71–90.
Hayes, S.L. et al. (2012) Collaboration between local health and local government agencies for health improvement, *Cochrane Database of Systematic Reviews*, CD007825.
Himmelmann, K. et al. (2005) The changing panorama of cerebral palsy in Sweden. IX. Prevalence and origin in the birth-year period 1995–1998, *Acta Paediatrica*, 94(3): 287–94.
Homer, C.J. et al. (2008) A review of the evidence for the medical home for children with special health care needs, *Pediatrics*, 122(4): e922–37.

IHME (2012) *Global Burden of Disease*. Institute for Health Metrics and Evaluation. http://www.healthmetricsandevaluation.org/gbd/visualizations/gbd-heatmap [accessed 23 June 2013].

Jaudes, P.K. and Mackey-Bilaver, L. (2008) Do chronic conditions increase young children's risk of being maltreated? *Child Abuse and Neglect*, 32(7): 671–81.

Jones, J. (2006) *Parents' Views about 'Team around the Child' How your feedback is helping to shape 'Team around the Child' in the future*. Telford: Mindful Practice, Telford and Wrekin Council, Shropshire County Council.

Kodner, D.L. and Spreeuwenberg, C. (2002) Integrated care: meaning, logic, applications, and implications – a discussion paper, *International Journal of Integrated Care*, 2: e12.

Kuh, D. et al. (2003) Life course epidemiology, *Journal of Epidemiology and Community Health*, 57(10): 778–83.

Lollar, D.J., Hartzell, M.S. and Evans, M.A. (2012) Functional difficulties and health conditions among children with special health needs, *Pediatrics*, 129(3): e714–22.

Madden, R., Sykes, C. and Ustun, T.B. (2007) *World Health Organization Family of International Classifications: definition, scope and purpose*. Geneva: World Health Organization.

Mangione-Smith, R. et al. (2005) Measuring the effectiveness of a collaborative for quality improvement in pediatric asthma care: does implementing the chronic care model improve processes and outcomes of care? *Ambulatory Pediatrics*, 5(2): 75–82.

Marmot, M. (2010) *Fair Society, Healthy Lives: The Marmot Review*. London: The Marmot Review.

Marmot, M. et al. (2012) WHO European review of social determinants of health and the health divide, *The Lancet*, 380(9846): 1011–29.

Maslow, G.R. et al. (2011) Growing up with a chronic illness: social success, educational/vocational distress, *Journal of Adolescent Health*, 49(2): 206–12.

Mitchell, E.A. et al. (2005) A randomized controlled trial of an asthma clinical pathway for children in general practice, *Acta Paediatrica*, 94(2): 226–33.

Modi, N. et al. (2013) A healthy nation: strengthening child health research in the UK, *The Lancet*, 381(9860): 73–87.

Murray, C.J. et al. (2012) Disability-adjusted life years (DALYs) for 291 diseases and injuries in 21 regions, 1990–2010: a systematic analysis for the Global Burden of Disease Study 2010, *The Lancet*, 380(9859): 2197–223.

NCD Alliance (2011) *A Focus on Children and Non-Communicable Diseases (NCDs)*. Position paper, UN Summit on Non-Communicable Diseases (NCDs), New York, September 2011. http://ncdalliance.org/sites/default/files/resource_files/20110627_A_Focus_on_Children_and_NCDs_FINAL_2.pdf [accessed 23 June 2013].

NCDCHILD (2013) http://www.ncdchild.org (accessed 10 March 2013).

Newton, H. (2011) 'Very sore nights and days': the child's experience of illness in early modern England, c.1580–1720, *Medical History*, 55(2): 153–82.

Nolte, E. and McKee, M. (2008) *Caring for people with chronic conditions. A health system perspective*. Maidenhead: Open University Press.

O'Connor Duffany, K. et al. (2011) Community Interventions for Health (CIH): A novel approach to tackling the worldwide epidemic of chronic diseases, *CVD Prevention and Control*, 6: 47–56.

Ouwens, M. et al. (2005) Integrated care programmes for chronically ill patients: a review of systematic reviews, *International Journal for Quality in Health Care*, 17(2): 141–6.

Øvretveit, J.O. (2011) *Evidence: does clinical coordination improve quality and save money*. London: The Health Foundation.

Patterson, C.C. et al. and EURODIAB Study Group (2009) Incidence trends for childhood type 1 diabetes in Europe during 1989–2003 and predicted new cases 2005–20: a multicentre prospective registration study, *The Lancet*, 373(9680): 2027–33.

Pearce, N. et al. (2007) Worldwide trends in the prevalence of asthma symptoms: phase III of the International Study of Asthma and Allergies in Childhood (ISAAC), *Thorax*, 62(9): 758–66.

Pharoah, P.O. et al. (1990) Birthweight specific trends in cerebral palsy, *Archives of Disease in Childhood*, 65(6): 602–6.

Pharoah, P.O., Platt, M.J. and Cooke, T. (1996) The changing epidemiology of cerebral palsy, *Archives of Disease in Childhood: Fetal and neonatal edition*, 75(3): F169–73.

Reindal, L. and Øymar, K. (2006) Hospital admissions for wheezing and asthma in childhood – are they avoidable? *Journal of Asthma*, 43(10): 801–6.

RICHE (2012) *Research Inventory for Child Health in Europe*. Research Inventory for Child Health in Europe. http://www.childhealthresearch.eu [accessed 23 June 2013].

Robertson, C.M., Svenson, L.W. and Joffres, M.R. (1998) Prevalence of cerebral palsy in Alberta, *The Canadian Journal of Neurological Sciences*, 25(2): 117–22.

Rosen, R., Mountford, J. and Lewis, G. (2011) *Integration in action: four international case studies*. London: Nuffield Trust.

RCPCH (2012a) *Bringing Networks to Life – an RCPCH guide to implementing Clinical Networks*. London: Royal College of Paediatrics and Child Health.

RCPCH (2012b) *National paediatric diabetes audit. Report 2010–2011*. London: Royal College of Paediatrics and Child Health.

Sacher, P.M. et al. (2010) Randomized controlled trial of the MEND program: a family-based community intervention for childhood obesity, *Obesity (Silver Spring)*, 18(Suppl 1): S62–8.

Sartain, S.A. et al. (2002) Randomised controlled trial comparing an acute paediatric hospital at home scheme with conventional hospital care, *Archives of Disease in Childhood*, 87(5): 371–5.

Sepulveda, C. et al. (2002) Palliative Care: the World Health Organization's global perspective, *Journal of Pain and Symptom Management*, 24(2): 91–6.

Smibert, A. et al. (2010) School, community, and family working together to address childhood obesity: Perceptions from the KOALA lifestyle intervention study, *European Physical Education Review*, 16: 155–70.

Smith, S.M., Allwright, S. and O'Dowd, T. (2007) Effectiveness of shared care across the interface between primary and specialty care in chronic disease management, *Cochrane Database of Systematic Reviews*, CD004910.

Stanley, F.J. and Watson, L. (1992) Trends in perinatal mortality and cerebral palsy in Western Australia, 1967 to 1985, *BMJ*, 304(6843): 1658–63.

Strassburg, H.M. (2011) Sozialpaediatrische Versorgung in Deutschland. In: Kerbl, R. et al. (eds) *Kinder und Jugendliche im besten Gesundheitssystem der Welt*. Wien: Springer.

Surman, G., Newdick, H. and Johnson, A. (2003) Cerebral palsy rates among low-birthweight infants fell in the 1990s, *Developmental Medicine and Child Neurology*, 45(7): 456–62.

Svensson, B., Bornehag, C.G. and Janson, S. (2011) Chronic conditions in children increase the risk for physical abuse – but vary with socio-economic circumstances, *Acta Paediatrica*, 100(3): 407–12.

Szczepanski, R. (2010) Schulungen bei chronischen Erkrankungen. Editoral, *Kinder- und Jugendarzt*, 41: 361.

Tamburlini, G. (2012) Child health and child health services in Italy, *Medico e Bambino*, 31: 178–84.

Tsai, A.C. et al. (2005) A meta-analysis of interventions to improve care for chronic illnesses, *American Journal of Managed Care*, 11(8): 478–88.

United Nations (1989) *Convention on the Rights of the Child*. New York: United Nations.

Urbanus-van Laar, J.J. et al. 2008. Suboptimal asthma care for immigrant children: results of an audit study, *BMC Health Services Research*, 8: 22.

van der Lee, J.H. et al. (2007) Definitions and measurement of chronic health conditions in childhood: a systematic review, *JAMA*, 297: 2741–51.

van der Linden, B.A. (2001) *The birth of integration; explorative studies on the development and implementation of transmural care in the Netherlands 1994–2000*. Utrecht: Universiteit Utrecht.

van der Linden, B.A., Spreeuwenberg, C. and Schrijvers, A.J. (2001) Integration of care in The Netherlands: the development of transmural care since 1994, *Health Policy*, 55(2): 111–20.

Viner, R.M. et al. (2011) 50-year mortality trends in children and young people: a study of 50 low-income, middle-income, and high-income countries, *The Lancet*, 377(9772): 1162–74.

Wang, H. et al. (2012) Age-specific and sex-specific mortality in 187 countries, 1970–2010: a systematic analysis for the Global Burden of Disease Study 2010, *The Lancet*, 380(9859): 2071–94.

White, N.H. et al. (2001) Beneficial effects of intensive therapy of diabetes during adolescence: outcomes after the conclusion of the Diabetes Control and Complications Trial (DCCT), *Journal of Pediatrics*, 139(6): 804–12.

WHO (1986) *The Ottawa Charter for Health Promotion – First international conference on health promotion*. WHO/HPR/HEP95. Ottawa: World Health Organization.

WHO (2002) *Innovative care for chronic conditions. Building blocks for action. Global report*. Geneva: World Health Organization.

WHO (2011) *Global status report on noncommunicable diseases 2010*. Geneva: World Health Organization.

Winter, S. et al. (2002) Trends in the prevalence of cerebral palsy in a population-based study, *Pediatrics*, 110(6): 1220–5.

Wolfe, I. et al. (2011) Improving child health services in the UK: insights from Europe and their implications for the NHS reforms, *BMJ*, 342: d1277.

Wolfe, I. et al. (2013) Health services for children in western Europe, *The Lancet*, 381(9873): 1224–34.

Zwar, N. et al. (2006) *A systematic review of chronic disease management*. Sydney: Australian Primary Health Care Institute.

chapter four

Transition from children's to adults' services

Rose Crowley, Ingrid Wolfe

"For in every adult dwells the child that was, and in every child lies the adult that will be."

John Connolly
The Book of Lost Things, 2007

Introduction

Over the past two decades, evidence has mounted that the transition from paediatric to adult care for young people with chronic illness or disability is often poorly managed, with adverse health consequences in adolescence and later adult life. The importance of a smooth transition between paediatric and adult services, and the most effective way to achieve this, has become a subject of considerable debate. These discussions can be seen as part of a wider recognition of the limitations in current service provision for adolescents (Viner, 2001, 2008), and of the difficulties inherent in coordinating care between paediatric and adult services. The need to provide appropriate health services throughout adolescence and into young adulthood has followed the epidemiological shift towards chronic conditions that has taken place. This is a consequence of improved prevention and care resulting in increasing numbers of children surviving into adulthood with complex disabilities or chronic health needs, while the burden of infections and acute illnesses has declined. Despite this success, there has been mounting evidence that the period of transition to adult care may be associated with worse health outcomes, and with negative experiences for both patients and their families. Calls for improved services have come from the American Association of Paediatrics, the United Kingdom Department of Health and the Royal College of Physicians in Edinburgh, as well as subspecialty groups concerned with conditions as diverse as cystic fibrosis (Cowlard, 2003), spina bifida (Crevier and Mercier, 2008), inflammatory bowel disease (Desir and Seidman, 2003), mental health problems (Davis and Sondheimer, 2005) and for survivors of paediatric cancers (Kaatsch et al., 2005) and transplantation (Kaufman, 2006). The most effective way to achieve a smooth transition between paediatric and adult services remains unclear, as it requires a comprehensive programme that reflects and encourages the patient's physical, psychological and social development, rather than merely a transfer from paediatric to adult care.

This chapter will therefore outline some of the potential challenges in providing transitional care; describe how concerns over existing arrangements have developed historically; and highlight the specific issues raised by transition in a number of common or important conditions. The existing evidence base for generic features of successful transitional programmes will be discussed, before outlining current attitudes towards transitional care in different European countries, as described by the respondents to our questionnaire. A notable feature of these responses was that policies in a number of countries are at an early stage of development: the potential avenues for future research and service development are still being decided and the need for rigorous evaluation will be an important component.

Overview of the issues

Concerns over the adequacy of current provisions for transitional care have arisen from a number of groups, encompassing a range of chronic illnesses and disabilities. Poor management of the transition can result in: worsening of glycaemic control in those with diabetes mellitus (Wysocki et al., 1992); increased loss to follow-up and associated poor health outcomes for survivors of paediatric cancers or cardiac surgery (Rianthavorn and Ettenger, 2005; Yeung et al., 2008); and graft failure in transplant recipients (Watson, 2000). Qualitative research with young adults has confirmed that many experience the transfer to adult care as disjointed (Box 4.1), and find it difficult to adjust to the increased responsibility for care they are given in adult medicine (O'Connell, Bailey and Pearce, 2003; Dovey-Pearce et al., 2005; Anthony et al., 2009). Similar concerns have been raised in qualitative research with the parents of those with chronic illness and with professionals involved in their care. For these reasons, there has been a shift away from considering transition as a simple transfer between paediatric and adult services, towards understanding it as a comprehensive process that may take a number of years, representing just one component in the adolescent's achievement of adult independence. Programmes addressing transition have therefore involved not only changes in service delivery to improve continuity of care, but also specific patient development programmes, involving both disease-specific information and more generic psychological skills training and self-management. The flexibility needed in such a process, to adapt to the changing needs and circumstances of individual patients, provides a particular challenge for service delivery.

Box 4.1 Transition experience of a patient with Wegener's granulomatosis

> I didn't know it was going to be my last appointment at the children's hospital until midway through a routine consultation, when my doctor suddenly announced that he thought it was time for me to leave. I was shocked – I knew I'd have to leave the children's hospital soon, but I thought I'd get a little more warning than that. It felt like a very abrupt end to a relationship that had become an important part of my life.
>
> My condition is rare in childhood and I had never even met another person with the same condition as me. Suddenly, at the adult hospital, I was surrounded by other patients with the same condition and I wasn't prepared for this. I was the youngest person in the waiting room by far – everybody else was at least a decade or two older than me – and it made me wonder whether I was looking into my own future. This was a scary thought. There were patients attached to oxygen, patients who had lost their sight and patients using wheelchairs. The lifelong nature of my condition and its potential consequences were suddenly much more real to me than they had ever been at the children's hospital.
>
> *Source:* young adult patient, United Kingdom

Challenges in adolescent transitional care

The provision and coordination of transitional care present a number of distinct challenges to health and social care services. First, there are logistical difficulties: paediatric and adult services have separate staff, training and budgets, and are often geographically separate, making it all the more difficult to ensure continuity of care. Secondly, paediatric and adult medicine often have marked differences in their philosophy and in the degree of responsibility placed on the patient, so it is crucial that adolescents acquire the independence and self-care skills they will need in order to successfully negotiate this change, and function successfully as adult patients.

In most European countries, adolescent medicine is not recognized as a separate subspecialty, and a lack of sufficient focus on caring for this age group, in either paediatric or adult medicine training, has resulted in adolescents historically being a neglected group (Viner, 2003) (see Chapter 7). There is an inherent need for flexibility in arranging transitional care, reflecting the individual needs and rates of development of this patient group, rather than having a set age at which 'transfer' to adult medicine should occur. Adolescents are, of course, undergoing a period of profound physical, psychological and social change in their lives, and will be undertaking transitions in their educational, work and social environments, of which their transition to adult health services is only one small part. This is particularly true of those with complex health care needs or disabilities, where particular vocational support may be needed. Adolescents with chronic illness are often a particularly challenging group to engage, as they are asked to take on greater (adult) levels of responsibility just at a time when rebellion against authority is common amongst their peers.

A further level of complexity in consultations during the transition period arises from the need to sensitively coordinate not only the interactions between the young person and their paediatrician, adult physician, and all the other involved clinicians, but also between the patient and their parents.

Transitional care can be seen as a continuous process, occurring throughout the period of adolescence, with a gradually increasing emphasis on the adolescent acquiring the skills necessary to cope as an adult patient and a gradual reduction in parental support. As such, the process of 'transitional' encounters is likely to vary at different ages, with early discussions taking place in the paediatric setting with a parent present, while later consultations should ideally be between the patient, paediatrician and adult physician. A particular challenge is raised by conditions in which adult services are less well developed than paediatric services, so that arranging transfer, let alone a coordinated programme of transition, is difficult. Examples include cystic fibrosis, of which most adult respiratory physicians have little experience (Vega-Briceno, Guiraldes and Sanchez, 2006); grown-up survivors of congenital heart disease (who have very different needs to the majority of adult cardiology patients); and grown-up cancer survivors (over whom there is ongoing debate regarding the most appropriate location and pattern of follow-up). A recent survey of internal medicine specialists in the United States identified marked concerns about their lack of training in congenital and childhood-onset conditions (Peter et al., 2009). Adult services are very poorly developed for ADHD and autistic spectrum disorders, with no obvious adult equivalent of the community paediatrician role (Brown et al., 2005). Indeed, a recent survey of community paediatricians in the United Kingdom revealed that only 22% were aware of any adult services for ADHD in their area (Marcer, Finlay and Baverstock, 2008).

The evidence for worse health outcomes post transition

There has been accumulating evidence, across a broad range of conditions, that existing arrangements for the transition to adult services can be associated with deterioration in health outcomes and health-related quality of life. Such evidence includes both quantitative measures of attendance rates and disease outcomes, and qualitative research with patients and their families. For example, interviews with 22 adolescents with a range of chronic illnesses (including cystic fibrosis, sickle cell anaemia, juvenile idiopathic arthritis and inflammatory bowel disease), conducted over an 18-month period of transition, identified fears about the process of transfer to adult care; the need to form relationships with new physicians; and feeling unprepared for the move to a new clinic (Tuchman, Slap and Britto, 2008). The interviewees also voiced the desire for earlier discussion of transition, to give them more time to prepare for it, plus prior visits to their new clinic and introduction to health care teams. Post-transition qualitative interviews with young adults with diabetes (Dovey-Pearce et al., 2005), cystic fibrosis (Brumfield and Lansbury, 2004) or sickle cell disease (Nonnast-Daniel, 2005), revealed that they found the lack of consistency in staff, necessitating repetition of information and compromising rapport, a particularly disheartening element of the transition process. Patients have mentioned that the transfer often feels disjointed, and that they lack information or understanding about the process or new staff they will encounter (Zack et al., 2003). There is also some evidence that in haemophilia (Geerts, van de Wiel and Tamminga, 2008), cystic fibrosis (Craig, Towns and Bibby, 2007), and heart transplant recipients (Anthony et al., 2009), transition may be of even greater concern to parents than the patients, so negative consequences may be underestimated if only adolescents, rather than their caregivers, are interviewed.

A key theme linking the qualitative and quantitative evidence is a high rate of loss to follow-up when children are transferred to adult care, reflecting both failures of service delivery (complete failure of communication of transfer between paediatric and adult teams) and poor compliance with appointments by adolescents. The consequences of inadequate follow-up can be devastating; in those with corrected congenital heart disease, a lapse in care can result in a three-fold increase in the need for urgent cardiac intervention (Yeung et al., 2008). The most common reason for this lapse of care was the patient having been told they did not need follow-up, and improved patient knowledge about the importance of regular follow-up has been shown to result in better attendance rates post transfer (Reid et al., 2004). Failure of continued review has also been widely reported for those who have undergone neurosurgical procedures, with one series reporting a decline in attendance from 100% to 40% during transfer for those with a shunt in situ for hydrocephalus (Tomlinson and Sugarman, 1995), with serious consequences if complications are missed. A study in Germany demonstrated the negative impact on clinic attendance rates that transition had among 101 young adults with diabetes, although, of note, this did not result in any significant increase in HbA1c (Busse et al., 2007). It has been difficult to establish whether transition necessarily results in clinical deterioration in some conditions, with two cohorts of patients with cystic fibrosis showing no deterioration in lung function, frequency of complications or evidence of social functioning (Craig, Towns and Bibby, 2007; Dugueperoux et al., 2008). Although concerns about worse outcomes post transition have been raised in a large number of other paediatric subspecialties, such as renal medicine (Watson, 2005) and endocrinology (Volta et al., 2003), worse outcomes in these conditions have not been conclusively established. The duration of negative effects is also unclear, with no long-term follow-up establishing the effect of successful transition on long-term health outcomes in adulthood.

Transition in specific conditions

Diabetes

Much of the literature concerning adolescent transitional care has focused on the management of diabetes mellitus, which is in some respects a useful starting point for developing systems to evaluate and improve transitional care. Both type 1 and type 2 diabetes are increasing in prevalence in childhood, and the condition provides a range of both disease-specific and more general measures of adherence to treatment and clinical outcome. Glycosylated haemoglobin and frequency of diabetic ketoacidosis (DKA) admissions have been used in many studies to assess patient concordance with insulin therapy during adolescence, while failure to attend adult clinic appointments and health-related quality of life have been used as more general measures of health. Diabetes mellitus could also provide an opportunity to assess long-term adult outcomes, using the established associations between glycosylated haemoglobin levels and later microvascular and macrovascular complications. The importance of transition has been highlighted in the United Kingdom by the National Service Framework for Diabetes, which states that 'transition will be organised in partnership with each individual, and at an age appropriate to and agreed with them'. The evidence base for planning transitional practices in diabetic adolescents was the subject of a recent systematic review, which highlighted the dearth of studies comparing outcomes following different models of transitional care (Nakhla et al., 2008), while a review considering the barriers to successful transition in diabetes identified patient, parental and service factors that can hinder the transfer to adult services (Fleming, Carter and Gillibrand, 2002). Qualitative research with young people has stressed the importance of multidisciplinary teams during transition, with many valuing the advice of dieticians in acquiring self-management skills (Visentin, Koch and Kralik, 2006). There is also an increasing body of evidence surrounding strategies that may improve adherence throughout adolescence, a notoriously difficult time for achieving good glycaemic control, due to both physiological and psychological factors. These have shown improved concordance rates using problem skills training (Grey and Berry, 2004); self-management training (Knowles et al., 2006); family models of care (Laffel et al., 2003); and enhanced telephone support (Lawson et al., 2005), although none specifically targeted the period of transfer to adult care. A survey of patient satisfaction in Italy identified that 79% of those questioned considered 20 years to be the correct age for transfer from paediatric to adult care, considerably later than the age at which this generally happens (Vanelli et al., 2004).

Cystic fibrosis

Optimizing care for teenagers and young adults with cystic fibrosis is an area of increasing importance, as a growing proportion of those born with the disease are now surviving into adulthood. Currently, approximately one-third of patients with cystic fibrosis are over 18 years of age (Nasr, 2000). The question of how best to integrate existing well-developed, highly specialized paediatric services with adult respiratory medicine services needs to be addressed, as does the most effective way of training adult physicians in caring for patients with this condition. There has been considerable geographical variation in the strategies adopted within the United Kingdom and across Europe, with regard to the degree of centralization of services into highly specialized tertiary centres, and the degree of involvement paediatricians have with their 'grown-up' patients. Highly specialized cystic fibrosis centres have been established in many countries and, in some cases, patients continue to be under the care of paediatricians throughout their adult life. Qualitative studies have generally established overall satisfaction following transition, despite some anticipatory anxieties (Steinkamp et al., 2001; Craig, Towns and Bibby, 2007). In common with diabetes, self-management programmes have been developed for young people with cystic fibrosis (although not yet specifically during transition), and these have resulted in significant improvements in weight gain and cooperation with treatment (Cottrell et al., 1996). The rationale behind using such strategies in a disease in which effective treatment requires so much commitment from patients is clear.

Transplant recipients

The consequences of any decline in adherence with treatment during the transition period are profound for children who have received solid organ transplants, with graft failure during early adulthood being a recognized consequence of non-adherence for both kidney (Watson, 2000) and liver recipients (Bucuvalas and Alonso, 2008).

Congenital heart disease

Survivors of complex congenital heart disease provide a further example of the transition of highly specialized services for complex patients. Advances in paediatric cardiothoracic surgery have meant that increasing numbers of children with complex congenital heart disease are surviving into adulthood, and their specific health care needs, as distinct from the majority of adult cardiology patients, are increasingly being recognized (Webb, 2001, 2005). The discrepancy in provision between children's and adult services has been highlighted and there is a recognized need for adult cardiologists with particular expertise in the long-term management of survivors of congenital heart disease (Webb, 2005). Worryingly, a Canadian study of a single birth cohort of 360 patients with complex congenital heart disease (Reid et al., 2004) found that less than half of patients (47%) successfully transferred to adult care. One aspect of this loss to follow-up appears to be a lack of knowledge among patients about the importance of continuing to attend for regular check-ups despite feeling healthy; education about this needs to be integrated into a structured transition programme (Dore, de Guise and Mercier, 2002).

Oncology

Improved survival rates for a range of paediatric cancers have resulted in a large cohort of children requiring long-term follow-up. This includes monitoring throughout adulthood for the late effects of treatment, primary tumour recurrence and treatment-related secondary cancers, with profound implications for service provision and associated costs (Eiser et al., 2007). The question of who should best care for these patients provides a further level of complexity in the arrangement of transition care. Multiple models of care have been proposed, based on disease, treatment and local healthcare structures (Skinner et al., 2006), and it has even been argued that shared care between paediatric oncologists and adult physicians, throughout adulthood, is a feasible strategy (Blaauwbroek et al., 2008).

Disabilities

Young adults with disabilities need to transition effectively to adult health care, while also undergoing often complex educational and vocational transitions, particularly for those with complex health care needs. Such conditions therefore exemplify the issues surrounding multi-agency models of care, in which social care and educational support play key roles (Blomquist, 2006), and patients may benefit from extended psychological support and skills training (Evans, McDougall and Baldwin, 2006). A literature review of issues in spina bifida and cerebral palsy recommended that strategies focus on preparation, flexible timing, care coordination, transition clinic visits and identifying interested adult physicians, although there was little supportive empirical data (Binks et al., 2007).

Juvenile idiopathic arthritis is another condition that has received attention, with a particular problem highlighted that many young adults with rheumatological disease express concerns that they feel out of place in adult services, which deal predominantly with an elderly patient population. Rheumatology is therefore one of the areas in which young adult clinics have been proposed to be of increased importance to provide a sense of community with peers (McDonagh, Shaw and Southwood, 2006; McDonagh, 2008). There is evidence of improvement in practices, even if not yet in outcomes: a recent United Kingdom multicentre audit reported improved transition planning and support (Robertson et al., 2006), while 75% of young people in a United States survey reported being encouraged to assume responsibility for their health care (Escalante et al., 2004).

Mental health and learning difficulties

The importance of effective transition for those with mental health problems has only recently been widely discussed, but it provides a number of discrete problems, over and above those for physical illness (Davis, 2003; Clark et al., 2008). This has been reflected in guidance documents: for example, transition issues form part of the SIGN guidelines on autistic spectrum disorders (Scottish Intercollegiate Guidelines Network, 2007) and the NICE guidelines on ADHD (National Institute for Health and Care Excellence, 2008), the latter stating that 'there remain, however, difficulties regarding transitional arrangements between child and adult mental health services', with variation nationally in the age of transfer (between 16 and 19) and little coordination. A review of the situation for those with eating disorders (Arcelus, Bowman and Morgan, 2008) reiterated inconsistency in the referral process and a lack of agreement on age boundaries between child and adolescent mental health services, with the risk that patients could become 'lost' in the gap between them.

Transition programmes

Although the existing literature concerning transition has tended to focus on groups of patients with specific conditions, there are certain key themes that can be generalized for all adolescents with chronic health conditions. Although there is still little robust evidence to support this, there is a consensus of opinion about some of the areas transitional care practice should aim to deliver, in terms of structure and process. A systematic literature review of studies, which evaluated outcomes following transition programmes, identified ten studies and highlighted three broad themes for interventions, according to whether they focused on the patient, staff or on improving service provision/access (Crowley et al., 2011). Interventions aimed directly at the patient included both disease-specific education programmes and generic skills training; staff interventions incorporated the provision of a named transition coordinator and 'overlap' clinics, jointly staffed by paediatric and adult physicians; while service improvements included out-of-hours phone support and increased efforts to contact those who had missed an appointment, plus the creation of specific clinics for young adults within adult services. Although studies had been conducted to evaluate the full range of interventions, their overall methodological quality was poor, with the majority involving pre and post intervention measurement, without any control group. Analysis was complicated by the fact that many of the studies incorporated a number of features together in a single new transition programme, with only two evaluating an isolated intervention (an overlap clinic). Each intervention could also encompass a range of practices and these were often poorly described: for example, the role of 'transition coordinator' could describe both someone responsible simply for arranging appointments and someone responsible for delivering an entire individualized programme of educational and psychological support. Six studies demonstrated statistically significant improvements in outcomes following interventions during the transition period, with the majority of successful programmes involving patient education and/or specific transition clinics (either 'overlap' clinics jointly staffed by paediatric and adult physicians, or specific young adult clinics within adult services). It was notable that all six of the successful studies involved diabetes mellitus, and this is clearly the condition for which the greatest evaluation of services has taken place.

'Overlap' transition clinics or young adult clinics in adult services

The rationale behind having specific transition clinics, attended by both paediatric and adult physicians, is clear: such an approach should ensure greater continuity of care and allow patients to undergo a gradual introduction to adult services. In addition, in general adult clinics for some conditions (notably diabetes mellitus and arthritis), the majority of other patients will be much older. It has therefore been argued that young people may feel less 'out of place' in a targeted adult clinic for their age group.

Patient education programmes

The recognition that adolescence is often a time of diminished cooperation with treatment for young people with chronic disease has meant that specific educational programmes have been developed to improve understanding in a number of conditions. Alternatively, generic skills training and strategies to improve patient autonomy have been proposed for helping adolescents to become sufficiently psychologically mature to successfully manage their conditions as adults. Some transition programmes therefore incorporate generic skills training or programmes to ease navigation of the adult health care system. This focus on encouraging adolescents to develop autonomy in accessing health care has been combined with strategies to gradually reduce parental input during adolescence. An interesting development in this area has been the development of tools to assess transition readiness for individual patients, so that the speed of transition is adapted as they learn and develop (Annunziato et al., 2007); however, the impact of this in adult life has not yet been evaluated. Peer education programmes, led by young adults with chronic disease who have been through the process of transition, are also in development (Box 4.2). Patient education has also been successfully used in conjunction with individual transition plans, resulting in improved health-related quality of life (HRQoL) scores for adolescents with juvenile idiopathic arthritis; again, it remains to be seen what impact this will have after transfer (Remorino and Taylor, 2006).

Box 4.2 The 'Staying Positive' programme, United Kingdom

'Staying Positive' workshops, part of the United Kingdom's Expert Patient Programme, are self-management workshops designed to give young people living with chronic illnesses the skills and self-confidence they need to cope with their conditions. The set of three one-day workshops, delivered over six to eight weeks, includes activities on communicating with health care professionals; dealing with the side-effects of medication; and, importantly, coping with the transition from children's to adult services.

Transition is discussed in the workshops by asking the participants to imagine a journey they are going to make – perhaps to the South Pole or the Amazon rainforest. What do they need to do in preparation for their trip? Do they, perhaps, need to learn how to put up a tent, or how to start a fire?

Through discussing how to prepare for such an expedition, the young people begin to understand that transitioning from paediatric to adult services is like a journey. They are encouraged to start thinking early on about how the move might affect them and what they can do to prepare for it. Participants of the workshops range between the ages of 12 and 18 years old; hence, some may never have even considered the fact that they will have to leave children's services, while others may have already made the move. The young people share experiences, fears and advice, helping each other to deal with the prospect of becoming more independent in managing their conditions.

Like all facilitators for the Staying Positive workshops, I have a long-term medical condition. For me, one of the most important aspects of the workshops is simply giving the young people the chance to speak openly and honestly about the way their conditions affect them. Perhaps for the first time, participants feel able to express anger at having a condition or talk about upsetting feelings, knowing that somebody else in the room understands how they feel. Over the course of the three workshops, I witness the young people growing in confidence. This self-confidence is crucial for the young people to use the skills they have learnt in the workshops to manage their conditions – not just as they move onto adult services but for the rest of their lives.

Fiona Price-Kuehne
Young facilitator for Staying Positive Expert Patient Programme Community Interest Company

Named 'transition co-ordinator'

The need for coordination between paediatric and adult services, which may be geographically separate and have distinct structures, processes and staff, has meant that many have argued for the importance of having a transition coordinator (Betz and Redcay, 2005). Such an individual would also be ideally placed to provide continuity of care and individualized support for patients over a prolonged transition period.

Out-of-hours phone support

Young people may require extra support as they adapt to the greater responsibility for their health care they must take as adult patients. In particular, diabetic patients may need advice about adapting their insulin regime in changing circumstances. Providing such support by phone, at times convenient to the adolescents, was identified in qualitative research with young adults as a feature they would have found helpful during transition.

Greater attempts to contact those who did not attend follow-up

Identification of those who have missed appointments may help to identify those in danger of disengaging from services, before there is complete loss of contact with health professionals.

Transition services: the European experience

The level of recognition of transition as a problem varies not only between conditions, but also between countries in Europe, Australia and the United States. This was demonstrated by a comparative analysis of the strategies in place for the transition of those with disabilities in Australia, Spain, the Netherlands and Switzerland in 1995 (Bowes et al., 1995). At that stage, a range of attitudes was clear: from there being 'little experience, or even interest, in transition issues' (Spain) to different models of transition support being discussed in the literature and national conferences (Australia). A more recent review of policies in Australia revealed multiple state and national policies and proposed models of care, demonstrating the patchy nature of provision and some lack of coordination (Steinbeck, Brodie and Towns, 2007). Within Europe, a 2009 survey highlighted the variation in the age range covered by paediatrics in different European countries (Ercan et al., 2009), but attitudes towards and strategies for transition in Europe have not previously been compared. The responses to the 'Child Health Services and Systems in Europe' questionnaire (Table 4.1) identified that the boundary between paediatric and adult care varies between 16 and 19 years old. The questionnaire was used to assess attitudes towards transitional care across a range of European countries, using clinical scenarios and policy questions to assess service provision, as part of a broad investigation of health conditions. A thematic analysis of the responses identified that transitional care was an area on which a range of viewpoints emerged, as outlined in Table 4.1. General themes included: recognition that transition may be more easily coordinated in smaller, more centralized paediatric subspecialties; the complex nature of transitioning patients with neurodevelopmental problems, particularly when adult services are poorly developed; and a discrepancy between provision for physical and mental health conditions.

It was clear from the questionnaire responses that the United Kingdom's Department of Health has produced a relatively large number of policy documents relating to transition, in comparison with other European countries. Transition is one standard in the National Service Framework for Children, which requires that 'All young people have access to age-appropriate services which are responsive to their specific needs as they grow into adulthood', and a similar requirement is made in the National Service Framework for Diabetes. The growing importance of transition issues is also demonstrated by educational programmes for adolescent health care: both the Adolescent Health Project Curriculum (produced by the Royal College of Paediatrics and Child Health [RCPCH]) and EuTEACH (European Training in Effective Adolescent Care and Health) include modules on transition. Although there is no overall guidance on transition from the RCPCH, it is included in their guidance on a range of conditions, including chronic fatigue syndrome/myalgic encephalomyelitis (CFS/ME) and diabetes mellitus.

Table 4.1 Themes identified from responses to the 'Child Health Services and Systems in Europe' questionnaire

Theme	*Issues raised by country respondents*
Age of transfer from paediatric to adult care	• Desire for paediatrics to include those up to age 19 (England, Israel, Norway) versus fixed transfer at age 16 (Netherlands) • Discrepancy between age ranges covered for physical and mental health conditions (England, Isle of Man) • Need for flexibility over age range in complex conditions e.g. cerebral palsy (Netherlands) • May be different for highly specialized conditions, e.g. cystic fibrosis, managed by paediatricians 'well into their twenties' (Israel)
Success of existing transition arrangements	• Some consensus that transition is better developed in smaller subspecialties (e.g. cystic fibrosis, immunodeficiency, congenital heart disease and metabolic disease in Norway, and cystic fibrosis in the Isle of Man) • Reported to be 'very poor' overall (Isle of Man) • 'Variable' (England, Norway) • 'Improving slowly' (England) • Not noted to be a problem (Netherlands) • 'Inadequate planning for transfer to adult specialists' (Israel)
Particular areas of concern	• Difficulty of arranging transfer for conditions in which adult services are poorly developed (ADHD mentioned by England, rehabilitation services by Norway) • Complexity of transitional arrangements for complex needs/disability (England) • Poor arrangements for mental health transition (Isle of Man) • Complex neurodevelopmental disorders – 'frequently will have fragmented care and will find help mainly from voluntary organizations i.e. not good' (Israel)
Geographical variation in service delivery	Variation in arrangements for asthma care (Isle of Man)
Existing publications on transition	England: *Transition: getting it right for young people* (2006) and *Transition: moving on well* (2008), DVD made by young people recounting their experiences of transition (2006)
Plans for future development	• 'Adolescent Medicine' conference planned with transition as a key theme (Norway) • RCPCH are producing an e-learning tool for paediatricians on adolescent health, including transition (England) • Department of Health, England, is funding research into models of multi-agency transition for young people with disabilities or autistic spectrum disorders

Future challenges

The issues surrounding transitional care have been in discussion for many years, across a broad range of both physical and mental health conditions. Despite many calls for service improvement, implementation has been patchy and evaluation of existing programmes very limited, making recommendations for evidence-based policy problematic. The heterogeneity of interventions, conditions and outcomes in existing studies makes it difficult to directly compare practices and there have been no long-term follow-up studies of the impact of transition programmes in determining adult health outcomes. A key question mark remains over how sustainable any observed changes in health outcomes may be and this is clearly a priority area for future research. In certain conditions, there is a known link between short- and long-term outcomes: for example, between glycaemic control and diabetic complications. The impact of adolescent experiences in long-term outcomes for disabilities or arthritis is less clear, with more empirical data needed to establish the effectiveness and cost-effectiveness of transition interventions.

A further question raised by the existing studies is whether there is any way of identifying which patients are most in need of, or likely to benefit from, enhanced transition support. Two studies of diabetic patients (Holmes-Walker, Llewellyn and Farrell, 2007; Lane et al., 2007) showed greater gains from the transition programme in the subgroup of patients with the highest pre-transition HbA1c. However, it can certainly be argued (see, for example, Kennedy et al., 2007) that transition considerations are one of the key elements of adolescent health care and should therefore be incorporated into the management of all young people with a chronic condition, rather than being targeted at any specific group. Although in the recent systematic review that aimed to include disabilities and mental health conditions, it was notable that no truly evaluative studies of transition programmes in these conditions were found (Crowley et al., 2011). The importance of transition in these conditions, and the particular challenges they provide, has been a subject of debate, but they have lagged far behind chronic physical illnesses in the development and evaluation of transition programmes. Further research is also needed to determine over what period transition should take place, and if, as many have argued, it needs to be a flexible process adapted to the needs of the individual, using tools to assess transition readiness and develop individual transition plans. The study (cited previously) of adult survivors of congenital heart disease in Canada (Reid et al., 2004) that found that only 47% successfully transferred to adult care, reported that the probability of this was increased if the last paediatric clinic visit took place at a later age.

Potential avenues for research are also highlighted by related studies that aimed to improve adherence during adolescence (although not specifically during the transition to adult care), including text messaging to improve communication (Franklin et al., 2003) and a negotiated telephone support system to improve self-management (Howells et al., 2002). The use of new technology to engage adolescents (for example, websites providing patient information or facilitating peer support) is also notable. Similarly, approaches to service development and evaluation can be identified from analogous programmes in different patient groups (for example, the use of individual care coordinators in cancer services, the development of the Expert Patient Programme in chronic disease management, and the use of tools to assess readiness for the transition between hospital and community care in HIV-positive youth (Wiener et al., 2007). Such approaches may be used to expand approaches to transitional care, but there remains much that needs to be done both in research and in advocacy.

The International and Interdisciplinary Health Care Transition Research Consortium (IIHCTRC) was formed in early 2009, in response to the evident lack of evidence-based, literacy- and culturally-appropriate models and validated tools to monitor the process of health care transition. This consortium is based in the United States but has collaborations in European and other countries, as shown in Box 4.3. Membership includes emerging adults with chronic disease and disability, their siblings and parents, and clinicians and

Box 4.3 The International and Interdisciplinary Health Care Transition Research Consortium

The vision and mission of the IIHCTRC are:

Vision: To achieve a well planned, culturally and literacy-appropriate health care transition from pediatric to adult-focused care for all adolescents and emerging adults with chronic medical conditions or disabilities.

Mission: Develop and evaluate health care transition programs implemented in a variety of clinical settings using standardized assessment of processes and outcomes of care at the individual, health system and population-level. The research will improve the patient health outcomes and the health care delivery of adolescents and emerging adults with chronic medical conditions by maximizing their individual strengths through literacy-appropriate and culturally appropriate interventions.

The work program of the consortium is conducted by three trans-disciplinary subgroups: Health Education, Transition Readiness and Advocacy.

The health education subgroup is identifying and disseminating provider education curriculums and interventions designed for health providers to learn about the process of health care transition.

The transition-readiness/outcomes subgroup is conducting a study using two transition assessment instruments: the TRAQ4 Readiness Assessment and the STARx Questionnaire.

The advocacy subgroup's efforts are focused on bringing adolescents/ emerging adults and their parents together to share their stories, successes, and challenges with health care professionals. This in turn will help develop patient and family-centered health care transition programs. This group also advocates for policy changes to ensure that all emerging adults with chronic medical conditions and disabilities (CMCD) receive appropriate health care transition services and support. Finally, this subgroup developed the consortium's website, which can be accessed at http://healthcaretransitionresearch.org

Sources: Maria Ferris, David Wood, and Cecily Betz.personal communication; Ferris, M. et al. (2010); Sawicki, G.S. et al. (2011); Pham, V. (2008).

health researchers in medicine, nursing, psychology and other health care disciplines.

Future work throughout Europe should focus on improving the evaluation of existing programmes across the spectrum of chronic illness and disability, in support of developing more effective transition to adult care for the increasing numbers of young people with ongoing conditions.

Acknowledgement

We are grateful to the young people who contributed anonymous accounts of their experiences of health services, and to Fiona Price-Kuehne, Maria Ferris, David Wood, and Cecily Betz, of The International and Interdisciplinary Health Care Transition Research Consortium, for their contributions.

References

Annunziato, R.A. et al. (2007) Adherence and medical outcomes in pediatric liver transplant recipients who transition to adult services, *Pediatric Transplantation*, 11(6): 608–14.

Anthony, S.J. et al. (2009) Perceptions of transitional care needs and experiences in pediatric heart transplant recipients, *American Journal of Transplantation*, 9(3): 614–19.

Arcelus, J., Bouman, W.P. and Morgan, J.F. (2008) Treating young people with eating disorders: transition from child mental health to specialist adult eating disorder services, *European Eating Disorders Review*, 16(1): 30–6.

Betz, C.L. and Redcay, G. (2005) Dimensions of the transition service coordinator role, *Journal for Specialists in Pediatric Nursing*, 10(2): 49–59.

Binks, J.A. et al. (2007) What do we really know about the transition to adult-centered health care? A focus on cerebral palsy and spina bifida, *Archives of Physical Medicine and Rehabilitation*, 88(8): 1064–73.

Blaauwbroek, R. et al. (2008) Shared care by paediatric oncologists and family doctors for long-term follow-up of adult childhood cancer survivors: a pilot study [see comment], *Lancet Oncology*, 9(3): 232–8.

Blomquist, K.B. (2006) Healthy and ready to work – Kentucky: incorporating transition into a state program for children with special health care needs, *Pediatric Nursing*, 32(6): 515–28.

Bowes, G. et al. (1995) Transition health services for youth with disabilities: a global perspective, *Journal of Adolescent Health*, 17(1): 23–31.

Brown, R.T. et al. (2005) Treatment of attention-deficit/hyperactivity disorder: Overview of the evidence, *Pediatrics*, 115(6): e749–57.

Brumfield, K. and Lansbury, G. (2004) Experiences of adolescents with cystic fibrosis during their transition from paediatric to adult health care: A qualitative study of young Australian adults, *Disability and Rehabilitation*, 26(4): 223–34.

Bucuvalas, J.C. and Alonso, E. (2008) Long-term outcomes after liver transplantation in children, *Current Opinion in Organ Transplantation*, 13(3): 247–51.

Busse, F.P. et al. (2007) Evaluation of patients' opinion and metabolic control after transfer of young adults with type 1 diabetes from a pediatric diabetes clinic to adult care [see comment], *Hormone Research*, 67(3): 132–8.

Clark, H.B. et al. (2008) Research on transition to adulthood: building the evidence base to inform services and supports for youth and young adults with serious mental health disorders, *Journal of Behavioral Health Services and Research*, 35(4): 365–72.

Cottrell, C.K. et al. (1996) The development and evaluation of a self-management program for cystic fibrosis, *Pediatric Asthma, Allergy and Immunology*, 10(3): 109–18.

Cowlard, J. (2003) Cystic fibrosis: transition from paediatric to adult care, *Nursing Standard*, 18(4): 39–41.

Craig, S.L., Towns, S. and Bibby, H. (2007) Moving on from paediatric to adult health care: an initial evaluation of a transition program for young people with cystic fibrosis, *International Journal of Adolescent Medicine and Health*, 19(3): 333–43.

Crevier, L. and Mercier, C. (2008) L'organisation de la transition enfant à adulte en neurochirurgie pédiatrique au Canada [The organization of the transition from childhood to adulthood in pediatric neurosurgery in Canada], *Neurochirurgie*, 54(5): 583–6.

Crowley, R. et al. (2011) Improving the transition between paediatric and adult healthcare: a systematic review, *Archives of Disease in Childhood*, 96(6): 548–53.

Davis, M. (2003) Addressing the needs of youth in transition to adulthood, *Administration and Policy in Mental Health*, 30(6): 495–509.

Davis, M. and Sondheimer, D.L. (2005) State child mental health efforts to support youth in transition to adulthood, *Journal of Behavioral Health Services and Research*, 32(1): 27–42.

Desir, B. and Seidman, E.G. (2003) Transitioning the paediatric IBD patient to adult care, *Baillière's Best Practice and Research in Clinical Gastroenterology*, 17(2): 197–212.

Dore, A., de Guise, P. and Mercier, L.-A. (2002) Transition of care to adult congenital heart centres: what do patients know about their heart condition? *Canadian Journal of Cardiology*, 18(2): 141–6.

Dovey-Pearce, G. et al. (2005) Young adults' (16–25 years) suggestions for providing developmentally appropriate diabetes services: a qualitative study, *Health and Social Care in the Community*, 13(5): 409–19.

Duguépéroux, I. et al. (2008) Clinical changes of patients with cystic fibrosis during transition from pediatric to adult care, *Journal of Adolescent Health*, 43(5): 459–65.

Eiser, C. et al. (2007) Follow-up care for young adult survivors of cancer: lessons from pediatrics, *Journal of Cancer Survivorship*, 1(1): 75–86.

Ercan, O. et al. (2009) Demography of adolescent health care delivery and training in Europe, *European Journal of Pediatrics*, 168(4): 417–26.

Escalante, C.P. et al. (2004) Outcomes of treatment pathways in outpatient treatment of low risk febrile neutropenic cancer patients, *Supportive Care in Cancer*, 12(9): 657–62.

Evans, J., McDougall, J. and Baldwin, P. (2006) An evaluation of the "Youth en Route" program, *Physical and Occupational Therapy in Pediatrics*, 26(4): 63–87.

Ferris, M. et al. (2010) Toward Evidence-Based Health Care Transition: The Health Care Transition Research Consortium. International Journal of Child and Adolescent Health (2010) Volume 3, Issue 4.

Fleming, E., Carter, B. and Gillibrand, W. (2002) The transition of adolescents with diabetes from the children's health care service into the adult health care service: a review of the literature, *Journal of Clinical Nursing*, 11(5): 560–7.

Franklin, V. et al. (2003) "Sweet Talk": text messaging support for intensive insulin therapy for young people with diabetes, *Diabetes Technology and Therapeutics*, 5(6): 991–6.

Geerts, E., van de Wiel, H. and Tamminga, R. (2008) A pilot study on the effects of the transition of paediatric to adult health care in patients with haemophilia and in their parents: patient and parent worries, parental illness-related distress and health-related Quality of Life, *Haemophilia*, 14(5): 1007–13.

Grey, M. and Berry, D. (2004) Coping skills training and problem solving in diabetes, *Current Diabetes Reports*, 4(2): 126–31.

Holmes-Walker, D.J., Llewellyn, A.C. and Farrell, K. (2007) A transition care programme which improves diabetes control and reduces hospital admission rates in young adults with Type 1 diabetes aged 15–25 years, *Diabetic Medicine*, 24(7): 764–9.

Howells, L. et al. (2002) A randomized control trial of the effect of negotiated telephone support on glycaemic control in young people with Type 1 diabetes, *Diabetic Medicine*, 19(8): 643–8.

Kaatsch, P. et al. (2005) Das langzeit-follow-up in der Deutschen pädiatrischen onkologie als basis für die durchführung von studien mit langzeitüberlebenden [Follow up of long-term survivors after childhood cancer in Germany], *Klinische Padiatrie*, 217: 169–75.

Kaufman, M. (2006) Transition of cognitively delayed adolescent organ transplant recipients to adult care, *Pediatric Transplantation*, 10(4): 413–17.

Kennedy, A. et al. (2007) Young people with chronic illness: the approach to transition, *Internal Medicine Journal*, 37(8): 555–60.

Knowles, J. et al. (2006) The development of an innovative education curriculum for 11–16 yr old children with type 1 diabetes mellitus (T1DM), *Pediatric Diabetes*, 7(6): 322–8.

Laffel, L.M.B. et al. (2003) Impact of ambulatory, family-focused teamwork intervention on glycemic control in youth with type 1 diabetes, *Journal of Pediatrics*, 142(4): 409–16.

Lane, J.T. et al. (2007) Glycemic control over 3 years in a young adult clinic for patients with type 1 diabetes, *Diabetes Research and Clinical Practice*, 78(3): 385–91.

Lawson, M.L. et al. (2005) A randomized trial of regular standardized telephone contact by a diabetes nurse educator in adolescents with poor diabetes control, *Pediatric Diabetes*, 6(1): 32–40.

Marcer, H., Finlay, F. and Baverstock, A. (2008) ADHD and transition to adult services – the experience of community paediatricians, *Child: Care, Health and Development*, 34(5): 564–6.

McDonagh, J.E. (2008) Getting it right for young people: Developing adolescent rheumatology services, *Future Rheumatology*, 3: 133–41.

McDonagh, J.E., Shaw, K.L. and Southwood, T.R. (2006) Growing up and moving on in rheumatology: development and preliminary evaluation of a transitional care programme for a multicentre cohort of adolescents with juvenile idiopathic arthritis, *Journal of Child Health Care*, 10(1): 22–42.

Nakhla, M. et al. (2008) Translating transition: a critical review of the diabetes literature, *Journal of Pediatric Endocrinology and Metabolism*, 21(6): 507–16.

Nasr, S.Z. (2000) Cystic fibrosis in adolescents and young adults, *Adolescent Medicine*, 11(3): 589–603.

National Institute for Health and Care Excellence (2008) Attention Deficit Hyperactivity Disorder: Diagnosis and Management of ADHD in children, young people and adults, NICE clinical guideline 72 (http://www.nice.org.uk/nicemedia/live/12061/42059/42059.pdf accessed June 2013).

Nonnast-Daniel, B. (2005) Spezielle probleme der transplantationsnachsorge bei adoleszenten [Special problems of post-transplantation care in adolescents], *Transplantationsmedizin: Organ der Deutschen Transplantationsgesellschaft*, 17: 22–5.

O'Connell, B., Bailey, S. and Pearce, J. (2003) Straddling the pathway from paediatrician to mainstream health care: transition issues experienced in disability care, *Australian Journal of Rural Health*, 11(2): 57–63.
Peter, N.G. et al. (2009) Transition from pediatric to adult care: internists' perspectives, *Pediatrics*, 123(2): 417–23.
Pham, V. Development and validation of a patient-directed transition-readiness measure for adolescents with chronic kidney disease: a pilot study. Dissertation. Chapel Hill: NC: Univ of North Carolina at Chapel Hill, 2008.
Reid, G.J. et al. (2004) Prevalence and correlates of successful transfer from pediatric to adult health care among a cohort of young adults with complex congenital heart defects, *Pediatrics*, 113(3 Pt 1): e197–205.
Remorino, R. and Taylor, J. (2006) Smoothing things over: the transition from pediatric to adult care for kidney transplant recipients, *Progress in Transplantation*, 16(4), 303–8.
Rianthavorn, P. and Ettenger, R.B. (2005) Medication non-adherence in the adolescent renal transplant recipient: a clinician's viewpoint, *Pediatric Transplantation*, 9(3): 398–407.
Robertson, L.P. et al. and British Society of Paediatric and Adolescent Rheumatology (2006) Growing up and moving on. A multicentre UK audit of the transfer of adolescents with juvenile idiopathic arthritis from paediatric to adult centred care, *Annals of the Rheumatic Diseases*, 65(1): 74–80.
Sawicki, G.S. et al. (2011) Measuring the transition readiness of youth with special healthcare needs: validation of the TRAQ-Transition readiness assessment questionnaire, *J Pediatr Psychol.* 2011 Mar; 36(2):160–71
Scottish Intercollegiate Guidelines Network (2007) Assessment, diagnosis and clinical interventions for children and young people with autism spectrum disorders, Guideline No. 98 (http://www.sign.ac.uk/guidelines/fulltext/98/contents.html, accessed June 2013).
Skinner, R. et al. and UK Children's Cancer Study Group Late Effects Group (2006) Long-term follow-up of people who have survived cancer during childhood, *The Lancet Oncology*, 7(6): 489–98.
Steinbeck, K.S., Brodie, L. and Towns, S.J. (2007) Transition care for young people with chronic illness, *International Journal of Adolescent Medicine and Health*, 19(3): 295–303.
Steinkamp, G. et al. (2001) Transition of adult patients with cystic fibrosis from paediatric to adult care – the patients' perspective before and after start-up of an adult clinic, *European Journal of Medical Research*, 6(2): 85–92.
Tomlinson, P. and Sugarman, I.D. (1995) Complications with shunts in adults with spina bifida, *BMJ*, 311(7000): 286–7.
Tuchman, L.K., Slap, G.B. and Britto, M.T. (2008) Transition to adult care: experiences and expectations of adolescents with a chronic illness, *Child: Care, Health and Development*, 34(5): 557–63.
Vanelli, M. et al. (2004) Effectiveness of an uninterrupted procedure to transfer adolescents with Type 1 diabetes from the Paediatric to the Adult Clinic held in the same hospital: eight-year experience with the Parma protocol, *Diabetes, Nutrition and Metabolism – Clinical and Experimental*, 17(5): 304–8.
Vega-Briceno, L.E., Guiraldes, C.E. and Sanchez, D.I. (2006) [Cystic fibrosis: facing patient transition from the pediatrician to the internist][Article in Spanish], *Revista Medica de Chile*, 134(3): 365–71.
Viner, R. (2001) Barriers and good practice in transition from paediatric to adult care, *Journal of the Royal Society of Medicine*, 94 (Suppl 40): 2–4.
Viner, R. (2003) Bridging the gaps: transition for young people with cancer, *European Journal of Cancer*, 39(18): 2684–7.

Viner, R.M. (2008) Transition of care from paediatric to adult services: one part of improved health services for adolescents, *Archives of Disease in Childhood*, 93(2): 160–3.

Visentin, K., Koch, T. and Kralik, D. (2006) Adolescents with Type 1 diabetes: transition between diabetes services, *Journal of Clinical Nursing*, 15(6): 761–9.

Volta, C. et al. (2003) Transition from pediatric to adult care of children with chronic endocrine diseases: a survey on the current modalities in Italy, *Journal of Endocrinological Investigation*, 26(2): 157–62.

Watson, A.R. (2000) Non-compliance and transfer from paediatric to adult transplant unit, *Pediatric Nephrology*, 14(6): 469–72.

Watson, A.R. (2005) Problems and pitfalls of transition from paediatric to adult renal care, *Pediatric Nephrology*, 20(2): 113–17.

Webb, G. (2005) Improving the care of Canadian adults with congenital heart disease, *Canadian Journal of Cardiology*, 21(10): 833–8.

Webb, G.D. (2001) Care of adults with congenital heart disease – a challenge for the new millennium, *Thoracic and Cardiovascular Surgeon*, 49(1): 30–4.

Wiener, L.S. et al. (2007) Transition from a pediatric HIV intramural clinical research program to adolescent and adult community-based care services: assessing transition readiness, *Social Work in Health Care*, 46(1): 1–19.

Wysocki, T. et al. (1992) Diabetes mellitus in the transition to adulthood: adjustment, self-care, and health status, *Journal of Developmental and Behavioral Pediatrics*, 13(3): 194–201.

Yeung, E. et al. (2008) Lapse of care as a predictor for morbidity in adults with congenital heart disease, *International Journal of Cardiology*, 125(1): 62–5.

Zack, J. et al. (2003) Perspectives of patients with cystic fibrosis on preventive counseling and transition to adult care [see comment], *Pediatric Pulmonology*, 36(5): 376–83.

chapter five

Child public health

Ingrid Wolfe, Giorgio Tamburlini, Pieter Auke Wiegeresma, Matthew Thompson, Peter Gill, Simon Lenton

> It is easier to build strong children than repair broken men
>
> *Frederick Douglass 1818–95*
>
> *American social reformer, born a slave, became an orator, writer, statesman*

Concepts in child public health

Child public health is about the lives of children living in families and communities. The health, well-being and development of children is determined by their personal and collective circumstances and by political, social and economic forces. Public health knowledge and advocacy can represent children's lives and realities to those in power in order to improve their social and economic conditions and improve their health.

The history of public health is littered with arguments about definitions. The tension between individual and population-based approaches to concepts of health can be counter-productive, with arguments about the relative merits of one or the other, when in fact neither is sufficient on its own and both are necessary. Indeed, John Ryle, who founded the discipline of social medicine at the University of Oxford in the 1940s, was thought to have considered social medicine as an extension into the community of the holistic approach he adopted with individual patients (Holland and Stewart, 1998). Social medicine more closely derives from clinical experience, defining its concerns as being: epidemiology; the study of the medical and health needs of society; the study of the provision and organization of health services; and the study of the prevention of disease (Society for Social Medicine, 2012). The mission statement of the International Society for Social Pediatrics and Child Health (ISSOP) is 'health professionals acting locally and globally to improve the health and wellbeing of children and young people' (ISSOP, 2008). Thus, the social epidemiology of childhood is about poverty, environment, family, globalization, economics and politics.

The current practice of public health is shaped by its history. Public health, focused on sanitation, was the first great global health movement and made enormous progress in reducing infant and child mortality. The pace of child health improvement accelerated from the beginning of the 20th century, with the control of major childhood infectious diseases, such as diphtheria and pertussis, and later measles. Preventive medicine was the next major step in public health. The Lalonde Report (Lalonde, 1974) marked the start of the health promotion era and the Ottawa Charter in 1986 set out its key principles (WHO, 1986). Vaccination was a technological development directly resulting from progress in scientific thinking. Advances in living conditions in general, and communicable disease prevention in particular, led to an epidemiological shift such that NCDs came increasingly to dominate childhood illness. Health promotion and disease prevention comprise the second great global health movement. Understanding the importance of social determinants, followed naturally from the rise of health promotion, and was accelerated through the work of Marmot and others, helped give rise to a third global health movement: health systems strengthening. This movement is driven by the epidemiological transition and shaped by social and economic forces. There is upward pressure on health care costs and cost-containment has been a major driver for system reform, even before the current financial crisis. Ongoing reforms have many diverse components, often reflecting the prevailing political philosophy in each country, but one common element is the aim to reduce demand for care through health improvement (Figueras and McKee, 2012). This can be seen in measures to enhance the elements of prevention and health promotion within health care, and especially primary care, and to strengthen public health services.

This chapter begins with a brief description of the main determinants of health in childhood and beyond, focusing especially on distal factors grouped into four broad (and largely interlinked) areas:

- political, social and economic forces
- physical environment
- individual and family factors
- health services

This section is followed by a discussion of the strategies and interventions through which public health action can influence the determinants of child health, in four main categories:

- health promotion and risk reduction
- political, social and economic policy
- health services public health
- mechanisms of accountability for child health.

The determinants of child health

Child health is important not only because of its immediate consequences for the child, but also because of the long-term effects on population health. Research in recent decades strongly suggests that many diseases and conditions that arise in childhood, and even much later along the life-course, may have causes that start in the earliest years of life. Exposure to inadequate nutrition, to chemical and physical pollutants, to social and psychosocial adverse conditions, to infectious or other harmful agents or processes, may interfere with early organ and system development, disrupt metabolic pathways, modify disease susceptibility and have profound effects on outcome at birth, on health during infancy and childhood, and throughout the entire life-course. Indeed, there is a growing body of evidence that there are periods of development when children and young people are especially sensitive to risk and to protective factors, when such influences can have particularly pronounced effects. Thus, public health investments should be increasingly directed at improving the environment in which children are conceived and grow (Cattaneo et al., 2012).

This has led many countries to adopt policies that are shaped by a life-course approach to health, recognizing that a child's life trajectory is influenced by a wide range of determinants acting at different times and places. Some increase risks while others are protective. Interventions should reduce the former and enhance the latter. Importantly, since beneficial and harmful influences can have a cumulative effect along the life-course, early interventions produce the greatest dividends (WHO, 2008) (Figure 5.1).

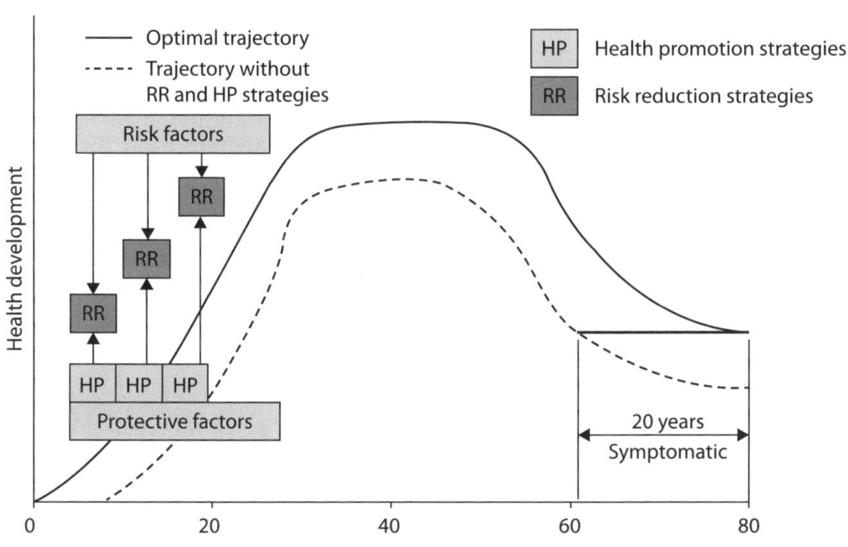

Figure 5.1 How risk reduction and health promotion strategies influence health development

Source: Adapted from Halfon, 2012

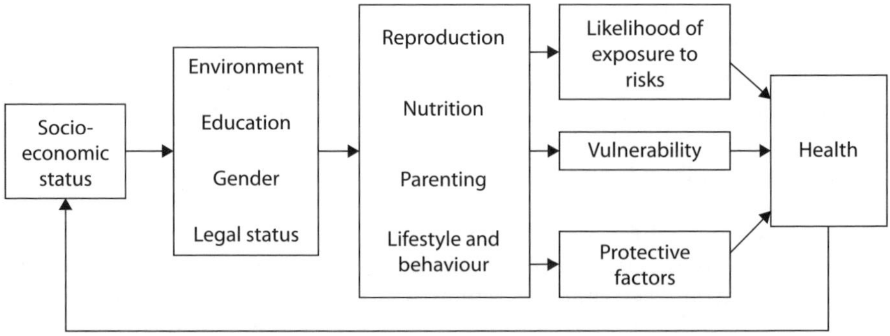

Figure 5.2 A causal web illustrating how socioeconomic factors relate to health

Source: Adapted from Cattaneo et al., 2012

Social and economic determinants are the most important factors shaping children's health and life chances in Europe (WHO Regional Office for Europe, 2009a), interacting in a complex web of direct and indirect causality, as illustrated in Figure 5.2.

Political, social, and economic determinants

Poverty, deprivation and inequalities

Child poverty is commonly defined as the proportion of children living in households with an income less than 60% of the average national income, so rates are highly subject to national fiscal policy. Countries can augment family income through redistributive policies, tax exemptions, and social benefits and services (Bradshaw, 2006). The cost of bringing up children means that in some countries they are more likely to be living in poverty than the general population (TÁRKI Social Research Institute, 2010), however fiscal and social policy can redistribute resources equitably across age groups, as shown in Table 1.1. While the situation does vary according to national welfare policies, with the lowest rates of child poverty and deprivation generally in the Nordic countries and highest rates in southern and eastern European countries, in most countries children living in lone-parent households are at increased risk of poverty, as are children from migrant families and those from minority and Roma populations, as shown in Figure 5.3 (UNICEF CEE/CIS, 2007; Cattaneo et al., 2012).

Inequalities in overall child mortality according to family income have been documented in many countries, but most work has been undertaken in the United Kingdom and Scandinavia (TÁRKI Social Research Institute, 2010). The mortality gap is widest for deaths from injuries and violence (UNICEF Innocenti Research Centre, 2005). These inequalities are mirrored in measures of risk, disease incidence and prevalence; for example, child overweight and obesity are related to adverse social and economic conditions (Cattaneo et al., 2012); rates of asthma are higher among children from low-income families

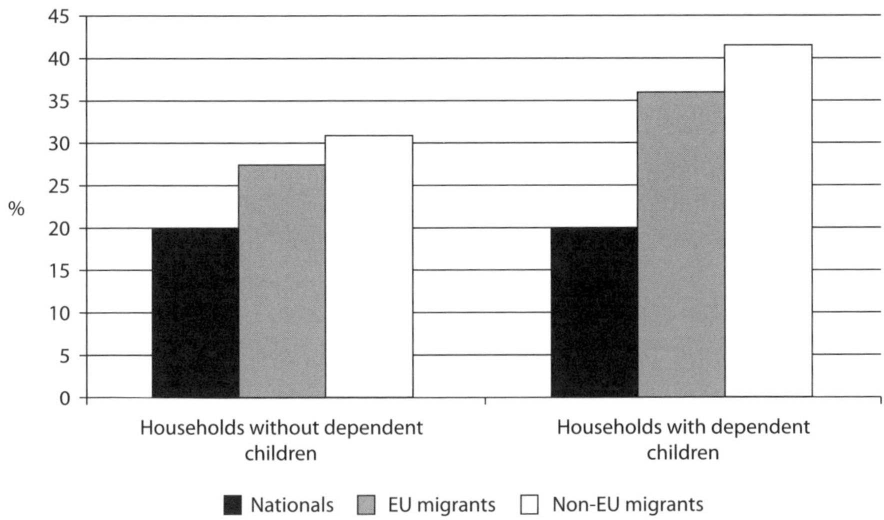

Figure 5.3 Population at risk of poverty

Source: Eurostat 2008

(Cattaneo et al., 2012); as are many other conditions including cerebral palsy (Hjern and Thorngren-Jerneck, 2008), disability (Blackburn, Spencer and Read, 2010), general well-being (Cattaneo et al., 2012), and all forms of mental health problems (except autism, although this may be due to ascertainment bias) (WHO, Regional Office for Europe 2009a). See also Chapter 8 for a discussion of the risks of social inequalities and mental health.

Overweight and obesity

Tackling the rising prevalence of child obesity must be a priority given its contribution to disease and disability in childhood (type 2 diabetes, fatty liver disease, endocrine disorders and musculoskeletal complaints), and because children grow up to be obese adults with risks for developing a variety of problems such as cardiovascular disease, diabetes and cancers. An estimated 14 million children in the 25 pre-2004 European Union Member States were overweight, accounting for nearly one-fifth of the European population of schoolchildren. Of these, at least 3 million are obese, and this number is rising annually between 0.55% and 1.65% (Lobstein, Baur and Uauy, 2004). Prevalence rates for overweight and obesity in children under 4 years of age range from 11.8% in Romania to 33.2% in Spain; countries in between this range vary but, in general, Mediterranean countries tend to report higher prevalences than northern and eastern Europe (Cattaneo et al., 2010). Among schoolchildren between 6–9 years of age, on average 24% are overweight or obese (Cattaneo et al., 2012).

It is too simplistic to consider obesity as merely a problem of imbalance between energy intake and expenditure, a view that largely underpins the individualist medical approach to its management. A growing body of evidence suggests the importance of risks from the earliest stages of development; for example, epigenetic changes may affect later susceptibility to obesity (Gluckman et al., 2009). Incontrovertibly, the increasing prevalence of overweight and obesity reflects the changing environments that children inhabit, dominated by energy-dense food and drink, which in many countries is intensively marketed to children (Cairns, Angus and Hastings, 2009) and, to a much lesser degree, fewer opportunities to exercise (Swinburn et al., 2011).

Food and nutrition

A systematic review of determinants of children's intake of fruit and vegetables identified socioeconomic status and availability as important factors, as well as gender, age and parental intake. Many studies have shown that few children eat the WHO recommended daily allowance of fruit and vegetables (Jones et al., 2010). However, child nutrition starts in the womb and is influenced by maternal and placental health. The earliest indicator of the quality of antenatal nutrition is birth weight, with wide variations in rates of low birth-weight (LBW) babies across Europe, from under 5% of births (in Scandinavian countries) to over 8% (in eastern Europe) (OECD, 2011). Postnatally, breastfeeding is an important determinant of health, with many diverse protective effects (Table 5.1).

There is widespread agreement, reflected in policy recommendations in most countries, that breastfeeding should be the exclusive source of nutrition until 6 months of age and should be combined with other sources of food until 1–2 years. Definitions of exclusivity of breastfeeding and durations vary between countries, so interpretation of data is difficult. However, measures of exclusive breastfeeding at 6 months do seem to vary widely, from 1% in the United Kingdom, to over 30% in some Scandinavian countries (33% in Sweden) and eastern European countries (42% in Bulgaria) (Cattaneo et al., 2012).

Table 5.1 Health protective effects of breastfeeding

Health outcomes	*Average risk reduction*
Acute otitis media	50%
Gastrointestinal infections	64%
Lower respiratory tract infections	72%
Eczema	42%
Asthma	27%
Overweight and obesity	22%
Type 2 diabetes	38%
Acute leukaemia	19%
Sudden infant death syndrome	36%

Source: Cattaneo et al., 2012

Until the 1960s, the greatest concern about food and nutrition for older children in Europe was under-nutrition. Measures such as the European Community's Common Agricultural Policy and free trade agreements, coupled with increased global trade and advances in food production and distribution, radically changed the situation. By the 1980s, the food industry was increasingly dominated by large corporations that promoted energy-dense products at low prices (Hawkes, 2006). The inevitable consequence, especially when accompanied by an increasingly sedentary lifestyle, was an epidemic in child obesity, with poorer children particularly at risk (Sturm and Datar, 2005; Duffey et al., 2010). On average, 24% of Children aged 6–9 years in Europe are overweight or obese (Lobstein et al., 2004). Self-reported data from older children in the Health Behaviour of School-age Children study show wide variation between countries and regions. Boys are more likely to be overweight or obese than girls; self-perception of overweight or obesity is greater than that defined by BMI in western and central Europe but not eastern Europe, suggesting body-image concerns in the West; and there are associations between high prevalence of overweight and lower socioeconomic status in some countries (Currie et al., 2012).

Tobacco and alcohol

Tobacco is responsible for more (adult) deaths in the EU than any other single cause (Peto et al., 2012). Smoking behaviour usually becomes established in early life; most adults had their first cigarette in adolescence (Lamkin and Houston, 1998) and, despite widespread awareness of risks, smoking prevalence remains high among adolescents in many countries (Cattaneo et al., 2012; Currie et al., 2012). On average, 30% of 15-year-olds report first smoking at the age of 13 or younger, although there is wide variation between European countries, ranging from 7% to 65% (WHO Regional Office for Europe, 2008). There is evidence to suggest risk clustering; for example, early onset of smoking predicts alcohol-related problems later in adolescence or early adulthood (Riala et al., 2004). On average, 1% of 11-year-olds in Europe smoke at least once a week, 6% of 13-year-olds, and 19% of 15-year-olds, but again there are wide variations between countries. There has been a trend towards increasing smoking rates, especially in 13 to 15-year-olds, and smoking rates among girls are higher than among boys (WHO Regional Office for Europe, 2008).

Alcohol use causes damage to children, young people and unborn children. It affects health, well-being, educational attainment, employment and personal security. The social cost of alcohol is estimated to be around US$300–400 per capita, per year (Anderson, 2013). Rates of alcohol consumption increase markedly with age between 11 and 15 years; while 2% of 11-year-olds have been drunk at least twice, a third of 15-year-olds have done so, and 21% drink alcohol at least once a week (Currie et al., 2012).

Physical environment

Injuries

Injuries are one of the leading causes of disability and death among children and young people (Chapter 1). Just over 9000 children under the age of 20 years die in the European Union every year; over two-thirds are unintentional injuries and up to 90% of all injuries are thought to be preventable (ECSA, 2012a). They are much more frequent in central and eastern Europe than in western Europe but also vary greatly within countries, leading to stark geographic and socioeconomic inequalities (Armour-Marshall et al., 2012). The WHO Children's Environment and Health Action Plan for Europe (CEHAPE) has set out a goal to 'prevent and substantially reduce health consequences from accidents and injuries and pursue a decrease in morbidity from lack of adequate physical activity, by promoting safe, secure and supportive human settlements for all children'. National governments have committed to implement a variety of actions to achieve this goal, including the provision of safe play spaces, implementation of effective road safety measures (Sethi, 2007), transport planning, and safe school and home environments.

Physical activity for health

Low levels of physical activity in children are associated with higher weight, higher blood pressure and lower high-density lipoprotein (HDL) cholesterol levels (WHO Regional Office for Europe, 2006b). Moreover, children who are more physically active are thought to cope with symptoms of anxiety better, to perform better academically at school, and to adopt other healthy behaviours such as avoiding drug and alcohol use (WHO, 2004). Around half of 11-year-olds in Europe do not engage in sufficient physical activity for health, and the proportion increases through adolescence (WHO Regional Office for Europe, 2010). The HBSC survey reported that 23% of 11-year-olds, 19% of 13-year-olds, and 15% of 15-year-olds engage in at least one hour of moderately vigorous physical activity per day (Currie et al., 2012), which is the recommended amount based on a review of the literature (Strong et al., 2005).

Environmental health

Infants and children are thought to be at increased risk of harm from environmental hazards, because they are especially vulnerable when developing and growing, and because they may experience increased levels of exposure to such hazards. As in many areas of child health, there are marked social inequalities in environmental health: children who live in deprived areas are at an increased risk of accidents and injuries, as well as of exposure to environmental hazards such as toxic chemicals, contaminated water, air, soil and food, and to environmental tobacco smoke, pollutants and noise (Bolte, Tamburlini and Kohlhuber, 2010). CEHAPE specifies goals to 'prevent and reduce respiratory disease due to outdoor and indoor air pollution' and to 'reduce the risk of disease and disability from exposure to hazardous chemicals, physical agents, biological agents and working environments'.

Homelessness and poor quality of housing are more likely among children already disadvantaged through poverty, and are associated with poorer health and development outcomes in childhood. A study in the United Kingdom, completed before the ongoing financial crisis, estimated that 14% of children lived in homes considered unfit for habitation, and 1% were homeless or living in temporary accommodation (Rice, 2006).

Individual, family and community factors

Mental health is becoming a key concern as up to 20% of children in Europe may have a mental or behavioural problem, ranging from a minor complaint to a severe disorder, although there are large variations in prevalence estimates across countries. Several biological, psychological and social risk factors are associated with mental health and the development of mental disorders from early childhood to adolescence. Many mental health problems in adults have their origin in childhood. There is therefore increasing awareness of the importance of improving preventive action and access to mental health services for children. Although evidence on effectiveness is still limited and experience insufficient to indicate precise public health strategies, effective interventions for preventing mental ill health are well described (Campion, 2012). See Chapter 8 for further discussion of mental health among children and young people.

The parent–child relationship is an important part of a child's life, influencing development in the early years (Sturge-Apple, Davies and Cummings, 2010), and helping to shape health, development and well-being later in childhood and in adult life. A large body of research has shown how relationships in the home (between adults, and between parents and children) affect social development, as well as mental and emotional health (and, although this association is less clear, physical health) in childhood, with effects persisting later in life, independent of socioeconomic status in adulthood (Morgan and Swann, 2004). The association is likely to be causal, given the consistency of the findings, in many different populations, at different times, the strength of the observed associations, and the evidence of dose–response relations.

Although social attitudes to family and children vary across Europe, and are related to culture and religion, many countries have seen profound changes in family structure, attitudes and parenting styles over recent decades (Cattaneo et al., 2012). These changes, as well as information on risk factors related to family and community, are discussed further in Chapter 1.

Conditions amenable to public health and health care services

Infectious diseases are a classic public health problem, amenable to improvements in social conditions, but also to public health services and care such as immunization and surveillance. Infectious diseases also require treatment and, furthermore, in some countries, public health is also involved in planning, procuring and evaluating health care services to meet the full spectrum of health needs.

Infectious diseases surveillance and prevention

Although the burden of disease is shifting away from infectious diseases (Figures 1.8 and 1.9), some communicable diseases remain common, such as diarrhoea and other gastrointestinal and respiratory infections (Cattaneo et al., 2012). These problems place a substantial burden on health services; for example, acute otitis media is one of the most common reasons for young children seeking medical attention (See Chapter 2 for a further discussion about primary health services and acute illness). However, even among vaccine-preventable diseases, there are continuing outbreaks of a handful of illnesses including measles, rotavirus and influenza. Despite national vaccination programmes throughout Europe, measles has remained endemic in many areas and there are periodic outbreaks.

An emerging threat is antimicrobial resistance, an increasing problem due to the widespread use of antibiotics at community and hospital levels, and to the massive use of antibiotics in animal breeding. The 2006 annual report of the European Antimicrobial Resistance Surveillance System (EARSS) describes the developments between 1999 and 2006 and demonstrates the continuous decline in the effectiveness of antibiotics across Europe (EARSS, 2007). The Chief Medical Officer of England published a report on the threats of antimicrobial resistance, with urgent and specific recommendations for all levels within the health system (Chief Medical Officer, 2011). These are equally applicable throughout Europe and beyond.

Health services as a population-level determinant of health

Health services are an important – and modifiable – determinant of child health. However, comprehensive evaluations of the quality of children's care are lacking in most countries. Nonetheless, there are sufficient indications of variability between countries, for example, in deaths from common diseases that are amenable to health care (such as pneumonia and asthma) to suggest that there is significant scope for improvement in many countries (Wolfe et al., 2013). National audits of quality and consistency of care for specific diseases (such as diabetes and epilepsy) and reviews of child deaths suggest that the quality of care delivered by children's health services is variable and in some instances poor (Pearson, 2008; Diabetes UK, 2011; RCPCH, 2012; NHS, 2012). Research in several European countries suggests that up to two-thirds of hospital admissions among children with asthma could have been avoided with better preventive care, such as the use of asthma action plans, education on prevention of exacerbations, and reduction of triggers and risk factors such as parental smoking (Reindal and Oymar, 2006; Fuhrman et al., 2011). On the other hand, although there is much variation across Europe in the institutions and organizations involved in implementing action for children and adolescents with mental health problems, it is estimated that only a small proportion of these children and adolescents receive help from existing services (WHO Regional Office for Europe, 2009b).

From risk to intervention

Child health, risk of disease and delayed development are shaped and influenced by factors from many different sectors in society, as illustrated in Table 5.2.

Child public health practice is about addressing these various determinants, through a variety of policies and interventions outlined in the following section.

Table 5.2 An overview of exposures and risk factors, and their impact on child health, over the first 12 years of life

Main exposure	*Main health risks*	*Embryo and foetal stages*	*Birth to 2 years*	*Pre-school (3–6 years)*	*School (7–12 years)*
Poor maternal health	Poor pregnancy outcomes, low birth weight	++++	+++	++	++
Inadequate nutrition during pregnancy and early years	Overweight/underweight, anaemia, infections, immune disorders	++	++++	++	++
Inadequate parenting	Psychosocial problems and behavioural disorders		++++	++	++
Discrimination and social neglect	Psychosocial problems	++	+++	++	++
Environmental toxins	Congenital anomalies, lung diseases, neurotoxicity, endocrine disorders, cancer	+++	+++	++	+
Unsafe home and outside environment	Injuries	+	++	+++	+++
Insufficient physical activity	Obesity, cardiovascular and metabolic risk in later life	+	+	++	+++
Alcohol and tobacco	Congenital anomalies (including fetal alcohol syndrome, low birth weight, respiratory disorders	++++	++	+	+(++)

Source: Cattaneo et al., 2012

Child public health policies and interventions: evidence and experience

This section explores four categories of policy or interventions, each illustrated with examples, through which public health can influence the health of children: health promotion and risk reduction; action on political, social and economic determinants; public health's influence on health care; and finally, accountability systems.

Health promotion and risk reduction

Both health promotion and risk reduction are key functions of public health. But where do they sit within the traditional health system model? And whose business are they? At the individual level, both functions are delivered by clinicians, teachers and parents; at the population level, intersectoral policies are needed to shape the living conditions of children and families towards promoting health. While risk reduction is more typical of health services, reduction of psychosocial risk in individuals and communities implies the collaboration of the health sector and the education and social protection sectors.

Countries vary in how they attempt to strike a balance between individual and population approaches to health promotion. At one end of the spectrum lies the German model of office-based paediatricians, often in sole practice, among whose many responsibilities is health promotion, which may be one factor in its relatively low priority (Busse and Riesberg, 2004). By contrast, countries with comprehensive primary care systems that are firmly integrated within the wider health system, such as Sweden (Anell, Glenngard and Merkur, 2012), seem to have been more successful at embedding health promotion in the health system.

Health promotion and risk reduction activities should take place at all levels of the system, from individual consultations, such as the 'Make Every Contact Count' initiative and the universal and targeted 'Healthy Child Programme' in the United Kingdom (Box 5.1), the organization-wide 'Health-Promoting Hospitals' initiative (WHO Regional Office for Europe, 2007), and population-wide interventions such as those described in Table 3.3, to reduce NCD risks.

Promoting health and preventing overweight and obesity through nutrition and physical activity

An effective response to the growing problem of child obesity necessitates action by individuals from different disciplines, organizations and sectors (Rutter, 2011). However, no country has managed to reverse or even make a substantial impact on the obesity epidemic through public health policy. Here there are lessons to be learned from public health successes in tobacco control policy, including a much better understanding of the multinational food and drinks corporations, which market foods that are calorie-dense and nutrition-poor to children (Federal Trade Commission, 2008). Clearly, they do not spend vast sums on advertising without knowing whether this is effective and there is an association between the prevalence of child overweight and the number of

Box 5.1 An overview of the Healthy Child Programme for 0–5-year-old children in the United Kingdom

Universal		*Targeted*

• Health and development reviews
• Screening and physical examination
• Immunizations
• Promotion of health and well-being, e.g.
  • Smoking
  • Diet and physical activity
  • Breastfeeding and healthy weaning
  • Keeping safe
  • Prevention of sudden infant death syndrome
  • Maintaining infant health
  • Dental health
• Promotion of sensitive parenting and child development
• Involvements of fathers
• Mental health needs assessed
• Preparation and support for parenthood and family relationships
• Signposting to information and services
	• Emotional and psychological problems addressed
	• Promotion and extra support with breastfeeding
	• Support with behaviour change (smoking, diet, keeping safe, SIDS, dental health)
	• Parenting support programmes, including assessment and promotion of parent – baby interaction
	• Promoting child development, including language
	• Additional support and monitoring for infants with health or developmental problems
	• Common Assessment Framework completed
	• Topic-based groups and learning opportunities
	• Help with accessing other services and sources of information and advice
		Higher risk
		• High intensity-based intervention
		• Intensive structured home visiting programme by skilled practitioners
		• Referral for specialist input
		• Action to safeguard the child
		• Contribution to care package led by specialist service

Be alert to risk factors and signs and symptoms of child abuse, and follow local safeguarding procedures where there is cause for concern.

SIDS: sudden infant death syndrome.

Source: Adapted from the 'Healthy Child Programme: pregnancy and the first five years of life', Department of Health, 2009.

advertisements for obesogenic foods per hour (Lobstein and Dibb, 2005). Sugar-sweetened drinks, which are very high in calories, are an especially important factor in the rise in childhood obesity (Malik, Schulze and Hu, 2006; Moreno and Rodriguez, 2007), and related diseases such as type 2 diabetes and cardiovascular disease (Malik et al., 2010). By contrast, diets that are high in fruit and vegetables bring numerous health benefits for children and young people, including reduced risk of obesity (McCrory et al., 1999), diabetes (Ford and Mokdad, 2001), cardiovascular disease (Joshipura et al., 2001), and some cancers (Willett and Trichopoulos, 1996). Fruit and vegetable intake is influenced by several factors, many of which are modifiable through policy; for example, healthy food can be subsidized and made more easily available through local town planning regulations (Cooke et al., 2004; Rasmussen et al., 2006; van der Horst et al., 2007; Jones et al., 2010). Furthermore, replacing 2% of dietary trans-fat with polyunsaturated fat, and reducing salt content in food, can help prevent chronic disease later in life (WHO, 2003; Chisholm et al., 2004; Laxminarayan, Chow and Shahid-Salles, 2006).

There are WHO policy recommendations on improving nutrition and promoting physical activity to counteract obesity (WHO Regional Office for Europe, 2006a); on ways to combat child obesity, for example, food pricing (tax and subsidy); and on agricultural policy to support healthy eating and discourage consumption of foods that are high in fat and sugar and of low nutritional value (Obesity Coalition, 2007; Engelhard and Dorn, 2009; Frieden, Dietz and Collins, 2010). Furthermore, the European Commission has established a 'Platform on Diet, Physical Activity and Health' to support countries attempting to prevent and reverse the obesity epidemic; however, there has been little implementation of this at country level (European Commission, 2005). This is a particularly important deficit since the influences of globalized food and advertising industries on shaping dietary choices is likely to be formidable, and protecting the health interests of children and young people is likely to require action at national and trans-national policy levels (Kovacic, 2008).

Physical inactivity, although less important than the consumption of energy-dense food, is an important factor in the development of obesity and thus chronic disease. By contrast, physical activity promotes health and well-being, reduces the risk of chronic disease, and can help in the management of existing conditions (WHO Regional Office for Europe, 2002; NICE, 2009). There are Europe-wide and country recommendations that children and young people should do at least one hour of moderate to vigorous physical activity each day, with policy guidance on how to achieve this, such as school activities and transport-related policy (European Commission, 2008).

Interventions are needed to change the obesogenic environment in which children live and grow; in order to make healthy choices the easy ones to make; and to shape behaviour through social marketing, health education and health promotion (Swinburn, 2011).

Preventing and reducing tobacco and alcohol use

Adolescents are targeted actively by those selling alcohol and tobacco, with considerable consequences for their health, both in adolescence and later life.

Consumption of both is driven, to varying degrees, by price, marketing and availability, and the health consequences are greatest in adolescents who are disadvantaged and vulnerable in other ways. Consequently, policy responses should target the main drivers, for example, through taxation, restriction on sales and measures to limit marketing.

The WHO Framework Convention on Tobacco Control obliges signatories to implement a range of tobacco control policies, summarized by the mnemonic MPOWER: Monitoring tobacco use and prevention policies; Protecting people from passive smoke in public places; Offering assistance to quit smoking; Warning about the harms of smoking; Enforcing bans on promotion, advertising and sponsorship; Raising taxes on tobacco to discourage smoking. Each of these areas is supported by evidence of effectiveness (Currie and Gilmore, 2013).

While the majority of countries have legal age limits for drinking alcohol, enforcement is variable (Currie et al., 2012). Alcohol consumption is highly sensitive to price and availability (Anderson, 2013), and there is a variety of effective policy options for country- and regional-level efforts to reduce alcohol consumption and harm, the most effective being price increases, limits on availability, and bans on advertising (WHO and World Economic Forum, 2011).

Promoting social resilience and supporting families

There are few comprehensive evaluations of child health promotion programmes but some projects have begun to demonstrate signs of success and may be able to provide some useful learning points for others. Many of these programmes feature elements of the 'Triple P – Positive Parenting Programme', a population-based public health intervention which was developed in Australia, is used throughout Europe, and has been extensively evaluated internationally (University of Queensland, 2012).

The 'Family Nurse Partnership' programme in England is based on the 'Nurse–Family Partnership' programme developed and evaluated in the United States, which showed strong evidence of improved social and emotional development in children (Olds et al., 2004; Kitzman et al., 2010). The English programme focuses on delivering preventive and supportive interventions to vulnerable first-time mothers and their partners. It began in 2007 and preliminary evaluation shows that the programme is well accepted and that health behaviour, such as smoking cessation in pregnancy, and breastfeeding initiation rates may be improved (Barnes et al., 2011). RCTs are due to report in 2013. The English Family Partnership Model, with health visitors reaching out to vulnerable mothers and babies at risk of abuse and neglect in their homes, has been linked to possible improvements in maternal attitudes and infant cooperativeness, but effects were not sustained beyond 3 years (Barlow et al., 2008). Parents valued the relationships they established with the home visitors, reporting increased confidence, better parenting skills and stronger relationships (Kirkpatrick et al., 2007). This model has been evaluated as part of the European Early Promotion Project (EEPP), which comprises universal and targeted home visiting programmes for mental health promotion. A large multicentre (five-country) European trial found significant improvement in mother–child interaction, such as more responsive relationships, more use of appropriate play and less reliance on punishment (Puura et al., 2005).

There are numerous examples of programmes promoting health and social resilience in families, which are considered to be examples of good practice, and for which there are early evaluations suggesting possible success in outcomes, ranging from parental acceptability of services to improved child behaviour. See also chapter 6, on school health, for discussion on school-based interventions to promote resilience. In common with many public health interventions, there is a tension inherent in the balance between universal and targeted approaches to providing services. Rose described this difficulty as a dichotomy between a high-risk strategy and a population strategy, and acknowledged that a combined approach is a realistic way forward in many instances (Rose, 1985). Examples from each type of approach are included in Boxes 5.2 to 5.4 (Eurochild, 2012; Schrader-McMillan, Barnes and Barlow, 2012), and discussed further in Chapter 6. While it is not possible to conclude which approach delivers the best outcomes, Sweden has a long history of success through a universal approach to public health services as part of a population welfare model.

Box 5.2 SPIL centres in Einthoven, The Netherlands: services targeted for families in need

The concept of SPIL centres was derived from the recognition that the needs of children and families were not a high enough priority; that this applied especially to families at risk; and that complex situations required a more coordinated cooperative approach to solutions.

SPIL centres derive their name from the three core concepts involved: play, learning and integration. They began in 2002, and are being rolled out across the municipality with one planned for each neighbourhood and each designed according to local need. The aims are to identify children at risk early and to provide multidisciplinary services in one place, ideally linked to a school or day care centre, as the place where children and families spend most time. SPIL centres focus on children from birth to 12 years, and offer both universal and targeted services. The mantra is 'one family, one plan', indicating personalized services tailored to the particular child and their family's circumstances and needs.

SPIL centre activities include early childhood education, primary school, parenting support and health care. There is a life-course approach to services: from 0 to 2 years, the focus is on caring, childrearing, and education; from 2+ to 6 years, play and learning are the dominant elements; and from 6 to 12 years, education and learning are the focus. Parenting support is a thread running through all years, and in all programmes, and this element can include general support and teaching about parenting and child development, or more specific topics, such as dealing with behavioural problems or emotional difficulties.

Early evaluation of the programme revealed some difficulties with implementation, leading to gaps in provision and the suggestion that families with the greatest needs might still be experiencing difficulties in receiving appropriate support, but generally the service coverage was good. Measures of effectiveness and cost-effectiveness are currently being developed but data are not yet available.

Box 5.3 Family support programme in Stenungsun, Sweden: emphasis on universal services

The Stenungsun programme provides support for parents. It is a resilience-building programme with its roots in the Ottawa Charter. It is set in an area of Sweden that has a history of progressive social policy, with strong links between health and social care sectors. It arose as a local response to a national policy to promote mental health by supporting parents.

The programme adopts a universal approach, providing services for all expectant couples and parents of children from birth to 17 years, but tailors services according to life-stage. The programme begins in the antenatal period, with parental training and support from multiprofessional teams, including midwives, teachers, counsellors and social workers, working closely with parents. All school-age children receive universal services, such as Family Workshops (Familjeverkstan) but there are also targeted programmes for at-risk families. These include parents under 20 years old, single mothers, those without work, or with a history of mental illness or drug abuse. These groups are offered targeted intensive support. Teaching and support of parenting skills continues through school-age years. Services and support can be accessed directly, via telephone, or through a range of alternative means, such as Facebook groups and other web-based sites.

Box 5.4 Family Partnership Model in London, United Kingdom: from supporting parents to empowering communities

The Family Partnership Model is an approach to working with children and families, which uses a structured portfolio of services focusing on home visiting with the child and mother, extending outwards to empowering communities. The aims are to promote psychological and social well-being among children, and to improve outcomes for them, their families and communities. The model relies on trained nurses to deliver specific and intense supportive interventions to mothers at home during the first 18 months of a baby's life, and is associated with more positive outcomes, such as maternal sensitivity and infant cooperation, than the less structured and less intensive support in other programmes such as Home Start. Positive outcomes reported from a small number of studies include improved social and emotional well-being of vulnerable children.

Support for parenting also involves the provision of services such as day care centres and other school services. In all European countries, some form of child care or early childhood education is provided, however enrolment rates vary widely. For children from birth to age 3 years, enrolment exceeds 50% only in Denmark and Iceland, despite evidence of the benefits for health, development and school readiness (OECD, 2009).

Programmes and interventions to promote social resilience, and to support parents and families, are popular with the public and with politicians. However, there is insufficient reliable evidence of effectiveness for most services. Research efforts should be focused in this area to avoid unanticipated adverse consequences or wasted resources.

Assessing and promoting child development

In the past, screening for developmental disabilities and children's emotional and behavioural disorders was very popular, even though it rarely met established criteria for screening (Wilson and Jungner, 1968). This is still the case in the United States (Radecki, Sand-Loud and O'Connor, 2011) and, although a wide array of screening and assessments instruments are available, several problems have emerged (Sices et al., 2009).

First, all screening tests are judged by their sensitivity (how well they identify children truly in need of follow-up) and their specificity (how well they eliminate those who do not need follow-up), but it is exceedingly difficult to design a developmental screening test that is both highly sensitive and specific, given the high variability of child development. In fact, all tested instruments have relatively low sensitivity and specificity.

Secondly, they do not take into account the family environment and its effects on development, thus frequently misdiagnosing as abnormal development what is actually a result of parental neglect or inadequate rearing practices.

Thirdly, screening is acceptable only if effective treatment is available, which is only partially true, for several developmental and behavioural problems.

Nevertheless, child health professionals should be capable of assessing development, identifying environmental risk factors and, most importantly, advising parents on how to improve and stimulate development, both physical and cognitive, and improve their relationship with the child. The diagnosis of developmental and behavioural problems, particularly in the wide grey area of subtle abnormalities or delays, is much improved if parents are given a chance to improve their behaviour and the child is reassessed after a short period of time to see how he/she has reacted.

Home visiting programmes and also well-child visits should therefore put increasing emphasis on promoting development, for example, by encouraging parents to read aloud to their children, at the same time as promoting exclusive and prolonged breastfeeding and recommending vaccination (Tamburlini, Manetti and Toffol, 2011).

Screening for congenital anomalies and genetic diseases

The purpose of screening is to identify children who are more likely to be helped than harmed by detection and subsequent treatment of the risk factor or disease. Screening is an important element of public health, from pre-conception to adulthood. It offers the potential to detect genetic disorders, including inborn errors of metabolism and congenital malformations, most of which are curable or amenable to a much better course and prognosis through early intervention.

Screening in European countries is organized in many different ways and consequently practice varies widely. The United Kingdom has a single national body (the National Screening Committee), which considers screening practice, reviews evidence and determines policy, plus a separate Newborn Screening Programme. This is unusual; in most countries screening services are devolved, so practice varies considerably both within and between countries.

Universal screening is aimed at all children within a certain age range, while targeted screening focuses on children at higher risk for certain conditions, using some form of risk stratification. Although the latter may seem more cost-efficient, if identification of those at high risk is weak, then parents may be falsely reassured or children may be missed. There is considerable variation within Europe in what is screened for, at what ages, and at what intervals this should be repeated.

Also, in order for screening to be beneficial, there needs to be a benefit to identifying children with the condition being screened for. In other words, there has to be evidence that treatment is available and that the outcome for screen-detected abnormalities is better than it would have been without screening (Wilson and Jungner, 1968). A set of recommended child health screening programmes in each age group is available at the European level (Holland, Stewart and Maseria, 2006), although in practice there is considerable variation between countries in what is screened for, and at what ages and intervals.

Vaccination policy and practice

Immunization against infectious diseases has been an enormous public health success. Many vaccine-preventable diseases have declined greatly and, in the case of polio, could now be eradicated worldwide. Indeed, childhood vaccination is said to be one of the most cost-effective health interventions available (OECD, 2011). As with screening, there are some differences between countries, although to a lesser extent. There is a core group of diseases against which immunization is offered everywhere in Europe and another group for which practice varies (Table 5.3).

For the purposes of this chapter, vaccination coverage is important in two distinct ways. First, it tells us about the likely protection offered to the population and individual children. Secondly, it indicates quality of care and the functioning of a health system. Vaccination coverage in European countries is variable, with some large differences between countries. There are consequences for health, of course, but there are also clues from examining the

Table 5.3 Childhood immunizations offered in Europe

Immunizations offered by all European countries	*Additional immunizations offered by some European countries*
Diphtheria	Haemophilus influenza B
Tetanus	Hepatitis B
Pertussis	Meningococcal C
Mumps	Pneumococcal
Measles	Human papilloma virus
Rubella	Rotavirus
Polio	Tuberculosis

Source: WHO Vaccine Preventable Diseases Monitoring System

underlying health system as to why there may be problems and also what might be done to improve matters for children.

Measles is a helpful example in attempting to understand the influence of various types of public health service. Measles infection is highly transmissible and, although the disease is often mild, it can also be severe and even life-threatening. Vaccination is crucial and highly effective (99% efficacy) in individual children (van Boven et al., 2010); if around 95% or more of the population are vaccinated, then there are sufficiently few opportunities for transmission that a population-level effect (herd immunity) results, such that protection is extended to children who are unvaccinated, due, for example, to young age or a medical condition, such as immunodeficiency, precluding vaccination. Measles coverage rates in Europe are variable and so are incidence rates. Outbreaks of measles continue to occur in several European countries, including France, the United Kingdom and Ireland, countries with suboptimal vaccination coverage rates. France has long been known to have lower vaccine coverage rates than many comparable European countries and had the largest outbreak in 2011 (WHO, 2011). This may be related to the decentralized public health system in France, with much care being delivered by physicians in private practice, which can present difficulties for rapid, inexpensive and comprehensive large-scale public health interventions, ranging from information to vaccination. However, the answer does not always lie in a large centralized public health system either, since public confidence can be lost when a government-controlled service loses control of the message, as was seen in the United Kingdom during the measles, mumps, rubella (MMR) scare in the 1990s (Wolfe, 2013a).

Some of the lowest vaccination coverage rates are in wealthy countries with health systems that are otherwise functioning well. There may be clues in the way health services and systems are organized that can help explain, in part, the big differences between countries. Also, there is no EU-wide immunization policy. National public health systems responsible for vaccine delivery, call–recall systems and surveillance vary along a spectrum from centralized to decentralized. Finland and the Netherlands are examples of centralized systems, and achieve measles coverage rates of over 95%, whereas France and Germany have relatively decentralized systems, with local and regional areas sometimes operating almost independently (WHO, 2012). Centralized systems tend to purchase vaccines in bulk, and may be more efficient at providing information rapidly and consistently.

While vaccination has achieved much success, vaccines are not available for every infectious disease and, as previously discussed, European countries have different vaccination policies and varying success with uptake. Consequently, other means of communicable disease control remain crucial. Surveillance is of foremost importance because early identification of outbreaks is key to control. Indicators for routine communicable disease surveillance operate through an EU-wide system known as The European Surveillance System (TESSy), which covers an agreed list of diseases. Event-based surveillance is designed to detect events of possible importance in a less structured way. There is also an EU early warning system (EWS) in operation for outbreaks and public health threats throughout the European Economic Area (European Union, 1998). The European Centre for Disease Prevention and Control (ECDC) and the WHO Regional Office for Europe play dominant roles in regional surveillance and the control of public health threats.

Physical environment, accident and injury prevention

An interim evaluation of the CEHAPE goals has demonstrated some progress in implementing national action plans in most countries (WHO Regional Office for Europe, 2010). Most national strategies include health education and surveillance, backed by legislation. Legislation is key; laws to eliminate lead in petrol and paint, and to reduce the use of lead in industry, have led to a dramatic fall in children's blood lead levels. In the United Kingdom, for example, blood lead levels in children fell from 23 μg/dl in the 1960s to 1–3 μg/dl in the 1990s, and the United Kingdom has recently implemented a review of strategies to further reduce children's exposure to lead in drinking water, beginning with a surveillance study of raised lead levels in children (Health Protection Agency, 2009).

Lower exposure to environmental tobacco smoke among children, resulting from the ban on cigarette smoking in public places in England, is thought to have caused a reduction in children's hospital admissions for acute asthma. Previously, the rate of admission for children with acute asthma was increasing by 2.2% a year; immediately after the implementation of legislation banning smoking in public places there was an 8.9% reduction in admission rates. It is estimated that nearly 7000 fewer children were admitted to hospital in the first three years after the new law came into force (Millett et al., 2013).

Childhood accidents and injuries are considered by CEHAPE and also by the European Child Safety Alliance (ECSA), which produces Child Safety Action Plans and also publishes evaluations of national implementation of policies and rankings at regular intervals in the form of 'Report Cards' (ECSA, 2007). If all countries in Europe matched the country with the lowest child injury mortality rate (the Netherlands), there would have been over 3800 fewer deaths among children and adolescents in 2010 (ECSA, 2012b).

Action on political, social and economic determinants of health

Poverty and inequality reduction: macroeconomics, fiscal policy and social protection

Material deprivation and poverty are not inevitable. Governments make choices about how they distribute resources. Different types of government and various interpretations of the welfare state concept have an important influence on health systems policy and therefore health. An analysis of OECD countries suggested that those with Social Democratic-type governments have lower levels of poverty, smaller income inequalities and lower infant mortality rates than Conservative-leaning governments (Navarro and Shi, 2001).

Some governments make the reduction of childhood poverty a priority, while others do not. For example, Austria, Belgium and the United Kingdom, which have universal non-means tested child benefit (although the United Kingdom has recently abolished this) provide for at least 40% of children's needs through social support, while Italy, Portugal and Spain, which do not have universal non-means tested child benefits, provide less than 20% (Figari, Paulus and Sutherland, 2007; Spencer, 2010). Indeed, the relative child poverty rates in countries before and after taking account of financial support from governments is revealing; Sweden achieves a reduction in relative child poverty from nearly 40% to 10% through social support, whereas the United Kingdom relative child poverty rate is similar to that in Sweden before support (between 35% and 40%) but only reduces it to between 20% and 25% after social support (Spencer, 2010). This demonstrates the scope for further improvement in countries such as the United Kingdom, which could potentially achieve greater reductions in relative child poverty through more redistributive welfare policies.

Countries vary in their approach to policies on socioeconomic equity; thus, in Sweden and Poland, equity features throughout broad aspects of policy that impact on health and welfare, such as transport and the environment. By contrast, Norway and Denmark have sections on inequalities within their overall health policy portfolio (Moberg, 2008). The role of targets is important too; England led the way here, with a comprehensive policy and specific targets for reducing health inequalities in the early 21st century, a model rejected by the new Coalition Government that took office in 2010, although a general commitment to make progress remains (Department of Health, 2012).

The links between policy, social spending and health outcomes, such as mortality, are complex, however, and may be related to the relative proportions of benefits given as cash or benefits in kind. See Figure 1.7.

The overall consequences of social spending on child survival can be seen in Figure 5.4, which shows how those countries with higher levels of social spending have fewer childhood deaths. Redistributive policies can help to overcome social inequalities that might lead to disadvantage. Thus, while single parenthood is, in many countries, a risk factor for childhood poverty and consequent poor health, such as in the United Kingdom, this is not the case in Sweden, where children born to Swedish single mothers have health outcomes that are similar to children born to married middle-class mothers in the United

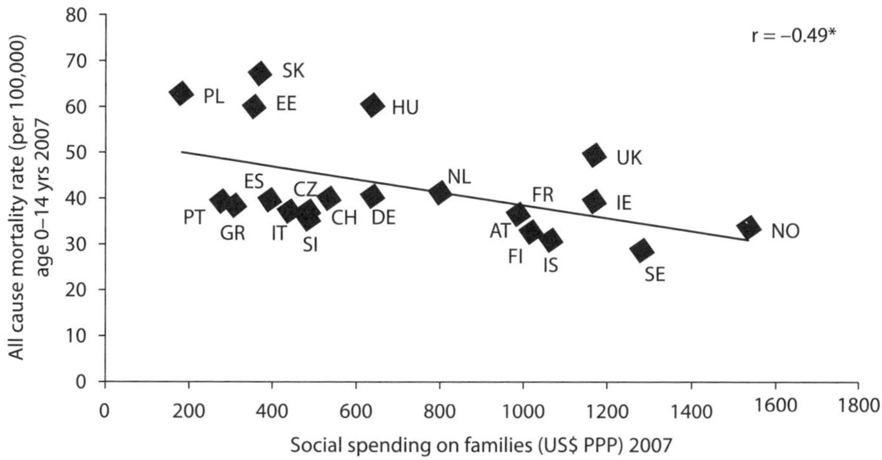

Figure 5.4 Association between social spending on families and child mortality

Note: *= correlation coefficient
Source: WHO, 2012; OECD, 2013
Key: AT Austria; BE Belgium; CH Switzerland; CZ Czech republic; DE Germany; DK Denmark; EE Estonia; ES Spain; FI Finland; FR France; GR Greece; HU Hungary; IE Ireland; IS Iceland; IT Italy; LU Luxembourg; NL Netherlands; NO Norway; PL Poland; PT Portugal; SE Sweden; SI Slovenia; SK Slovakia; UK United Kingdom

Kingdom. Indeed, the lowest rates of relative poverty are achieved in the Scandinavian countries (UNICEF Innocenti Research Centre, 2007).

In the same way, the well-being of children living in countries with strong social protection policies, such as the Scandinavian countries, is higher, while those from countries with less social protection, such as the United Kingdom, have lower well-being scores (UNICEF Innocenti Research Centre, 2007).

Since the United Kingdom's 'Black Report' was published in 1980, followed by the WHO's 'Health for All' initiative in 1984, many European countries have developed an interest in reducing social and health inequalities, but this is expressed more clearly through policies in some countries than others. The first country to introduce policies to reduce health inequalities was the Netherlands (Mackenbach and Bakker, 2003), followed by Italy, England and Finland, and most others have followed to a greater or lesser extent, with varying levels of success (Hogstedt et al., 2008). The different emphasis given to the various factors contributing to inequalities may partly explain the varying levels of success in different countries. Crombie and colleagues describe four broad types of factors that governments invoke to explain the causes of social inequalities, the choice of which influences the policies they institute to address the problems: social and economic conditions; individuals' history and circumstances, such as education and employment; social and community factors, such as inclusion; and lifestyle choices, such as diet and smoking (Crombie et al., 2005). Sweden's policies on reducing social inequalities include all aspects but focus especially on structural factors while, by contrast, Denmark emphasizes personal choice and individual behaviour (Vallgarda, 2001).

The role of public health in health care services for children

Health services are planned in different ways, reflecting the organization of broader health systems, which in turn are shaped by politics as well as historical and cultural influences. Health care public health is about the rational planning of services to meet needs, but the ability to do so is entirely contingent on the information available. Health needs information is often (perhaps usually) derived from patterns of use of existing services. This constrains service reconfigurations. Moreover, the way in which services are arranged determines workforce training, numbers and distribution. Thus, a flawed system that is not designed around the needs of children and families becomes self-perpetuating. Effective health care public health should address this issue by undertaking rigorous health needs assessment (providing such data are available) and designing services on the basis of need, then evaluating and improving them thereafter.

Although universal health coverage is usually considered to be an issue of low- and middle-income countries, there are also problems in the high-income countries of Europe, particularly around equity and access to health care services (Cattaneo et al., 2012). Thus, universal health access, meaning coverage of health care supply plus the influence of social determinants, may be a more appropriate term. Furthermore, in some countries it is becoming clear that the current financial crisis is being seen as an opportunity by those ideologically opposed to the welfare state and are seeking to find excuses to weaken it (McKee et al., 2013). However, health care public health should play a pivotal role in health systems' accountability; indeed, the lack of accountability mechanisms may account for at least some of the gulf between policy, implementation and health outcomes that exists in many European countries. If universal health access and health systems strengthening – the third global health movement – are to be realized fully in Europe, health care public health will need to play a leading role.

Accountability systems; monitoring, reviewing and remedying

Monitoring is an essential public health function, providing data on the health of children in the population, patterns of protective and risk factors, and the burden of disease, all of which are necessary for designing and evaluating health care and public health services. Families, health professionals and policy-makers seeking to improve health services are frequently held back by the lack of useful information. Unfortunately, children are often an afterthought when health information systems are created. What is measured should be meaningful for the child and his or her family. For example, a child with a serious chronic disease, such as cystic fibrosis, may spend much time attending appointments and be frequently admitted to hospital. Consequently, school attendance will be an important indicator of the success of disease management. Poor performance on such a measure can point to appropriate policy responses, shaping services more appropriately and ensuring close links between health and education, for example, through a hospital school service.

It is not, however, straightforward to devise child health indicators, with the usual challenges compounded as children's lives are, in many ways, more complex than adults. For example, child health can differ dramatically according to developmental stage; what matters to a newborn baby is quite different from a young school-age child or adolescent. Children are dependent on their parents and carers, in different ways at different stages: for example, in interpreting what ails them; explaining their behaviour; bringing them to the attention of health professionals; giving them medicines; supporting their behaviour change, and so on. The demography of the child population differs too; the young (like the very old) are especially vulnerable to the effects of poverty. Finally, child disease epidemiology varies from that in adults; congenital and developmental conditions, infectious diseases, and patterns of risks and injuries are all examples of these distinctions.

Figure 5.5 sets out a conceptual model of the relations between policy, determinants and child health outcomes, and illustrates the complexities of devising an effective comprehensive system for child health monitoring.

There are some notable examples of progress in devising child health indicators, discussed in detail in Chapter 11.

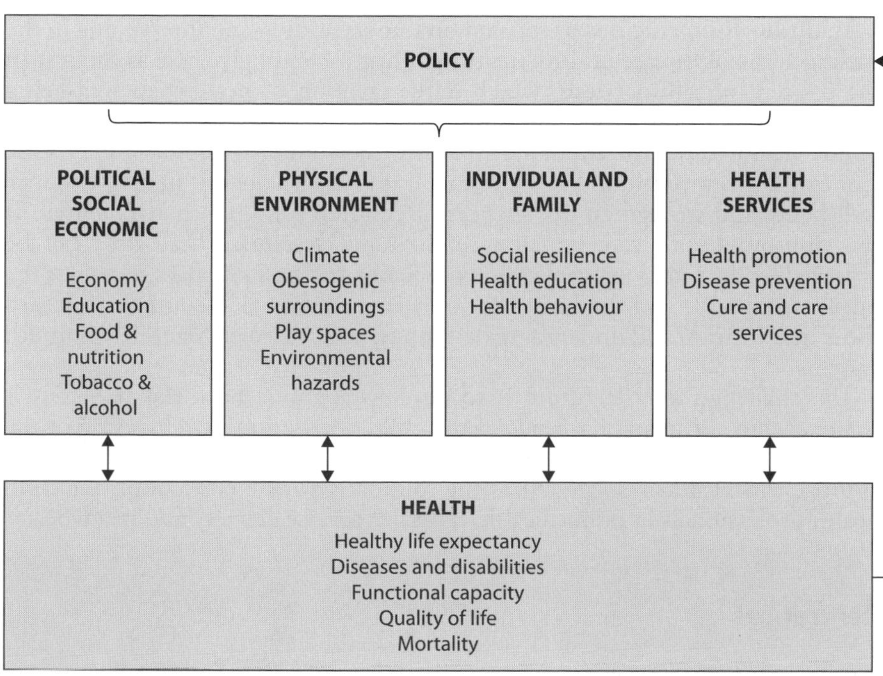

Figure 5.5 A conceptual model of the relations between policy, determinants and child health outcomes

Child health information systems in European countries are thought to vary widely, although there is little reliable comparative information. A comprehensive set of child health indicators, with reliable and uniform systems for data collection and analysis, is needed across Europe. This would allow tracking of progress against goals, and meaningful comparisons between countries. Monitoring systems should allow child health measurement and tracking of progress; however, to deliver on policy, a process of review and remedying action should follow. National oversight mechanisms for child health with formal responsibility, for example, at ministerial level, could help ensure that appropriate remedying action is taken when monitoring systems pick up problems (Wolfe et al., 2013b).

Future challenges

Public health lies at the junctions between biology and society and between the individual and the population. The challenge facing public health services in the 21st century is to create mechanisms that can prevent conditions occurring and treat them effectively and equitably. This means that those providing services for children and their families should be seen not as isolated, disconnected institutions, but as parts of an integrated system, which itself has a clarity of purpose, shared values and can provide a 'joined-up model of delivery', within a research-driven context to foster evidence-based improvement.

Traditionally, medicine has focused on understanding and intervening in the pathogenesis of disease and its treatment, but increasingly there is interest in the concept of salutogenesis, which is the creation of health and well-being (Antonovsky, 1987). Through a life-course health development approach, public health can save children's lives, by the million (Centers for Disease Control and Prevention, 1999). It can improve the quality of life, enhance well-being and strengthen the chances of children fulfilling their potential. It can improve health care practice, services and systems. These aims can be achieved by the judicious application of science and best practices to reduce the burden of disease and disability, not only in currently rich countries but also those in transition and undergoing development from poverty and failed health systems.

The challenge for the future is to develop a public health system that is responsive to the changing needs of the child population. A refocusing of the interests of all those concerned with child health is needed; a rights-based approach to health is suggested as the foundation for a curriculum for child health professionals in public health, in health service delivery and in advocacy.

References

Anderson, P. (2013) Alcohol. In: Mackenbach, J. and McKee, M. (eds) *Successes and failures of health policy in Europe. Four decades of diverging trends and converging challenges*. Maidenhead: Open University Press.

Anell, A., Glenngård, A.H. and Merkur, S. (2012) Sweden health system review, *Health Systems in Transition*, 14(5): 1–159.
Antonovsky, A. (1987) *Unraveling the Mystery of Health: How people manage stress and stay well.* San Francisco, CA: Jossey-Bass.
Armour-Marshall, J. et al. (2012) Childhood deaths from injuries: trends and inequalities in Europe, *European Journal of Public Health*, 22(1): 61–5.
Barlow, J. et al. (2008) *The Oxfordshire Home Visiting Study: Three Year Follow-Up.* Warwick: University of Warwick.
Barnes, J. et al. (2011) *The Family-Nurse Partnership Programme in England: Wave 1 implementation in toddlerhood and a comparison between Waves 1 and 2a implementation in pregnancy and infancy*. London: Department of Health.
Blackburn, C.M., Spencer, N.J. and Read, J.M. (2010) Prevalence of childhood disability and the characteristics and circumstances of disabled children in the UK: secondary analysis of the Family Resources Survey, *BMC Pediatrics*, 10: 21.
Bolte, G., Tamburlini, G. and Kohlhuber, M. (2010) Environmental inequalities among children in Europe – evaluation of scientific evidence and policy implications, *European Journal of Public Health*, 20(1): 14–20.
Bradshaw, J. (2006) *A review of the comparative evidence on child poverty*. York: University of York.
Busse, R. and Riesberg, A. (2004) *Health care systems in transition: Germany*. Copenhagen: WHO Regional Office for Europe, on behalf of the European Observatory on Health Systems and Policies.
Cairns, G., Angus, K. and Hastings, G. (2009) *The extent, nature and effects of food promotion to children: a review of the evidence to December 2008*. Geneva: World Health Organization.
Campion J., Bhui, K., Bhugra D. (2012) European Psychiatric Assocation (EPA) guidance on prevention of mental disorders. *European Psychiatry*, 27: 68–80.
Cattaneo, A. et al. (2012) *Child Health in the European Union*. Luxembourg: European Commission.
Cattaneo, A. et al. (2010) Overweight and obesity in infants and pre-school children in the European Union: a review of existing data, *Obesity Reviews*, 11(5): 389–98.
Centers for Disease Control and Prevention (1999) Ten great public health achievements – United States 1900–1999, *Morbidity and Mortality Weekly Report*, 48(12): 241–3.
Chief Medical Officer (2011) Annual report of the Chief Medical Officer. Volume II, Infections and the rise of antimicrobial resistance. Department of Health, 2013.
Chisholm, D. et al. (2004) Reducing the global burden of hazardous alcohol use: a comparative cost-effectiveness analysis, *Journal of Studies on Alcohol and Drugs*, 65(6): 782–93.
Cooke, L.J. et al. (2004) Demographic, familial and trait predictors of fruit and vegetable consumption by pre-school children, *Public Health Nutrition*, 7(2): 295–302.
Crombie, I. et al. (2005) *Closing the Inequalities Gap: An international perspective.* Copenhagen: WHO Regional Office for Europe.
Currie, C. et al. (eds.) (2012) *Health Policy for Children and Adolescents, No 6. Social determinants of health and well-being among young people. Health Behaviour in School-aged Children (HBSC) study. International Report from the 2009–10 Survey.* Copenhagen: WHO Regional Office for Europe.
Currie, L. and Gilmore, A. (2013) Tobacco. In: Mackenbach, J. and McKee, M. (eds) *Successes and failures of health policy in Europe. Four decades of diverging trends and converging challenges*. Maidenhead: Open University Press.
Department of Health (2012) *NHS Outcomes Framework 2013–14: Equality Analysis.* London: Department of Health.

Diabetes UK (2011) *National Diabetes Audit*. London: Diabetes UK.
Duffey, K.J. et al. (2010) Food price and diet and health outcomes: 20 years of the CARDIA Study, *Archives of Internal Medicine*, 170(5): 420–6.
EARSS (2007) *Annual Report 2006*. Bilthoven: Dutch National Institute for Public Health and the Environment.
ECSA (2007) *Action Planning for Child Safety: a strategic and coordinated approach to reducing the number one cause of death for children in Europe*. Amsterdam: European Child Safety Alliance.
ECSA (2012a) *Child safety report cards Europe summary 2012*. Brussels: European Child Safety Alliance.
ECSA (2012b) *How safety conscious are European countries towards children? Europe summary for 31 countries*. Birmingham: European Child Safety Alliance.
Engelhard, C.L. and Dorn, S. (2009) *Reducing obesity: policy strategies from the tobacco wars*. Washington DC: Urban Institute.
Eurochild (2012) *Compendium of Inspiring Practices: Early intervention and prevention in family and parenting support*. Brussels: European Community Programme for Employment and Social Solidarity PROGESS (2007–2013).
European Commission (2008) *EU Physical Activity Guidelines. Recommended policy actions in support of health-enhancing physical activity*. http://ec.europa.eu/sport/library/documents/c1/eu-physical-activity-guidelines-2008_en.pdf [accessed 24 June 2013].
European Commission (2005) *EU Platform on Diet, Physical Activity and Health*. Luxembourg: European Commission.
European Union (1998) Decision No 2119/98/EC of the European Parliament and of the Council of 24 September 1998 setting up a network for the epidemiological surveillance and control of communicable diseases in the Community, *Official Journal of the European Communities*, L 268/01–L268/07.
Federal Trade Commission (2008) *Marketing food to children and adolescents. A review of industry expenditures, activities, and self-regulation. A report to Congress*. Washington DC: Federal Trade Commission.
Figari, F., Paulus, A. and Sutherland, H. (2007) *Research note: Supporting families through taxes and benefits*. Brussels: European Commission.
Figueras, J. and McKee, M. (2012) *Health systems, health, wealth and societal well-being: Assessing the case for investing in health systems*. Maidenhead: McGraw-Hill/Open University Press.
Ford, E.S. and Mokdad, A.H. (2001) Fruit and vegetable consumption and diabetes mellitus incidence among U.S. adults, *Preventive Medicine*, 32(1), 33–9.
Frieden, T.R., Dietz, W. and Collins, J. (2010) Reducing childhood obesity through policy change: acting now to prevent obesity, *Health Affairs (Millwood)*, 29(3): 357–63.
Fuhrman, C. et al. (2011) Hospitalizations for asthma in children are linked to undertreatment and insufficient asthma education, *Journal of Asthma*, 48(6): 565–71.
Gluckman, P.D. et al. (2009) Epigenetic mechanisms that underpin metabolic and cardiovascular diseases, *Nature Reviews Endocrinology*, 5(7): 401–8.
Halfon, N. (2012) Addressing health inequalities in the US: a life course health development approach, *Social Science and Medicine*, 74(5): 671–3.
Hawkes, C. (2006) Uneven dietary development: linking the policies and processes of globalization with the nutrition transition, obesity and diet-related chronic diseases, *Global Health*, 2: 4.
Health Protection Agency (2009) *A children's environment and health strategy for the UK*. London: Health Protection Agency.

Hjern, A. and Thorngren-Jerneck, K. (2008) Perinatal complications and socio-economic differences in cerebral palsy in Sweden – a national cohort study, *BMC Pediatrics*, 8: 49.

Hogstedt, C. et al. (eds) (2008) *Health for All? A critical analysis of public health policies in eight European countries*. Stockholm: Swedish National Institute for Public Health.

Holland, W., Stewart, S. and Masseria, C. (2006) *Screening in Europe. Policy Brief.* Copenhagen: European Observatory on Health Systems and Policies.

Holland, W.W. and Stewart, S. (1998) *Public health: the vision and the challenge*. London: Nuffield Trust.

ISSOP (2008) *Mission statement*. International Society for Social Pediatrics and Child Health http://www.essop.org [accessed 23 June 2013].

Jones, L.R. et al. (2010) Influences on child fruit and vegetable intake: sociodemographic, parental and child factors in a longitudinal cohort study, *Public Health Nutrition*, 13(7): 1122–30.

Joshipura, K.J. et al. (2001) The effect of fruit and vegetable intake on risk for coronary heart disease, *Annals of Internal Medicine*, 134(12): 1106–14.

Kirkpatrick, S. et al. (2007) Working in partnership: user perceptions of intensive home visiting, *Child Abuse Review*, 16(1): 32–46.

Kitzman, H.J. et al. (2010) Enduring effects of prenatal and infancy home visiting by nurses on children: follow-up of a randomized trial among children at age 12 years, *Archives of Pediatrics and Adolescent Medicine*, 164(5): 412–18.

Kovacic, W.E.C. (2008) *Marketing food to children and adolescents: a review of industry expenditures, activities, and self-regulation*. Washington DC: Federal Trade Commission.

Lalonde, M. (1974) *New perspective on the health of Canadians*. Ottawa: Health and Welfare of Canada.

Lamkin, L.P. and Houston, T.P. (1998) Nicotine dependency and adolescents: preventing and treating, *Primary Care*, 25(1): 123–35.

Laxminarayan, R., Chow, J. and Shahid-Salles, S.A. (2006) Intervention cost-effectiveness: overview of main messages. In: Jamison, D.T. et al. (eds) *Disease control priorities in developing countries*. New York: Oxford University Press.

Lobstein, T., Baur, L. and Uauy, R. (2004) Obesity in children and young people: a crisis in public health, *Obesity Reviews*, 5(Suppl 1): 4–104.

Lobstein, T. and Dibb, S. (2005) Evidence of a possible link between obesogenic food advertising and child overweight, *Obesity Reviews*, 6(3): 203–8.

Mackenbach, J.P. and Bakker, M.J. (2003) Tackling socioeconomic inequalities in health: analysis of European experiences, *The Lancet*, 362(9393): 1409–14.

Malik, V.S. et al. (2010) Sugar-sweetened beverages, obesity, type 2 diabetes mellitus, and cardiovascular disease risk, *Circulation*, 121(11): 1356–64.

Malik, V.S., Schulze, M.B. and Hu, F.B. (2006) Intake of sugar-sweetened beverages and weight gain: a systematic review, *American Journal of Clinical Nutrition*, 84(2): 274–88.

McCrory, M.A. et al. (1999) Dietary variety within food groups: association with energy intake and body fatness in men and women, *American Journal of Clinical Nutrition*, 69(3): 440–7.

McKee, M. et al. (2013) Universal health coverage: a quest for all countries but under threat in some, *Value Health*, 16(1 Suppl): S39–45.

Millett, C. et al. (2013) Hospital admissions for childhood asthma after smoke-free legislation in England, *Pediatrics*, 131(2): e495–501.

Moberg, H. (2008) Comparative studies of policies on health inequalities – a literature review. In: Hogstedt, C. et al. (eds) *Health for All? A critical analysis of public health policies in eight European countries*. Stockholm: Swedish National Institute for Public Health.

Moreno, L.A. and Rodriguez, G. (2007) Dietary risk factors for development of childhood obesity, *Current Opinion in Clinical Nutrition and Metabolic Care*, 10(3): 336–41.

Morgan, A. and Swann, C. (2004) *Social capital for health: issues of definition, measurement and links to health*. London: Health Development Agency.

Navarro, V. and Shi, L. (2001) The political context of social inequalities and health, *Social Science and Medicine*, 52(30): 481–91.

NHS (2012) NHS Atlas of Variation in Healthcare for Children and Young People: reducing unwarranted variation to increase value and improve quality. NHS, March 2012.

NICE (2009) *Promoting physical activity, active play and sport for pre-school and school-age children and young people in family, pre-school and community settings*, NICE Public Health Guidance 17. London: National Institute for Health and Care Excellence.

Obesity Coalition (2007) *Obesity Prevention: Priorities for action*. Carlton, Victoria: Obesity Coalition.

Olds, D.L. et al. (2004) Effects of home visits by paraprofessionals and by nurses: age 4 follow-up results of a randomized trial, *Pediatrics*, 114(6): 1560–8.

OECD (2009) *Education today: the OECD perspective*. Paris: Organisation for Economic Co-operation and Development.

OECD (2011) *OECD Health at a Glance 2011*. Paris: Organisation for Economic Co-operation and Development.

Pearson, G. (2008) *Why children die: a pilot study 2006; England (South West, North East, West Midlands), Wales and Northern Ireland*. London: Centre for Maternal and Child Enquiries.

Peto, R. et al. (2012) *Mortality from smoking in developed countries 1950–2005*. Oxford: Clinical Trial Service Unit.

Puura, K. et al. (2005) The outcome of the European Early Promotion Project: Mother–Child Interaction, *International Journal of Mental Health Promotion*, 7(1): 82–94.

Radecki, L. et al. (2011) Trends in the use of standardized tools for developmental screening in early childhood: 2002–2009, *Pediatrics*, 128(1): 14–19.

Rasmussen, M. et al. (2006) Determinants of fruit and vegetable consumption among children and adolescents: a review of the literature. Part I: Quantitative studies, *International Journal of Behavioral Nutrition and Physical Activity*, 3: 22.

Reindal, L. and Øymar, K. (2006) Hospital admissions for wheezing and asthma in childhood – are they avoidable? *Journal of Asthma*, 43(10): 801–6.

Riala, K. et al. (2004) Teenage smoking and substance use as predictors of severe alcohol problems in late adolescence and in young adulthood, *Journal of Adolescent Health*, 35(3): 245–54.

Rice, B. (2006) *Against the odds: An investigation comparing the lives of children on either side of Britain's housing divide*. London: Shelter.

Rose, G. (1985) Sick individuals and sick populations, *International Journal of Epidemiology*, 14(1): 32–8.

RCPCH (2012) *Epilepsy 12 National Report: United Kingdom collaborative clinical audit of healthcare for children and young people with suspected epileptic seizures*. London: Royal College of Paediatrics and Child Health.

Rutter, H. (2011) Where next for obesity? *The Lancet*, 378(9793): 746–7.

Schrader-McMillan, A., Barnes, J. and Barlow, J. (2012) *Primary study evidence on effectiveness of interventions (home, early education, child care) in promoting social and emotional wellbeing of vulnerable children under 5. Commissioned expert report for Social and emotional wellbeing: early years*. London: National Institute for Health and Care Excellence.

Sethi, D. (2007) *Youth and road safety in Europe*. Copenhagen: WHO Regional Office for Europe.
Sices, L. et al. (2009) PEDS and ASQ developmental screening tests may not identify the same children, *Pediatrics*, 124(4): e640–7.
Society for Social Medicine (2012) *Constitution of the Society*. http://www.socsocmed.org.uk/constitution1.htm [accessed 24 June 2013].
Spencer, N.J. (2010) Poverty and child health. In: Koller, T. (ed.) *Poverty and social exclusion in the European Region: Health systems respond*. Copenhagen: WHO Regional Office for Europe.
Strong, W.B. et al. (2005) Evidence based physical activity for school-age youth, *Journal of Pediatrics*, 146(6): 732–7.
Sturge-Apple, M.L., Davies, P.T. and Cummings, E.M. (2010) Typologies of family functioning and children's adjustment during the early school years, *Child Development*, 81(4): 1320–35.
Sturm, R. and Datar, A. (2005) Body mass index in elementary school children, metropolitan area food prices and food outlet density, *Public Health*, 119(12): 1059–68.
Swinburn, B.A. et al. (2011) The global obesity pandemic: shaped by global drivers and local environments, *The Lancet*, 378(9793): 804–14.
Tamburlini, G., Manetti, S. and Toffol, G. (2011) Primary health care and early childhood development, *The Lancet*, 378(9807): e16.
TÁRKI Social Research Institute (2010) *Child Poverty and Well-being in the European Union*. Report for the European Commission, DG Employment, Social Affairs and Equal Opportunities Unit E2. Budapest: TÁRKI Social Research Institute.
UNICEF CEE/CIS (2007) *Romani children in South East Europe: the challenge of overcoming centuries of distrust and discrimination*. Belgrade: UNICEF.
UNICEF (2005) *Child poverty in rich countries*. Florence: UNICEF Innocenti Research Centre.
UNICEF (2007) *Child poverty in perspective*. Florence: UNICEF Innocenti Research Centre.
University of Queensland (2012) *Parenting and Family Support Centre*. http://www.pfsc.uq.edu.au/research/evidence [accessed 24 June 2013].
Vallgårda, S. (2001) Governing people's lives. Strategies for improving the health of the nations in England, Denmark, Norway and Sweden, *European Journal of Public Health*, 11: 386–92.
van Boven, M. et al. (2010) Estimation of measles vaccine efficacy and critical vaccination coverage in a highly vaccinated population, *Journal of the Royal Society Interface*, 7(52): 1537–44.
van der Horst, K. et al. (2007) A systematic review of environmental correlates of obesity-related dietary behaviors in youth, *Health Education Research*, 22(2): 203–26.
WHO (1986) *The Ottawa Charter for Health Promotion – First international conference on health promotion*. WHO/HPR/HEP95. Ottawa: World Health Organization.
WHO Regional Office for Europe (2002) *The European Health Report 2002*. Copenhagen: WHO Regional Office for Europe.
WHO (2003) *Choosing interventions that are cost effective (WHO-CHOICE)*. Geneva: World Health Organization.
WHO (2004) *Global strategy on Diet, Physical Activity and Health*. Geneva: World Health Organization.
WHO Regional Office for Europe (2006a) *European Ministerial Conference on Counteracting Obesity*. Conference Report. Copenhagen: WHO Regional Office for Europe.

WHO Regional Office for Europe (2006b) *Physical activity and health in Europe: Evidence for action*. Copenhagen: WHO Regional Office for Europe.

WHO Regional Office for Europe (2007) *The International Network of Health Promoting Hospitals and Health Services: Integrating health promotion into hospitals and health services. Concept, framework and organization*. Copenhagen: WHO Regional Office for Europe.

WHO Regional Office for Europe (2008) *Closing the gap in a generation: Health equity through action on the social determinants of health*. Geneva: World Health Organization.

WHO Regional Office for Europe (2008) *Health Policy for Children and Adolescents, No 5. Inequalities in young people's health. Health behaviour in school-aged children international report from the 2005/2006 survey*. Copenhagen: WHO Regional Office for Europe.

WHO Regional Office for Europe (2009a) *The European health report 2009: Health and health systems*. Copenhagen: WHO Regional Office for Europe.

WHO Regional Office for Europe (2009b) *Policies and practices for mental health in Europe: Meeting the challenges*. Copenhagen: WHO Regional Office for Europe.

WHO Regional Office for Europe (2010) *Health and environment in Europe. Progress Assessment*. Copenhagen: WHO Regional Office for Europe.

WHO (2011) *The Weekly Epidemiological Record, volume 86, number 49 (pp557-564)*.

WHO (2012) *European Health for All Database (HFA-DB)*. http://www.euro.who.int/en/what-we-do/data-and-evidence/databases/european-health-for-all-database-hfa-db2 [accessed 24 June 2013].

WHO (2013) Vaccine-preventable diseases: monitoring system. http://apps.who.int/immunization_monitoring/globalsummary/

WHO and World Economic Forum (2011) *From Burden to "Best Buys": Reducing the economic impact of non-communicable diseases in low and middle-income countries*. Geneva: World Health Organization and World Economic Forum.

Willett, W.C. and Trichopoulos, D. (1996) Nutrition and cancer: a summary of the evidence, *Cancer Causes Control*, 7(1): 178–80.

Wilson, J. and Jungner, G. (1968) *Principles and practice of screening for disease*. Public Health Papers No. 34. Geneva: World Health Organization.

Wolfe, I. (2013a) Child health. In: Mackenbach, J. and McKee, M. (eds) *Successes and failures of health policy in Europe. Four decades of diverging trends and converging challenges*. Maidenhead: Open University Press.

Wolfe, I. et al. (2013b) Children's health services in Europe, *The Lancet*, 381(9873): 1224–34.

chapter six

Schools and the health of children and young people

Arja Rimpelä, Woody Caan, Sven Bremberg, Pieter Auke Wiegersma, Ingrid Wolfe

Supporting school-age children to be healthy to learn and to learn to be healthy
(Save the Children Programme)

Introduction

Children's school years offer unique opportunities. The entire population of a specific age group is in one place at one time, providing ideal circumstances for promoting health, intervening when necessary, and for studying children's health.

This chapter covers two broad aspects to the topic: school health as a concept relating to the population, and health services provided by health professionals for children in schools. After a brief review of the history of school health, the chapter is divided into four main parts: population health; school health services; schools and children with special needs; and schools and population health research. A review of evidence and the European experience for each of these topics is presented, highlighting important challenges and lessons to support country efforts to improve the quality of, and access to, school health. Finally, the future challenges facing school health services and possible responses to them are examined.

History

The origins of school health in the United Kingdom probably stem from nineteenth-century employment law, which evolved from the interest Victorian philanthropists took in the living conditions, health and education of children at work in factories during the Industrial Revolution. School health services arose as a type of occupational health service for workers' children. Formal education in schools eventually became mandatory, as did the provision of some health care by employers. Medical inspections exposed poor hygiene conditions and inadequate physical environments, and the poor health and developmental status of children became apparent. Examinations of schoolchildren in nineteenth-century Europe revealed that one-third suffered from chronic conditions and physical defects (Stewart, 1911). Indeed, it was the discovery that many children were so unhealthy and malnourished that they were unable to contribute to the labour force and armed services in later years that prompted the development of formal school health services and, eventually, health visiting services (Stewart, 1911; Blair et al., 2003; Gardner, 2008).

Medical officers or school physicians began to be appointed by the end of the 19th century in many European countries, but the systematic establishment of school health services began in earnest in the first decades of the 20th century. The German system, developed first in Wiesbaden, served as a model for many countries and its basic elements can still be seen in contemporary school health services. The model comprised 'not merely the supervision of the school buildings, but the systematic supervision of school children themselves, supplemented by individual examinations at stated intervals' (Stewart, 1911).

After the Second World War, European school health remained focused on securing the health of the next generation but by the mid-20th century, as clinical medicine approached its ascendancy, the medical model of school health began to dominate. Early detection of physical diseases and abnormalities, and individual treatment of disease were the main priorities. By the 1980s and 1990s, discussions on school health services were being shaped by two different forces: concerns about cost-effectiveness, and a growing understanding of the vital role that social determinants play in the health and well-being of children. Changing social contexts and advancing scientific knowledge about the determinants of health, and particularly education, also prompted a shift in the emphasis of school health. Several high-quality studies indicate that education is in itself health-promotive, even without any specific health activities at school (Schuller and Desjardins, 2007; Gakidou et al., 2010). The recognition that early life influences can significantly affect later health outcomes (the life-course explanation), together with a renewed focus on the social determinants of health, have significantly changed the approach to children's health throughout Europe. For example, in the United Kingdom, critics argued that routine medical screening of schoolchildren was a poor use of resources (Gardner, 2008). Consequently, school health in the 21st century has shifted away from 'seek and treat' to 'prevent and promote', focusing on enhancing children's resilience and maximizing their health and well-being (Blair and DeBell, 2011). Inevitably, there are tensions between the traditional medical model of school health services for individual children and multiprofessional and multisectoral activities for improving the health of the school-age population in a school setting. A critical view is outlined in Box 6.1. However, these different approaches are not mutually exclusive.

Box 6.1 A critical approach to school health services

School health services were implemented at a time when most children (and parents) had very poor access to health care and when their environment was rife with all kinds of health-endangering exposures: pollution, poor food, poor hygiene, and consequently an abundance of infectious diseases. In those days, school health services by medical doctors were an effective approach to enhancing the health of children, and can be compared with the activities of physicians that went out into communities to care for the poor and needy. However, in recent decades, the need for a separate medical service has diminished considerably, clearing the way for a broader public health approach: system-oriented and targeting populations, rather than focusing on individuals. Although traditional school health services have seen the patient–doctor relationship – and therefore individual contact – as their core activity, such services can have unforeseen negative consequences. Almost 40 years ago, in his controversial book *Medical Nemesis*, Illich pointed out how health care services generate their own demand (Illich, 1976). As a consequence, people may transfer responsibility to health professionals, leading teachers and parents (and even pupils) to ignore 'signals of distress' or health-endangering behaviour of students, because these problems seem to be adequately dealt with by the (preventive) activities of school health services. The infrequent contacts with school health services cannot hope to make up for this deficiency.

Accordingly, many public health advocates argue that where school health services are still monodisciplinary, output-driven services, heavily focused on individual care, there should be a shift towards a multidisciplinary, proactive service that specializes in the development and evaluation of collective preventive activities, based on an understanding of the characteristics of the child population. A rigorous evaluation of the tasks traditionally carried out in school health services, many of which lack a scientific basis, is also called for. Finally, it is argued that school health services should change their approach, reaching out to address the dangers that jeopardize children's health and, consequently, the health of the whole population.

Source: chapter author (PAW)

The WHO approach to health promotion recognizes these complexities and considers well-being and ill health, focusing on learning, lifestyles, school conditions and creating networks with stakeholders and community, as well as on the participation and involvement of schoolchildren (Lee et al., 2006; Stewart-Brown, 2006). This holistic view on health gave rise to a new idea – the 'Health Promoting School' (HPS) (WHO, 1998, 2011). WHO took the concept further through the 'Global School Health Initiative' (United Nations World Food Programme, 2010), which strengthened links between public health and education across the world. The report articulated the need for research to improve school health programmes, an idea adopted by UNESCO and UNICEF, which embarked on an interagency initiative, FRESH (Focusing Resources on Effective School Health). The basis of FRESH is that 'a child's ability to attain her or his full potential is directly related to the synergistic effect of good health, good nutrition and appropriate education' (United Nations World Food Programme, 2010). The WHO Regional Office for Europe reiterated the importance of a multifaceted approach, reporting failures in child health promotion programmes that focus on children's health deficits rather than on assets for health and development (WHO 1998, 2011). Indeed, past approaches to school health that emphasized the medical input from clinicians missed the many non-clinical activities that promote positive health. For example, negative body image, and even self-hatred, are increasingly commonly reported issues and are associated with health-compromising behaviour in adolescence (McGee and Williams, 2000; WHO Regional Office for Europe, 2008). Non-governmental organizations (NGOs) have led the way in engaging with well-being issues, for example, an initiative to build a positive sense of body image by Girlguiding UK (Girlguiding UK, 2007). The environment in which children learn can be used to promote resilience and self-understanding, as in the growing European movement to hold some classes in a 'Forest School' (Knight, 2011).

School health in the United States was in some ways a precursor of developments in Europe. In 1972, Anderson proposed three action areas for school health with many similarities to the WHO HPS concept that would emerge more than two decades later: health services, health instruction and healthful living (Anderson, 1972). A comprehensive school health programme (Allensworth and Kolbe, 1987), now known as the 'Coordinated School Health Program', was developed jointly by the American School Health Association and Centers for Disease Control and Prevention (American School Health Association, 2011; Centers for Disease Control and Prevention, 2011) (Table 6.1).

Both the United States model and the WHO HPS concept are wider in scope than earlier versions of traditional school health services, yet some of the components are similar to those described in the 19th century. Both approaches recognize the importance of non-medical members of multidisciplinary teams. Today, school health services for children have come full circle, echoing their origins in employment law. School health once again has a dual purpose (the health of individual children and the well-being of the institution as a whole), just as in adult workplace occupational health services.

Population health for school children

Education and health are intimately related; children need to be healthy and well in order to learn, and education is a key determinant of health and well-being. John Stewart, in a report to the Canadian Medical Association in 1911, said that:

> During recent years and in almost all civilized countries there has been a steadily increasing conviction that no system of education is complete which

Table 6.1 Elements of a comprehensive school health programme

Theme	*Health Promoting School (WHO 1998, 2011)*	*Coordinated School Health Program (American School Health Association, 2011; Centers for Disease Control, 2011)*
School environment	Safe and healthy physical and psychosocial environment	Healthy and safe environment, including physical conditions, psychosocial environment and aesthetic surroundings
Health services	Access to health services	Nursing and other health services that students need in order to stay in school
Health education	Effective skill-based health education	Health education on a range of developmentally appropriate topics taught by knowledgeable teachers
Health promotion	School policies and practices to support health, such as nutrition programmes, physical education and recreation	Nutritious and appealing school meals and opportunities for physical activity, including physical education
Psychosocial	Programmes for counselling, social support and mental health promotion	Counselling, psychological and social services that promote healthy social and emotional development and remove barriers to students' learning
Teachers, staff and parents	Programmes strive to improve health of school personnel, families and community members as well as students	Health promotion for school faculty and staff
Community	Engages health and education officials, teachers, students, parents and community leaders to improve health	Family and community involvement are integral to the approach
Philosophy	Respects individuals' well-being and dignity, provides opportunities for success, and acknowledges good efforts and intentions	

> does not provide for medical inspection and supervision of schools and school children. All great writers on education of modern times lay stress on the importance of bodily health and vigour, and in their various systems, make provisions for physical training and school hygiene (Stewart, 1911).

Observational studies indicate that regular attendance at school may, in itself, be good for health since educational success in school (and beyond) has a positive effect on long-term physical health in adulthood (Kuh and Wadsworth, 1993). An experimental study design permits causal inferences, demonstrating that one additional year of schooling may result in lower mortality in middle age (Lager and Torssander, 2012). Better educational attainment when young may promote healthy ageing decades later (Steptoe et al., 2011). One hypothesis from research on healthy ageing is that education promotes problem-solving skills in young people that enable constructive responses to stressors later in life.

Children who experience poor health go on to have poor educational attainment, poor adult health and lower social status, irrespective of parental factors including income, education and social class (Case, Fertig and Paxson, 2005). However, timely intervention may change the trajectory completely. Children who have health problems at 7 years old but recover before the age of 16 may avoid a recurrence. In his life-course perspective on a child's potential for adult well-being, Wadsworth (Wadsworth, 1997) looked for positive factors that 'make it possible to escape' from the effects of adversity in early life. He reported that those children who had experienced multiple adversities before school entry (who would be expected to have poor lifelong health) could have good life chances for the next 50 years if they had positive experiences of education between the ages 5 to 11 years (Caan, 2004).

School health services need to ensure that they meet children's evolving health needs, just as all other types of health services currently struggle to do. Fewer than half (41%) of the countries in the WHO European Region report that their school health services respond to local priority health needs, defined as lifestyle-related issues, mental health and behavioural problems – and, at best, they respond only partially (Baltag and Levi, 2010). Building resilience; promoting health; a national curriculum of health education to increase children's understanding of their health and factors affecting their health; and screening for risks or diseases, are all examples of population-level interventions in schools. School environmental health is about ensuring a healthy sustainable environment for learning, health and well-being. National strategies to meet children's health needs rely on getting these population-level interventions right.

Building social resilience and reducing risky behaviour

The Netherlands has made notable progress in describing the relationship between the health of schoolchildren and the social environment in which they live. As part of the HBSC study, a survey of over 1700 Dutch adolescents identified factors predicting health risk behaviour, such as tobacco smoking, binge drinking of alcohol, cannabis smoking and early sexual activity. Predictive factors included socioeconomic and demographic characteristics, but also some more readily modifiable elements, such as parental permissiveness and peer influences (Harakeh et al., 2012), suggesting that interventions based on these influences may be beneficial. Patterns of alcohol use between ages 14 to 17 years are associated with multiple school problems, including bullying, truancy, shoplifting, antisocial behaviour and, especially, poor examination results, followed by unemployment after leaving school (Green and Ross, 2010). Reducing alcohol misuse by young people and reducing hospital admissions for self-harm are priorities in England (Glasper, 2012), as in other European countries, and school health teams are expected to contribute to this. Various programmes have been advocated to improve health-related behaviour, some focusing entirely on skills and others linked to wider programmes, such as early intervention projects (see Chapter 5). However, there have been few robust evaluations and, when assessed in RCTs, they have often been found to be ineffective. Examples include the D.A.R.E. (Drug Abuse Resistance Education) project (West and O'Neal, 2004; Pan and Bai, 2009), 'Strengthening Families Program' (Gorman, Conde and Huber, 2007) and Project ALERT (Ringwalt et al., 2010). There is a clear need for better evaluations of interventions targeting alcohol and drug use, smoking and other risky behaviours. However, there are several programmes that show promise, although caution is required as contextual factors may affect the trial results. Often, success seems to hinge on the enthusiasm of teachers. Further research should replicate the most promising studies and pay particular attention to content and context factors in rigorous evaluations (Foxcroft and Tsertsvadze, 2012). School-based resilience building programmes, such as those in the UK based on the Penn Resiliency Program (PRP) from the USA, have demonstrated hopeful results as in the original US-based strudies which showed some effectiveness in reducing anxiety and depressive symptoms in adolescents (Challen et al., 2009). See chapter 5 for more on social resilience.

Life skills programmes

Catalano et al. (2012) report good outcomes in reducing alcohol misuse from the 'Strengthening Families Program', which involves groups of young adolescents and their parents (Caan, 2009). The 'Seattle Social Development Project', which combines work with teachers, primary schoolchildren and parents, also reports success in preventing alcohol misuse. Foxcroft and Tsertsvadze (2011) conducted a systematic review on the prevention programmes available for children and adolescents in schools. They identified studies that showed no effects of preventive interventions, as well as studies that demonstrated statistically significant effects. There was no easily discernible pattern of characteristics that would distinguish trials with positive results from those with no effects.

Coaching and mentoring

There is a great deal of interest in Europe and the United States in health coaching and the mentoring of school-age children. In most survey countries, some element of health coaching or counselling features in school health services, often as part of routine examinations, but little is known about the content or type of these activities. In the Netherlands, an ecological case-referent study of Dutch youth health care was unable to demonstrate any positive result as measured by children's alcohol, tobacco and drug use or eating habits in a group that received more health counselling and well-care visits (Huijsman and Wagenaar, 1983; Zielhuis, 1985; Wiegersma, 1999; Wiegersma, Hofman and Zielhuis, 2001). Mentoring is a widely used intervention and several small studies report beneficial outcomes, such as improved behaviour and school attendance (St James-Roberts and Samlal Singh, 2001). A review of over 70 mentoring studies conducted in the decade to 2010 suggests modest effects in improving outcomes across a range of behavioural, social and educational outcomes. It is not clear, however, whether these beneficial effects are sustained, or whether mentoring is more effective than other behavioural school-based interventions. Finally, there is little evidence on the potential effects of mentoring on health outcomes, such as obesity prevention (Du Bois et al., 2001).

Health education

Education about health can be part of the national school curriculum, either as a subject on its own (for example, in England and Finland) or integrated into other subjects, and the role of health professionals involved varies accordingly. England has a Personal Social Health Education (PSHE) curriculum, although this is not currently compulsory (PSHE Association, 2012). In Finland, health education is compulsory; for grades 7 to 9 (ages 13 to 16) it is a separate subject and for younger children it is integrated with other subjects. Teachers of this subject are required to have an academic training in health education. In many Finnish schools, a health nurse (or occasionally other school health personnel) participates in planning lessons and often assists with teaching. In France, school nurses and doctors work in a service called 'mission de promotion de la santé en faveur des élèves' (mission of health promotion for students) as technical advisers. Teachers usually deliver the health education, but often in cooperation with health professionals, most often nurses, who may assist with lesson planning and teaching, especially of specialist or sensitive subjects such as sexuality and contraception.

Social and emotional learning

A whole-school intervention widely implemented in the United Kingdom is the 'Social and Emotional Aspects of Learning' (SEAL) programme for schools (NICE, 2008a). This forms part of a wider approach involving activities supported through a specific curriculum for practical learning and skills development in personal, social and health education (Department for Education, 2010) (Box 6.2).

Similar whole-school interventions have worked in other countries (Snyder

Box 6.2 The SEAL programme

SEAL is a British programme which comprises a 'comprehensive whole-school approach to promoting the social and emotional skills that underpin effective learning, positive behaviour, regular attendance, staff effectiveness and the emotional health and well-being of all who learn and work in schools'.

SEAL has a three-stage model of intervention to tailor the programme according to need. The programme has been implemented in 90% of primary schools (ages 4 to 11) and 70% of secondary schools (ages 11 to 18), and aspects of the implementation and impact of the programme have been evaluated. The results were mixed; numerous problems were identified with implementation and no convincing positive impact was found. It is possible that if implementation were more thorough, positive results would ensue, but this has yet to be demonstrated. Moreover, the basic assumptions underlying the programme have been questioned (Craig, 2007).

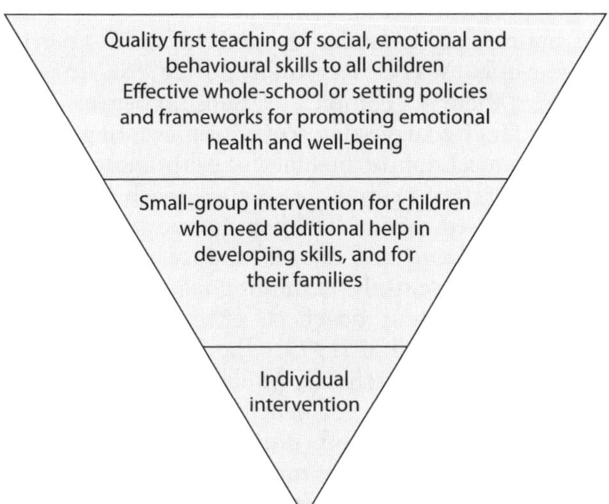

Source: Humphrey, Lendrum and Wigelsworth, 2010.

et al., 2012), with teachers, parents and students reporting improvements in well-being, participation and learning, and reductions in problems like bullying. The EU 'Lifelong Learning Programme' has recently funded the Emotional Literacy in Action (ELIA) project for teachers of vocational courses to improve adolescents' behaviour, motivation and employability.

The use of familiar characters and references can help to promote emotional resilience in young children. Classroom discussions using popular cartoon characters are one example (Cougar Hall and West, 2012). The Dutch psychologist Streng (2009) has created a series of popular board games to help schoolchildren develop resilience after common but challenging life events, such as bullying, bereavement or parental divorce. One of the most radical uses of everyday assets in school is the 'Roots of Empathy' programme, in which the visit of a baby to the class triggers discussion of pro-social behaviours among the pupils (Schonert Reichl et al., 2012). Some projects strengthen links with the local environment; for example, involving schoolchildren in nature conservation work is designed to engender 'connection, restoration, and respect for self and planet' (Burls and Caan, 2005).

Mental health promotion

Mental health is vital for optimal child development but is a growing concern among children and young people; indeed 50% of lifetime mental illness (excluding dementia) begins before the age of 14 years old (Kim-Cohen et al., 2003; Kessler et al., 2005) (see also Chapter 8). The most common causes of NCDs and conditions in children under 14 years old are neuropsychiatric and, in this category, depression is the most common single cause (Lim et al., 2012). Suicide is a major problem among young people in the EU, causing 0.2 per 100,000 deaths among children under 15 years old, and 7.4 per 100,000 deaths among 15–29-year-olds (WHO Regional Office for Europe, 2010). For some schoolchildren, there is a complex relationship between self-poisoning or self-injury and later fatality, suggesting scope for preventing suicides (Gilbert et al., 2009). Primary prevention of mental ill health and promotion of mental well-being form core parts of a comprehensive approach to the health of school-age children. School-based mental health promotion for children and young people can improve well-being and reduce conduct problems (NICE, 2008b). However, one ecological case study, examining regions with open consultation hours at schools did not find beneficial effects in terms of suicide rates (Wiegersma, Hofman and Zielhuis,1999). The EU's Dataprev project assessed mental health interventions in schools, publishing a systematic review of 52 studies. This shows clear evidence of beneficial effects of a variety of mental health promotion interventions, both universal and targeted, on the mental health of children and young people as measured by: positive mental health and pro-social behaviour; mental ill health; behavioural disorders; violence and bullying behaviours. Positive outcomes were most common in children who were at higher risk and who received targeted interventions. However, the effect sizes generally range from small to moderate and may diminish with time. A meta-analysis demonstrated that primary preventive mental health interventions at school were between 8% and 46% more successful than controls (Durlak and Wells, 1997), and that most programmes achieved reductions in problem behaviour as well as increases in competencies. A 2011 meta-analysis of 213 programmes offering universal school-based social and emotional learning, reported an 11% improvement in achievement in school tests, a 10% decrease in disruptive classroom behaviour, and a 25% improvement in social and emotional skills; these effects persisted for the 6 months follow-up of the study (Durlak et al., 2011). A selected summary of evidence on what works in school-based mental health promotion is shown in Box 6.3.

Box 6.3 What works in school-based mental health promotion?

- A whole-school approach, whereby mental health promotion and interventions to prevent mental ill health are a core part of the school environment and ethos, is more effective than a curriculum-based set of interventions.
- Greater benefits result when there is more integration of the mental health intervention with the academic curriculum.
- Combining universal and targeted approaches to interventions appears to be more effective than either on its own.
- Start in the early school years and continue long term.
- Well-trained specialists working closely with school staff.
- Interventions that develop children's skills, for example, cognitive behavioural therapy.
- The SAFE Approach: Sequenced instruction, Active learning strategies, Focus on developing social–emotional skills, Explicit targeting of specific social–emotional skills. Programmes adopting the SAFE approach were more successful than those that did not, achieving positive results in twice as many outcome categories (social and emotional learning skills, positive attitudes, positive social behaviours, conduct problems, emotional distress, academic performance).

Sources: Payton et al., 2008; Weare and Nind, 2011; Campion, Bhui and Bhugra, 2012.

Physical health promotion

There are many national policies for health promotion and education in school-aged children in European countries but, in practice, implementation of these appears to be patchy (Weichselbaum and Buttriss, 2011). In those countries where physical education lessons are part of the national curriculum (such as Norway and Finland), physical health promotion is integrated into everyday schoolwork. The school's physical environment sets some limits on what physical activities children can take part in during break-times but theme days and events are possible for every school. Another integrated health promotion action is free school meals, but these are not served in all European countries. Children need to be adequately nourished in order to achieve the full potential of school (Save the Children, 2011), and a nourishing school lunch can make a major difference, especially for hungry children from poor homes. Free school lunches are served in countries such as Sweden and Finland, where they follow healthy nutrition guidelines.

Many health promotion programmes aim to teach children and young people life skills to support their emotional development and promote their confidence and ability to refuse offers of drugs and refrain from dangerous behaviour. Thus, there is considerable overlap with resilience-building services and the distinction can be somewhat arbitrary. For example, school health promotion programmes can prevent or delay alcohol and tobacco use (Botvin and Griffin, 2007). The 'Healthy Schools' programme in England focuses entirely on supporting the health and well-being of children through behaviour change, such as promoting emotional literacy, providing guidance about healthy eating habits, and forming clubs that promote physical activity. The benefits from the physical activity of school sports, combined with the pleasure to be derived from taking part in games, make a 'Sport Strategy for Young People' an obvious component in education planning (Department of Health, 2009). Since 1999, the United Kingdom has adopted a simplified version of the WHO 'Health Promoting School', the 'National Healthy Schools Programme', two essential criteria being healthy eating and physical activity in each school. However, many individual British school health promotion programmes have been small-scale and shown only modest effects. For example, after a year of the APPLES behaviour change project in 10 schools, the only difference between children with and without the intervention was a mean increase in vegetables consumed of 0.3 portions per day, with no difference at all in BMI (Sahota, 2003). 'The Lancaster Model' (www.thelancastermodel.co.uk) is an exception and takes a more comprehensive strategic approach. This model is based on each school developing a structured public health plan, within which evidence-based prevention practice is organized around four overall themes: lifestyle choices; emotional health and well-being; personal, social, and health education; and sexual health behaviour. It has had a strong influence on broader developments in British school health services development. The Lancaster experience drew on a series of national consultations through the British Youth Council and the online network Netmums, culminating in a national strategy: 'Getting it right for children, young people and families' (Department of Health, 2012). The Czech Republic's Ministry of Education, Youth and Sports has had a 'healthy schools' programme since 1991, with some notable successes. For example, in a Czech physical activity programme, where boys and girls could choose some of their own gender-specific activities and were not overly limited by class and play schedules, none of the children were obese at the end of the programme, compared to 22% of girls and 23% of boys receiving traditional physical education (Sigmund, El Ansari and Sigmundova, 2012).

Grass-roots community-based initiatives may offer useful adjuncts to government-led policies to engage schoolchildren in improving diet and physical activity; for example, football and rugby clubs reaching into schools through 'Clubs that Count' (Adshead, 2007) or campaigns like 'Every School a Food-Growing School' (The Children's Food Campaign, 2010) may be effective at capturing the imagination of young people. Ambitious national programmes may begin with the best of intentions, like the 'School Breakfast Program' in the United States, but their impact on those most in need, such as children from ethnic minorities growing up in poor urban neighbourhoods, may be determined by very local issues for implementation, such as whether children can take breakfast to the classroom to eat before lessons (Basch, 2011a).

A school-based obesity prevention programme known as 'Planet Health' was evaluated in a RCT in the United States. The intervention comprised lessons on reducing television viewing time and the consumption of fatty foods, while increasing physical activity and fruit and vegetable intake. The trial was partially successful, producing cost savings in girls although no effect was seen in boys. Among female school students, the trial predicted there would be 1.9% fewer overweight adults, with a gain of 4.1 quality adjusted life years (QALYs), a reduction of approximately US$15,887 in medical care costs, and a gain of US$25,104 resulting from averted lost productivity. The net estimated cost of the intervention was US$4305 per QALY gained, saving US$7313 to society. A variety of scenarios was considered and the intervention was believed to remain cost-effective (Wang et al., 2003). The 'Planet Health for Obesity Prevention' programme has also been shown to reduce disordered weight control behaviour (DWCB), such as purging and abuse of dieting medicines among young girls. The Planet Health programme has been shown to be both effective and efficient in reducing DWCB: schools that achieved high levels of student participation in lessons promoting reduction in television viewing had lower odds of DWCB at follow-up (OR 0.8; CI 0.74–0.85); students from schools with active staff teams were less likely to have DWCB (OR 0.76; CI 0.66–0.86); and programmes that combined television viewing goals with active staff were the most effective, with odds ratios of students developing DWCB of 0.38 (CI 0.28–0.53) (Austin et al., 2012).

School health services

Health examinations are undertaken by school health services in most countries, although content varies and responsibility for environmental health often rests elsewhere. School health services can have beneficial effects on an entire school, in improving health and educational outcomes and in supporting educational staff to concentrate on their main roles. Baisch et al. (2011) showed that schools with school nurse programmes had higher immunization rates and more accurate health records. Furthermore, school nurses enable other staff to concentrate on their main functions, teaching and running the school.

Systems of governance, structures and organizations

School health services are integral to both the health and education sectors, but often fall into the gaps between these two sometimes quite distinct arenas. School health services may be delivered by health professionals, but they work in education environments, so effective governance is crucial. However, finding the optimal balance between governance and autonomy is challenging; for example, health service managers may require data for payment by episode of care that are not readily compatible with school information systems. Pooled budgets across health and education sectors, and programme budgeting (whereby payment is for a programme of care for a specified population), are two options that may help.

In many countries, health ministries are ultimately responsible for school health services but have devolved the responsibility to relatively autonomous local health or education authorities, which organize, fund and prioritize (or not) school health services. The division of responsibility between health and education is sometimes blurred, making it even more important, and indeed difficult, to ensure that the structures, funding and content of school health services are fit for purpose. Indeed, nearly 80% of respondents to a WHO European regional survey on school health stated that inadequate funding was a main challenge and one-third reported uneven access to school health services within their country (Baltag and Levi, 2010). For example, France manages school health services through the ministry of education, but numerous challenges are reported, with services fragmented (partly due to funding coming from a variety of different sources) and a lack of clarity over responsibilities for services (Chevreul et al., 2010). These findings have led to reforms in some countries, highlighting the importance of information for advocacy. For example, in Finland, large differences between local authorities prompted recent legislation to oblige municipalities to organize and produce services in an equitable manner (Wiss et al., 2007). Notably, Poland has persistent inequities in the provision of preventive health care, disproportionately affecting pupils from rural schools, basic vocational schools and special schools (Jodkowska et al., 2010).

Most European countries have school health services based within schools (56% of the WHO European region) (Baltag and Levi, 2010), but school health services are organized in a variety of different ways, with many countries spreading their services between schools and primary health care settings (Table 6.2).

Table 6.2 Characteristics of selected school health systems

Country	*Governance authorities*	*Financing*	*Responsibility for workforce*	*Organization of school health services*
Austria	Ministry of education	Regional or municipal authorities	Ministry of education	School based
Finland	Municipalities and ministries of social affairs and health	Municipalities and ministries of social affairs and health	Primary health care of the municipality	School health services are part of the health service, but distinct and are school based. Some services (e.g. school environment inspection) are offered by primary health care
France	Ministry of education	Multiple sources	Ministry of education	School based

Israel	Ministries of health and education and local health	Ministries of health and education and local health, via independent provider organization	Ministries of health and education and local health	School health services are part of the health service, but distinct. School health services visit schools
Italy	Ministries of health and education and local health and education services	Ministries of health and education, via regional health administration, which is responsible for delivering health services	Regional health authority via local health services	School health environment is taken care of by the local health authority; at the individual level, there are no special services as children's health is taken care of by the family paediatrician
Netherlands	Ministry of health and local health and education	Ministry of health and local health		School health services are part of the health service, but distinct. School health services visit schools. Also see youth health services (Box 6.4)
Norway	Ministry of health	Other	Other	School based
Poland	Ministry of health	National Health Fund and local government	Ministries of health and education	School health services are part of the health service, but distinct. School based. Some services offered by primary health care
Sweden	Ministry of health and local health and education	Local education (municipality)	Local health and local education	School based
United Kingdom	Local health	Local health	Local health	School health services are part of the health service, but distinct. School health services visit schools

Source: Child Health Services in Europe survey: Baltag and Levi, 2010; Pommier et al., 2010; Sagan et al., 2011

Health examinations of school-aged children

Health examination of an individual student may include screening for specific diseases and health problems, wider assessment of health status, health counselling, and delivering preventive measures such as vaccinations and fluoride supplementation. Individual health plans can be made during examination visits, designed to guide further support, treatments and follow-ups with health and other professionals. When parents are invited, they have an opportunity to discuss concerns and worries, and health professionals can gain an insight into the functioning of the child's family and its possible effects on the child's health and learning. Health examinations are performed in nearly all countries but their timing and content vary (Table 6.3).

Evaluations of school-entry examinations by physicians in the United Kingdom (Barlow, Stewart-Brown and Fletcher, 1998), and a review of yearly physical examinations in adolescence (Stickler, 2000), revealed that few new serious medical problems were detected by routine screening through general health examination (Yankenauer and Lawrence, 1955; Hall, 1996). However, policy decisions are influenced by many factors, including patient and parental expectations, and cultural and professional pressures. Moreover, the conclusions reached in cost-effectiveness studies may not be generalizable between countries, as school health service programmes are highly variable.

Recently, some countries have begun to focus on restoring routine health examinations to school health services but adapting the model to ensure that examinations correspond more closely to the current needs of school-aged children and a contemporary more holistic view of health. Early evaluations of these comprehensive health examinations (Box 6.5) in Finland suggested that 40–60% of assessed children had problems that needed attention (Strid, 1996; Salonen et al., 2004; Hietanen-Peltola, 2007), with family and emotional problems common. Based on an interview and medical examination, further action was considered necessary for 40% of children. The most common were: a follow-up visit; laboratory investigations; medication; physiotherapy or physical training. Specialist referral was made in 5% of cases, with a referral to a psychologist in 4%. Chronic diseases such as asthma had generally been identified already but medication often needed to be checked. In addition to interviewing children or parents, questionnaires were used to assess mental health, physical health and health-related behaviours. Among those found to be at risk for depression (6% of children), subsequent interventions ranged from discussion with parents to referral to a family counselling clinic and repeated meetings with the school doctor; only a few were already in care. Parents have participated effectively (90% among parents of 11 to 12-year-olds), even when working full-time. Teachers may be involved, for example, by administering questionnaires such as the 'Strength and Difficulties Questionnaire' (SDQ, 2013) for assessing individual children. Teachers seemed to recognize bullying and learning difficulties better than parents; however, involving teachers was found to be a challenge.

Table 6.3 Health examinations by country, age (grade) and health professional

Country	*Age (grade)**	*Health professional*
Austria	Once per school year beginning at school entry	Physician. No treatments or prescriptions are allowed
England/Scotland	Occasional	
Finland	Comprehensive health examination (and separate oral health examination) at 1st (7 years), 5th (11 years) and 8th (14 years) grades; basic examination once per academic year at all other grades from 2nd to 9th. 1st year of secondary education (16–17 years) by nurse; 2nd year by doctor	Comprehensive health examination by nurse and physician; basic health examinations by nurses and dentists
France	Ages 4, 6, 9, 12, 15 years	Initial screening by nurse, referring to a physician when needed
Netherlands	Several well-care visits during school years, mostly grades 2 (5–6 years) and 7 (10–11 years) in primary school; and grade 2 (13–14 years) in secondary education, according to national guidelines. In some regions there is an 'exit examination' for grade 4 in secondary education	Physicians, (specialized) nurses, physician assistants No treatments, prescriptions, or referrals to secondary care are allowed
Norway	Preschool (5 years), and at 3rd (8 years) and 8th (13 years) grades	Screening tests by nurses and referrals to physician when needed
Poland	Preschool, and at 3rd grade primary (9 years); 1st grade lower secondary (13 years); 1st (16 years) and last (18–19 years) grades of upper secondary	Physicians, with screening tests by nurse
Sweden	Health visits at 1st (7 years), 5th (11 years), 8th (14 years) and 11th (17 years) grades but other schedules may be applied	Routine visits, mainly by nurses. Physicians are involved in selected cases. The system varies between municipalities
Italy	School health service were abolished when the Italian NHS was established. Routine physical examinations are conducted by primary care paediatricians in office-based practices	

* There may be variations inside the countries or the guidelines are not fully implemented

Screening for diseases in school-aged children remains controversial and country programmes are not always firmly grounded in evidence. WHO's criteria for screening suggest that it should result in improved health of the population by detecting disorders in the early phase, followed by early treatment (Wilson and Jungner, 1968). Thus, the detection of disorders alone is not enough. Screening for scoliosis of the spine, for example, does not fit the WHO criteria and is no longer routine practice in some countries, such as the United Kingdom, although nearly one-third of countries in the WHO European region continue to do so (Baltag and Levi, 2010).

Little agreement on the best way forward, plus substantial variation in the timing and number of screening tests, remain in European countries (Table 6.4). Indeed, screening remains the most common school health service activity in European countries, followed by vaccination, then health promotion (Baltag and Levi, 2010). The most common screening tests are: height and

Table 6.4 Screening tests performed in school health services in selected countries

Country	*Screening test*						
	Height	*Weight*	*Vision*	*Hearing*	*Blood pressure*	*Dental health*	*Other*
Austria	✓	✓	✓	✓	✓	✓	STI, heart, lung
Finland	✓	✓	✓	✓	✓	✓	Growth, development and well-being
France	–	–	–	–	–	–	–
Israel	✓	✓	✓	✓			STI
Italy			✓			✓	Orthopaedics, anaemia
Netherlands	✓	✓	✓	✓			Physical development, speech and language, psychosocial
Norway	None						
Poland	–	–	–	✓	–	–	–
Sweden	✓	✓	✓	✓			BMI, scoliosis
United Kingdom	✓	✓	✓	✓			

Key: ✓: service provided; cell left blank: not provided, –: no information available

BMI: body mass index; STI: sexually transmitted infection

Source: Baltag and Levi, 2010

weight (84% of European countries); visual acuity (81%); hearing status (73%); dental (68%); blood pressure (46%); STIs (16%); and other conditions (49%). Mental health was hardly mentioned. Vaccinations were performed by 89% of the countries during screening visits.

School health services in the Netherlands are provided mostly by youth health professionals and mainly comprise screening and health counselling (Box 6.4). In Sweden, regular examinations undertaken by the school health services were previously known as health controls but are now called health visits, this name change signaling the shift away from screening and towards an emphasis on health promotion. In Finland, the comprehensive health examination (CHE) was introduced in 2009 and comprises several new elements (such as health promotion) in addition to physical examination and screening. The CHE includes a thorough assessment of pupils' health and well-being, of their family situation and (together with input from the teachers) of the child's well-being and learning capacity in the classroom (Box 6.5).

Box 6.4 School Health Services in The Netherlands: Youth Health Care (YHC)

Since the first school-based Youth Health Care activities were initiated in the Netherlands, more than a century ago, YHC has grown into a nationwide and labour-intensive service, employing hundreds of physicians, nurses and medical assistants working in primary and secondary schools. By the time they leave school, all children in the Netherlands will have been exposed to a wide variety of preventive health and health promotion activities, administered by many different YHC workers. The services are most often delivered on the school premises and may include health promotion programmes, screening for specific physical abnormalities, wellness visits and (freely accessible) consultation hours. The more individually oriented tasks are carried out by YHC physicians (who must refer onwards if a prescription is required), with others conducted by nurses and medical assistants. The schedule of activities in the YHC programme is contained in a 'Basic Range of Duties' document, which is widely accepted, although loosely grounded in evidence. For example, there might be evidence to support screening for overweight and obesity as an important risk factor for cardiovascular disease; however, there is little or no rationale for the 16 to 18 times this screening process happens in children. School health in the Netherlands continues to be the subject of active research and debate.

Source: Huijsman and Wagenaar, 1983; Zielhuis, 1985; Wiegersma, 1999.

Box 6.5 The comprehensive health examination (CHE) in Finland

The Finnish CHE is designed to assess schoolchildren in the context of their school and family. The child's health (including mental health and well-being) is assessed by a school nurse and a doctor. Both parents are invited to engage in the process, and are given the opportunity to discuss any concerns about their child's health and well-being, and to obtain information and advice. Well-being of the whole family is assessed when necessary, for example, if parents' health problems are thought to adversely affect the child's health, or learning and coping in school. At the examination, children can also meet health professionals confidentially and without their parents. The CHE includes a teacher's assessment on strengths and difficulties in the child's learning, relationships and coping in the class.

Summary statistics on the results of the CHEs of each class and grade are compiled so that school management and welfare teams can assess needs for health promotion and education, and for the organization of education and social and health services in the school.

Source: Ministry of Social Affairs and Health, 2009.

Specific disease prevention measures undertaken at schools include vaccination and dental care. Universal school-based prevention programmes, delivered on an individual basis, include vaccination programmes, such as the recently introduced human papilloma virus vaccine for adolescent schoolgirls in England and some other European countries. In Poland, school nurses are involved in a caries prevention programme for elementary school pupils, administering fluoride gel applications and teaching tooth-brushing techniques. See Chapter 5 for further discussion on vaccination.

Environmental health at school

Although the poor physical environment that children endured in factory schools in the 19th century triggered the development of school health services, leading to improvements in children's living and working conditions, the physical environment in many schools today remains far from satisfactory. Adults' workplace environments improved substantially during the 20th century, largely following legislative changes mandating regular health and safety inspections of all workplaces (including schools as workplaces for teachers), but the same laws may not apply to children's learning environments in schools. Sweden is one exception; the same legislation applies to health and safety of the working environment for teachers as for schoolchildren. School environmental health includes concerns for safety, noise, ventilation and air quality, as all of these can affect the school experience of children and are amenable to improvement.

Safety at school is a significant concern. Injuries at school, or during travel to and from school, are common. School health services can play an important role, not just in injury prevention and in providing urgent care when injuries occur, but also in collecting information to learn from accidents and injuries in order to improve preventive measures. In Sweden, school nurses systematically collect information on all injuries at school requiring medical attention, and interview students to understand what may have caused the injury and to identify any preventive measures that should be taken. This information is presented at regular meetings with the headmaster, teacher representatives, and sometimes students' representatives, and appropriate further action is decided upon during these sessions.

Excessive noise or stuffy atmospheres can limit the ability of students to learn. Noise can be decreased by providing support to the teacher in creating a calmer, quieter classroom, or by physical adjustments to classrooms, such as sound-absorbing material in ceilings.

Finally, the psychosocial environment of schools is now recognized as being an important aspect for children's health, well-being and potential for learning. Many schools have instituted rigorous policies on bullying, for example. In Sweden, such policies are mandatory by law.

Clinics at school

Open-door, low-threshold school clinics can help address pupils' urgent health needs during the school day (Table 6.5). The role and tasks of low-threshold clinics depend very much on how these are integrated with primary health care and hospitals, such as whether medicines can be prescribed, or whether there is responsibility for follow-up of some chronic diseases and disabilities. School nurses consider that psychosocial problems are the most common reasons for children and young people seeking urgent assistance through school health services (Clausson, Peterson and Berg, 2003).

In the United States, school-based health centres (SBHC) have been established to address the health needs of school-aged children in many states during the last two decades, although they still cover a small proportion of the population. Most of the available research comparing school-based clinics focuses on SBHC. Research in which these are matched with control schools demonstrates positive effects, such as a decrease in hospitalization and emergency department visits for children with asthma, with demonstrable cost savings (Guo et al., 2005); and increases in the proportion of students who receive mental health care, with possible improvements in psychosocial quality of life (Guo, Wade and Keller, 2008). A longitudinal study suggests an increase in health-related quality of life reported by students who had access to SBHC (Wade et al., 2008). However, the context differs from Europe because the United States lacks universal health coverage. The only European study on open-access school clinics (which also provide well-child care and health counselling) used an ecological case-referent study design. The results suggested a corrolation between alcohol, and tobacco use, and obesity, and access to YCH with open consultation hours compared with those who were allocated to YCH offering no open hours (Wiegersma, Hofman and Zielhuis, 2000).

Table 6.5 School health services: clinics at school

Country	*School-based clinics*	*Remarks*
Austria	No	Medical treatment by school doctor is restricted to first aid
England/Scotland	Nurses in some schools, some times	Gradual diminishment of school-based medical and nursing staff
	Paediatricians may hold clinics for children with long-term conditions in schools	Shift towards 'prevention and promotion' paradigm of school health
Finland	Yes, school nurses	School doctors are usually visited through school nurse only
France	A direct contact with nurse or doctor can be possible	Usually school doctors are visited through nurses or other school professionals only
Netherlands	Yes, by doctors, although they are increasingly being replaced by nurses	Free consultation hours for parents and teachers, too No curative activities or prescriptions are allowed
Norway	Yes, school nurses	
Poland	No	
Sweden	Yes, school nurses	
Italy	No school health services, all primary health care with office-based paediatricians	

Source: Child Health Services in Europe survey and Pommier et al., 2010

Workforce

The school nurse is the key member in the school health services workforce, but teams may comprise doctors, psychologists and counsellors, social workers, dentists, and others, such as nutrition specialists. Most countries in western Europe report staff shortages in school health services; indeed, only the Netherlands reports adequate numbers, and 35% of countries participating in the WHO survey expressed a need for clearer division between the responsibilities of school nurses, school doctors and GPs/family doctors (Baltag and Levi, 2010). The nurse is seen as an advocate, liaising with primary health care and with education, and may also have a function in referring directly to specialist care (Brownjohn, 2003). Children and young people valued both the clinical knowledge and confidentiality of these services and 'often preferred discussing sensitive issues with a nurse rather than a teacher' in PSHE sessions (Chase et al., 2010).

As workforce development and training begin, one of the challenges for school health teams is to balance ongoing work at the class or school level with the need for episodes of one-to-one support for some individuals, for example, when a child with juvenile-onset diabetes makes the transition between primary and secondary education. In England, the same school nurse is likely to bridge the secondary school and primary schools that provide its intake.

A significant barrier to access to school health services is the wide variation between countries in the provision of school health professionals (Baltag and Levi, 2010). For example, in Sweden the recommended resources are 40 hours of health professional staffing per week, with a recommended ratio of one nurse for 400 students, and one doctor for 10,000 students. Swedish legislation in 2010 ensures that school health services are part of the school welfare and health promotion teams, bridging the gap between population health and a more medical model. These teams also provide an individualized approach to school health services; the teams include school doctors, school nurses, school psychologists, school social workers and special education teachers, who will meet to discuss individual students. For example, a school nurse might identify depressive symptoms in a 14-year-old girl: the school health services team, including social workers and psychologists, would then discuss the case and formulate a comprehensive plan for providing support for the girl, both within and outside school. In Norway, the recommendation is one person-year per 1000 pupils; in Austria, it is one weekly hour per 60 pupils; in Finland, one nurse per 600 pupils and one doctor per 2100 pupils; and, in Poland, 800 pupils per nurse. There is, however, little information available on variation within countries, but this is likely to be substantial. In Finland, for example, the variation in the number of pupils per school nurse ranges from 300 to 1217, and per school doctor 1250 to 20,000 (Wiss et al., 2007). Such variations are not likely to reflect differences in need, with some notable exceptions like the city of Helsinki, which uses demographic characteristics of school catchment areas (such as deprivation and the proportion of immigrants in the population) in allocating resources for school health services. In England, local authorities and primary health services collaborate on joint strategic needs assessments (JSNAs) (Blair and DeBell, 2011). New interagency structures, called Health and Wellbeing Boards, are expected to use JSNAs to develop plans and allocate resources for improving child health (May, 2012). However, recent changes to the English NHS leave the role of school health unclear, despite attempts to align the purchasing of services (commissioning) with specific health outcomes.

In the early days of school health services, care was largely delivered by physicians, while more recently nurses have become the dominant school health services professionals. However, taking into account the profound changes in children's lives since those days; the increased knowledge of the effects learning difficulties have on children's health and well-being; and the understanding of the relationship between health and school performance, it is clear that doctors and nurses alone cannot provide the comprehensive health expertise that schools and schoolchildren need. Doctors and nurses are represented in most countries in the WHO European Region: 76% of the countries have school doctors and 65% have school nurses, however only 43% have psychologists, 24% a social worker, 22% a dentist, 8% physiotherapists and health care assistants, and 22% other professionals (Baltag and Levi, 2010). A wider approach has been taken by France, Sweden and Finland, which have multiprofessional school welfare teams, within which learning and health problems are discussed in regular meetings with representatives from both health and education professions.

Since schools are where children spend most of their time, there is under-exploited potential to hold multidisciplinary clinics for children with chronic problems. This could benefit the children, minimizing school absences and disruption. Moreover, the clinic staff can benefit from the insights and advice of school staff, who know the children from a different perspective and can provide useful monitoring and follow-up.

Schools and children with special needs

One episode of childhood illness causing only three weeks of school absence can have lasting consequences (Kuh and Wadsworth, 1993). Indeed, certain groups of children may gain life-changing benefits from participation in school. Historically, both children with disabilities and children 'looked after' in local authority care have had inadequate learning support. Pupils' attendance was often inadequate and teaching environments were impoverished in terms of mental stimulation and emotional growth.

School health services can contribute to the management of children with special health, developmental, physical, mental or social needs during the school day. The coordination of care for health needs in schoolchildren is crucial for their overall development. In different places, this can be a medical or nursing role, while sometimes other professionals like speech therapists or psychologists may take the lead.

Special health needs

Children with special health needs have an increased risk of adverse educational outcomes (Forrest et al., 2011). Moreover, the nature of childhood disability is evolving: childhood chronic diseases are increasingly prevalent, and behavioural, emotional and neurological problems are more common than physical problems (Halfon et al., 2012). See also Chapters 1 and 5 for further discussion on the evolving health needs of the child population. Unfortunately, there has been little formal evaluation of school health services for children with chronic conditions, disability or learning difficulties (Parent, Woodrich and Hasan, 2009; Gustafsson et al., 2010).

The most common European model is for children with special health needs to attend mainstream schools with the provision of additional support. The consequences for school personnel can be profound; for example, in France, support and advice for teaching staff is a major activity for school nurses and doctors, and this has been increasing in recent years. Children with special needs may require medicines during the school day, which means extra concern and work for teachers, and may cause conflicts between parents and school personnel. There are examples of parents having to come to school in the middle of the day to give insulin injections to their young child when teachers do not want, or are unable, to do this themselves, and where there are no school health services available. Keeping control of a classroom that includes one or more children with mental health and/or behavioural problems demands an extraordinary effort from a teacher, which can lead to burnout for teachers and may disturb learning for other children in the classroom.

A small quasi-experimental study in Switzerland suggested that including children with learning difficulties in mainstream classrooms has no significant effect on the short-term academic outcomes of the children with or without disability (Sermier Dessemontet and Bless, 2013).

Special health needs in adolescence

Adolescents' special health needs are widely recognized, as is their need for youth-friendly models of primary care (Kleinert, 2007; Patel et al., 2007; Sawyer et al., 2007; Tylee et al., 2007) (see also Chapter 7).

With the onset of puberty and sexual maturation, counselling and services for sexual and reproductive health are needed. Adolescent girls who become pregnant are likely to leave education abruptly. Basch (2011b) reviews the key issues for schools around teenage pregnancy. A joint medical and nursing outreach service in Reading, England, which sees young people at the place of their choice (e.g. school, youth club, foster home or a local coffee bar) has shown a substantial reduction in teenage pregnancies (Hunt, 2011). Worried teenage girls often present with more than one concern, and the confidential multiagency lunchtime school drop-in service pioneered by Richardson Todd describes a flexible model of support that at least two professional bodies now recommend (Richardson Todd, 2003). In France, school nurses can deliver contraceptives in emergency situations. The multidisciplinary School Health Research Group (Caan, 2004) identified a number of imaginative developments, for example, sexual health outreach to young people reluctant to visit general practices (South Leeds NHS Primary Care Trust and Leeds City Council, 2003), using a confidential 'Teenage Health Bus' to visit neighbourhoods with high rates of truancy. See Chapter 7 for further discussion on youth health services.

Open-door clinics of school health services are an easy opportunity for counselling on sexual health and the provision of contraceptives, as offered in Finland, while Sweden and Norway have separate youth clinics. In Poland, there is no such service, while in the United Kingdom, some authorities offer outreach services for youth but there has been public disquiet about the provision of contraception in school.

Mental health in adolescence is important, partly just because it is a challenging time of life with many transitions and increasing responsibility, but also because many mental disorders begin in adolescence although they may not be diagnosed until later in life. Adolescence therefore presents a window of opportunity for mental health promotion, early detection of problems and intervention. School settings are well placed for these services, and are as yet not well developed in most countries.

Approximately one young person in ten has a chronic disease or uses medicine regularly, and psychosocial symptoms and risk behaviours are common. Many adolescents report barriers in accessing ordinary health care, so again schools present a useful setting for improving access to health care for adolescents.

Disabilities

When London was awarded the Olympic and Paralympic Games, their base in Stratford was chosen as the British demonstration site for integrated care of children with disabilities, especially 'complex' cases involving multiple problems. Even for complex disabilities, it was striking that in the United Kingdom, most were only detected after children entered school (Caan, Pittam and Lutchmiah, 2006). About 2000 families in this deprived urban area had struggled with no professional support until their child was 5 or 6 years old. School nurses, special educational needs coordinators and primary school head teachers played a key gatekeeper role in the initial stages of engaging children and families, but the 400 most severely disabled schoolchildren needed an urgent joint clinic assessment by health and social services (led by senior paediatricians), combined with a home assessment by a specialist health visitor from the child development service. The Children Act 2004 had introduced a new statutory role of 'lead professional' to be the easily accessible contact for families where a child has extra needs for support. This multiskilled role was pioneered for children with disabilities in Stratford (Caan, Pittam and Lutchmiah, 2006), beginning with that service's specialist health visitor.

Clearly, for many children, it is desirable to detect disability long before school entry. Provided designated staff have the appropriate skills, early years services such as Children's Centres (Northrop, Pittam and Caan, 2008) can identify needs, for example, for speech therapy or portage, and promote school readiness. Persistent behavioural problems frustrate learning in many primary schools around the world, and recent research on the 'Incredible Years Teacher Classroom Management Program' (Bywater, 2012) shows one way in which early intervention can reduce conduct disorder at school age. Some disabilities (like developmental coordination disorder) only become obvious during activities at school, such as handwriting or playing football, and the educational psychologist Portwood (1999) shows how combined guidance for teachers and parents can make a real difference to children's experience of education. School-age children with more disabling conditions benefit from multiprofessional, interagency teamwork (Caan et al., 2000), which in turn requires shared systems of training, staff supervision and partnership, working alongside parents. It is these shared systems that take much more time to set up than just agreeing a 'care pathway' on paper. As disabled children enter their teenage years, and parents and staff gradually plan their transition to adult life in the community, a 'health facilitator' may be helpful in proactively making links with local services. This is crucial, for example, in relation to school-leavers at risk of sudden unexpected death from epilepsy (NICE, 2002). In another deprived urban area (Dagenham, England), the World Bank's concept of 'linking social capital' was used to develop innovative health facilitation for schools (Thomson et al., 2007).

Social vulnerability

There are groups of children who are especially vulnerable, for example, children from migrant or transiently resident families, and children who are looked after by local authorities. For example, children living in migrant or transiently resident families tend to have lower educational success and to experience worse health. See Chapters 1 and 5 for further information about the health of vulnerable children. One group whose integration into school health systems has been challenging is the Roma (Leeming, 2011). Young asylum-seekers' experiences of migration may have included trauma and bereavement, as well as the insecurity and homesickness other young migrants feel. In Liverpool, Chiumento et al. (2011) describe a school-based service for refugee children that may have lessons for other cities in term of its acceptance by young people.

Children who are suffering abuse, neglect or exploitation are likely to find learning difficult and may develop withdrawn or antisocial behaviour in class. The United States Centers for Disease Control and Prevention reports the median age at which child maltreatment starts to be 6 years old (i.e. while they are attending primary school), and that the lifetime cost per victim of non-fatal maltreatment is over US$210,000 (Prevention Action, 2012). In one-sixth of British schools, school nurses spend over 70% of their time on child protection work (Coates, 2011). Many children are growing up in 'troubled and chaotic' families (Department for Work and Pensions, 2012), where truancy and early involvement in criminal activity go hand in hand with a pattern of maltreatment over generations. The United Nations 'Convention on the Rights of the Child' needs to be considered in policies to prevent child maltreatment: the major risk factors to individuals and communities are well known, but skilled and strategic action is required (Reading et al., 2009). For example, alcohol dependence in parents or carers is a risk factor for both abuse and neglect: child-centred social work that helps reduce parental drinking over time can safeguard their children (Caan, 2013). Some families that are suspicious of local authority social workers can be successfully engaged by trained 'child protection volunteers', with a marked improvement in the risks to their children and improved school attendance (Cooper, 2011). However, compared to countries like Norway, schools elsewhere may have much less grasp on how problems at home, such as excessive parental alcohol intake, can influence learning (Torvik et al., 2011).

School nurse outreach services with vulnerable young people in trouble with the criminal justice system led to participation in a variety of creative and therapeutic community art groups, a pattern of enabling peer support that was discovered in several places (Baldacchino, Caan and Munn Giddings, 2008). In the United Kingdom, school health services identified two problems that were common, but for which most staff felt inadequately trained: substance use (mainly alcohol but sometimes in combination with other drugs); and self-harm (especially when associated with repeated visits to hospital accident and emergency departments).

Schools and population health research

School health services present an ideal and under-used opportunity for furthering understanding of health and health needs through the routine collection of data from a universal population. Good trend and longitudinal data are not just of interest for research. Reliable, continuously updated observations on schoolchildren, such as the Municipal Public Health database for Rotterdam-Rijnmond, enabled the Netherlands to tailor interventions with the right timing and intensity for different children. As well as growth and physical health, these data cover sensitive areas like emotional distress and suicidal thoughts, where early intervention may be valuable (de Wilde et al., 2011). The Netherlands collects biometric data on children, as well as ecological measures of the wider obesogenic environment in which that child lives (Slingerland, Borghouts and Hesselink, 2012), simplifying the planning and evaluation of interventions to reduce child obesity. Few countries have managed such coordination; however, child health information in England may eventually improve, led by the ChiMat collaboration (www.chimat.org.uk). A national seminar on social care research capacity (Caan, 2006) confirmed that understanding the health needs of the most socially excluded young people was a priority. The United Kingdom strategy 'No Health Without Mental Health' stressed the need for better interventions early in the life-course, and the Department for Education has now introduced an 'Early Intervention Grant', which includes 'targeted mental health support for children and young people' (HM Government, 2011). In order to target timely support in the right way to the right children, it is necessary to understand the needs of 'vulnerable children'; Evans (2012) has reported on progress to monitor health needs in a spectrum of different, vulnerable children.

Every second year, Finland collects data from all schools in the country for the 8th and 9th grades (14 to 16 years) and upper secondary and vocational school 1st and 2nd grades (ages 17 to 19), by electronic surveys covering individual health and health behaviour (including sexual health), as well school health and health promotion (http://www.thl.fi/fi_FI/web/fi/tilastot/vaestotutkimukset/kouluterveyskysely). Information on educational outcomes, health and well-being is available at national and regional levels for research as well as planning services. The results are analysed by class, grade and school for municipalities and individual schools. Schools use the results for promotion of health in the school community, for multiprofessional teamwork and for health education lessons. Municipalities use them for strategic planning and evaluation of their health promotion measures. At the national level, the results serve policy planning and evaluation. School health ambassadors are appointed to enhance the use of data at local and regional levels.

To discuss issues at an aggregate level, compiled information on the class and school is needed. Health promotion surveys completed by pupils, or statistics compiled from health examinations, are important tools for welfare teams when focusing on the school or class as a whole. With computerized record systems, it is easier to compile information on class and school levels, but how well these systems work presently is not known.

Future challenges

Countries throughout Europe have adopted a variety of different approaches to the concept of school health, but many of the challenges faced are common to all, such as adapting to the changing health needs of children and young people. The variety of European school health systems offers a valuable opportunity to learn from each other.

Common challenges faced by European school health services include:

- **Leadership**: Strong and effective leadership and advocacy for school health services are important to ensure delivery of system-wide reforms, such as capacity-building and improving the quality of services.
- **Research and evaluation**: Research and evaluation of school health and health services are fundamental to drive improvements. Further international comparisons are needed. Data on the effectiveness of school health services enable effective advocacy. Guidelines on school health services organization, practice, standards and performance assessment could support countries in taking forward their efforts to improve health.
- **Workforce**: Most countries report insufficient staff, and training is often inadequate. A lack of clear divisions and lines of responsibility among team members is also a frequently reported problem.
- **Wider context**: It is unclear in most countries how school health services fit and interact within the wider health sector, and particularly the education sector. This causes problems of duplication and gaps in services, as well as inefficiencies and poor-quality care.
- **School health services to meet health needs**: Many countries report that the structure and content of school health services are not commensurate with schoolchildren's health needs.

The unique aspect of school health, bringing an entire age group within a population together at the same time and place, applies also to education in young adult life. Health services for students in higher education settings face many similar challenges to school health, compounded by the fact that many young people move to different regions and countries within and outside Europe to seek further education (European Union for School and University Health and Medicine, 2007).

Research on school health services, and its place in comprehensive school health, needs more descriptive and analytic data and further international comparisons. However, based upon the best evidence currently available in the literature and supplemented by the findings of our survey, we have constructed a framework for describing school health and health services. This framework offers a basis for further research on school health and ultimately may be useful for shaping evidence-based policy-making (Table 6.6).

The 'Promoting Health through Schools' (WHO, 1997) report urges all people to imagine a future in which schools in every nation have the healthy development of all young people as an essential part of their core mission, and a world where schools take this challenge on and implement new and exciting ways to coordinate the educational process, environmental conditions (both

Table 6.6 A School Health Framework

Activity	*Target group*	*Function*	*Role of health personnel*
Health examination	Pupils of the entire class/age group (could also be to selected groups of children e.g. with high risk)	Individually organized visits in order to: detect health, social and learning problems and risks; to guide and counsel in health matters; to make an individual health plan; to meet parents	Physicians, nurses, dentists, health assistants are the main actors
		Individual preventive measures (vaccinations, fluoride prevention)	
	School management (and community leaders)	Compiling statistical summaries of a class and school to assess well-being and manage problems or targeting interventions	As above with school management, school health/welfare teams
Need-based care	Pupils' perceived health needs	Open-door, low-threshold clinic for pupils (primary care, guidance and counselling e.g. on sexual health); first aid	Nurses, physicians are the main actors
	Children with special needs e.g. chronic disease, disability, social and family problem	Organizing and assisting in care, management of school days; assisting teachers; follow-up of individual health plans (e.g. medication, restrictions in physical education, family problems)	Nurses and physicians involved; teachers, school assistants, other staff
Health education and preventive measures	Teachers	Advising teachers about planning teaching content for health education	Nurses/physicians or other health personnel participants
	Class, group, school	Classroom or group teaching in health Fluoride prevention, vaccination	

School welfare and health promotion teams	Individual pupil, class (teacher)	Finding and managing problems of learning, bullying, disturbance of conduct, truancy, etc.	Health personnel participants
	The entire school community, parents	Planning and implementing school health/welfare policies (e.g. rules, recreation)	Multiprofessional teams
	School management, teachers	Organizing health promotion events, theme days etc.	
		Working with stakeholders (e.g. parents, community leaders)	
School health inspection	Physical environment in classrooms, and inner and outer areas	Inspection of buildings, recreation areas, working conditions e.g. ventilation, ergonomics, hygiene	Physicians, nurses are participants Health inspectors, staff, school managers
	Psychosocial environment	Assessment of psychosocial well-being of classes and school e.g. by questionnaires, compiling results from health examinations	Physicians/nurse are participants Teachers, school management

within and outside the school) and the range of available health services in order to enhance the educational achievement and health of young people. The essential message about schools and health is articulated in the WHO vision for Health Promoting Schools: 'The determinants of both education and health are indivisibly linked' (DeBell and Jackson, 2000).

References

Adshead, F. (2007) Young people and risky sexual behaviour. In: Independent Advisory Group on Sexual Health and HIV (eds) *Sex, Drugs, Alcohol and Young People*. London: Department of Health.

Allensworth, D.D. and Kolbe, L.J. (1987) The comprehensive school health program: exploring an expanded concept, *Journal of School Health*, 57(10): 409–12.

American School Health Association (2011) http://www.ashaweb.org [accessed 24 June 2013].

Anderson, C.L. (1972) *School Health Practice*. Saint Louis, MO: Mosby Company.

Austin, S.B. et al. (2012) Effect of the planet health intervention on eating disorder symptoms in Massachusetts middle schools, 2005–2008, *Preventing Chronic Disease*, 9(E171; quiz E171).

Baisch, M.J., Lundeen, S.P. and Murphy, M.K. (2011) Evidence-based research on the value of school nurses in an urban school system, *Journal of School Health*, 81(2): 74–80.

Baldacchino, A., Caan, W. and Munn Giddings, C. (2008) Mutual aid groups in psychiatry and substance misuse, *Mental Health and Substance Use*, 1: 104–17.

Baltag, V. and Levi, M. (2010) *Pairing Children with Health Services: The results of a survey on school health services in the WHO European Region*. Copenhagen: WHO Regional Office for Europe.

Barlow, J., Stewart-Brown, S. and Fletcher, J. (1998) Systematic review of the school entry medical examination, *Archives of Disease in Childhood*, 78(4): 301–11.

Basch, C.E. (2011a) Breakfast and the achievement gap among urban minority youth, *Journal of School Health*, 81(10): 635–40.

Basch, C.E. (2011b) Teen pregnancy and the achievement gap among urban minority youth, *Journal of School Health*, 81(10): 614–18.

Blair, M. and DeBell, D. (2011) Reconceptualising health services for school-age children in the 21st century, *Archives of Disease in Childhood*, 96(7): 616–18.

Blair, M. et al. (2003) *Child Public Health*. Oxford: Oxford University Press.

Botvin, G.J. and Griffin, K.W. (2007) School-based programmes to prevent alcohol, tobacco and other drug use, *International Review of Psychiatry*, 19(6): 607–15.

Brownjohn, N. (2003) How school nursing links with other services, *Child and Adolescent Mental Health in Primary Care*, 1: 15–16.

Burls, A. and Caan, W. (2005) Human health and nature conservation, *BMJ*, 331: 1221–2.

Bywater, T.J. (2012) Perspectives on the Incredible Years programme: psychological management of conduct disorder, *British Journal of Psychiatry*, 201: 85–7.

Caan, W. (2004) The School Health Research Group, a science odyssey. In: RCN (ed.) *RCN International Nursing Research Conference*. London: Royal College of Nursing.

Caan, W. (2006) Building capacity for social care research. PP 29–30 in Proceedings of a National Seminar on Social Care Research Capacity. London: Department of Health and King's College London.

Caan, W., Pittam, G., Northrop, M. and Lutchmiah, J. (2006) *Integrated Child Development Service. Report on Department of Health project for Newham PCT*. Chelmsford: Anglia Ruskin University.

Caan, W. (2009) Providing a comprehensive picture of the Parenting Programmes being run throughout Essex. Report for Essex Country Council. Chelmsford: Anglia Ruskin University.

Caan, W. (2013) Alcohol and the family, *Contemporary Social Science*, 8(1): 8–17.

Caan, W. et al. (2000) A joint health and social services initiative for children with disabilities, *British Journal of Community Nursing*, 5(2): 87–90.

Campion, J., Bhui, K. and Bhugra, D. (2012) European Psychiatric Association (EPA) guidance on prevention of mental disorders, *European Psychiatry*, 27(2): 68–80.

Case, A., Fertig, A. and Paxson, C. (2005) The lasting impact of childhood health and circumstance, *Journal of Health Economics*, 24(2): 365–89.

Catalano, R.F. et al. (2012) Worldwide application of prevention science in adolescent health, *The Lancet*, 379(9826): 1653–64.

Centers for Disease Control and Prevention (2011) *Adolescent and School Health. Coordinated school health*. http://www.cdc.gov/healthyyouth/cshp/index.htm [accessed 24 June 2013].

Challen, A. et al. (2009) UK resilience programme evaluation, interim report. London: London School of Economics.
Chase, E. et al. (2010) *Promoting the health of children and young people through schools: the role of the nurse*. London: Institute of Education.
Chevreul, K. et al. (2010) France: Health system review, *Health Systems in Transition*, 12: 1–291, xxi–xxii.
Chiumento, A. et al. (2011) School-based mental health service for refugee and asylum seeking children: multi-agency working, lessons for good practice, *Journal of Public Mental Health*, 10(3): 164–77.
Clausson, E., Petersson, K. and Berg, A. (2003) School nurses' view of schoolchildren's health and their attitudes to document it in the school health record – a pilot study, *Scandinavian Journal of Caring Sciences*, 17(4): 392–8.
Coates, M. (2011) School nursing, a priority for child-centred public health, *British Journal of School Nursing*, 6(9): 439–43.
Cooper, J. (2011) Child protection volunteers help children and save money study finds, *Community Care*, 29 November. http://www.communitycare.co.uk/articles/29/11/2011/117834/use-of-child-protection-volunteers-sees-risk-levels-fall.htm [accessed 24 June 2013].
Cougar Hall, P. and West, J.H. (2012) Boundin': responding to life challenges with resilience, *Journal of School Health*, 82(4): 196–200.
Craig, C. (2007) *The potential dangers of a systematic, explicit approach to teaching social and emotional skills (SEAL)*. Glasgow: Centre for Confidence and Well-being.
Currie, C. et al. (eds) (2012) *Health Policy for Children and Adolescents, No 6. Social determinants of health and well-being among young people. Health Behaviour in School-aged Children (HBSC) study. International Report from the 2009–10 Survey*. Copenhagen: WHO Regional Office for Europe.
DeBell, D. and Jackson, P. (2000) *School nursing within the public health agenda: a strategy for practice*. London: McMillan-Scott (London Division) on behalf of the Queens Institute of Nurses.
Department for Education (2010) *Customer voice (wave 9): aspirations of children in care*. Research Brief DFE RBX 10 03. London: Department for Education.
Department of Health (2009) *Healthy lives, brighter futures. The strategy for children and young people's health*. London: Department of Health.
Department of Health (2012) *Getting it right for children, young people and families. Maximising the contribution of the school nursing team: Vision and Call to Action*. Leeds: Department of Health.
Department for Work and Pensions (2012) *Social Justice: transforming lives*. London: Department for Work and Pensions.
de Wilde, E.J. et al. (2011) Self-report of suicidal thoughts and behavior vs. school nurse evaluations in Dutch high-school students, *Crisis*, 32(3): 121–7.
Du Bois, D.L. et al. (2001) How effective are mentoring programs for youth? A systematic assessment of the evidence, *Psychological Science in the Public Interest*, 12(2): 57–91.
Durlak, J.A. et al. (2011) The impact of enhancing students' social and emotional learning: a meta-analysis of school-based universal interventions, *Child Development*, 82(1): 405–32.
Durlak, J.A. and Wells, A.M. (1997) Primary prevention mental health programs for children and adolescents: a meta-analytic review, *American Journal of Community Psychology*, 25(2): 115–52.
European Union for School and University Health and Medicine (2007) *The Tampere Declaration on Student Health Care in Europe*. http://www.eusuhm.org [accessed 24 June 2012].

Evans, S. (2012) Assessing the health needs of vulnerable children, are the data fit for purpose? *Journal of Public Mental Health*, 11(3): 117–40.

Forrest, C.B. et al. (2011) School outcomes of children with special health care needs, *Pediatrics*, 128(2): 303–12.

Foxcroft, D.R. and Tsertsvadze, A. (2011) Universal school-based prevention programs for alcohol misuse in young people, *Cochrane Database of Systematic Reviews*, 5: CD009113.

Foxcroft, D.R. and Tsertsvadze, A. (2012) Universal alcohol misuse prevention programmes for children and adolescents: Cochrane systematic reviews, *Perspectives in Public Health*, 132(3): 128–34.

Gakidou, E. et al. (2010) Increased educational attainment and its effect on child mortality in 175 countries between 1970 and 2009: a systematic analysis, *The Lancet*, 376(9745): 959–74.

Gardner, P.A. (2008) A brief history of the rise and fall of the School Medical Service in England, *Public Health*, 122(3): 261–7.

Gilbert, R. et al. (2009) Burden and consequences of child maltreatment in high-income countries, *The Lancet*, 373(9657): 68–81.

Girlguiding UK (2007) *Looking at me: a resource to help 10–14 year olds build a positive sense of body image and self esteem*. London: Girlguiding UK.

Glasper, A. (2012) Promoting the role of the school nurse, *British Journal of School Nursing*, 7(4): 166–8.

Gorman, D.M., Conde, E. and Huber, J.C., Jr. (2007) The creation of evidence in 'evidence-based' drug prevention: a critique of the Strengthening Families Program Plus Life Skills Training evaluation, *Drug and Alcohol Review*, 26(6): 585–93.

Green, R. and Ross, A. (2010) *Young people's alcohol consumption and its relationship to other outcomes and behaviour: Research Brief DFE RB005*. London: Department of Health.

Guo, J.J. et al. (2005) Impact of school-based health centers on children with asthma, *Journal of Adolescent Health*, 37(4): 266–74.

Guo, J.J., Wade, T.J. and Keller, K.N. (2008) Impact of school-based health centers on students with mental health problems, *Public Health Reports*, 123(6): 768–80.

Gustafsson, J.-E. et al. (2010) *School, Learning and Mental Health: a systematic review*. Stockholm: Health Committee, Royal Swedish Academy of Sciences.

Halfon, N. et al. (2012) The changing landscape of disability in childhood, *Future Child*, 22(1): 13–42.

Hall, D. (1996) *The Child Health Surveillance Handbook*, 3rd edn. Oxford: Radcliffe Publishing.

Harakeh, Z. et al. (2012) Individual and environmental predictors of health risk behaviours among Dutch adolescents: the HBSC study, *Public Health*, 126(7): 566–73.

Hietanen-Peltola, M. (2007) Developing school health service, (in Finnish) *Yleislääkäri*, 22: 9–14.

HM Government (2011) *No health without mental health: A cross-government mental health outcomes strategy for people of all ages*. London: Deparment of Health.

Huijsman, R. and Wagenaar, T. (1983) *Youth Health Care for 4–16 year olds: Organisation and implementation*. Amsterdam: University of Amsterdam.

Humphrey, N., Lendrum, A. and Wigelsworth, M. (2010) *Social and emotional aspects of learning (SEAL) programme in secondary schools: national evaluation*. Report: DFE-RR049. Manchester: Department for Education and School of Education.

Hunt, L. (2011) Targeted sex education pays dividends, *Community Care*, 23 June: 20–1.

Illich, I. (1976) *Limits to Medicine: Medical nemesis – the expropriation of health.* London: Marion Boyars.
Jodkowska, M. et al. (2010) [Inequalities in access to preventive health care for school children][article in Polish], *Medycyna Wieku Rozwojowego*, 14(2): 179–88.
Kessler, R.C. et al. (2005) Lifetime prevalence and age-of-onset distributions of DSM-IV disorders in the National Comorbidity Survey Replication, *Archives of General Psychiatry*, 62(6): 593–602.
Kim-Cohen, J. et al. (2003) Prior juvenile diagnoses in adults with mental disorder: developmental follow-back of a prospective-longitudinal cohort, *Archives of General Psychiatry*, 60(7): 709–17.
Kleinert, S. (2007) Adolescent health: an opportunity not to be missed, *The Lancet*, 369(9567): 1057–8.
Knight, S. (2011) *Forest School for all.* London: SAGE.
Kuh, D.J. and Wadsworth, M.E. (1993) Physical health status at 36 years in a British national birth cohort, *Social Science and Medicine*, 37(7): 905–16.
Lager, A.C.J. and Torssander, J. (2012) Causal effect of education on mortality in a quasi-experiment on 1.2 million Swedes, *Proceedings of the National Academy of Sciences*, 109(22): 8461–6.
Lee, A. et al. (2006) Can Health Promoting Schools contribute to the better health and wellbeing of young people? The Hong Kong experience, *Journal of Epidemiology and Community Health*, 60(6): 530–6.
Leeming, C. (2011) Efforts to integrate Roma people in Manchester are under threat from cuts, *Society Guardian*, 27 April 2011.
Lim, S.S. et al. (2012) A comparative risk assessment of burden of disease and injury attributable to 67 risk factors and risk factor clusters in 21 regions, 1990–2010: a systematic analysis for the Global Burden of Disease Study 2010, *The Lancet*, 380(9859): 2224–60.
May, A. (2012) *Health and wellbeing boards and children, young people and families.* London: Children And Young People's Health Outcomes Forum. https://www.gov.uk/government/uploads/system/uploads/attachment_data/file/156070/CYP-Factsheet-Health-and-Wellbeing.pdf.pdf [accessed 24 June 2013].
McGee, R. and Williams, S. (2000) Does low self-esteem predict health compromising behaviours among adolescents? *Journal of Adolescence*, 23(5): 569–82.
Ministry of Social Affairs and Health (2009) *Maternity and child welfare clinics, school and student health care and preventive oral health care. Grounds and applications directives for Decree (380/2009).* Helsinki: Ministry of Social Affairs and Health.
NICE (2002) *National clinical audit of epilepsy-related death.* London: National Institute for Clinical Excellence.
NICE (2008a) *Promoting children's social and emotional wellbeing in primary education.* London: National Institute for Health and Clinical Excellence.
NICE (2008b) *Promoting children's social and emotional wellbeing in primary education. NICE Public Health Guidance 12.* London: National Institute for Health and Clinical Excellence.
Northrop, M., Pittam, G. and Caan, W. (2008) The expectations of families and patterns of participation in a Trailblazer Sure Start, *Community Practitioner*, 81(2): 24–8.
Pan, W. and Bai, H. (2009) A multivariate approach to a meta-analytic review of the effectiveness of the D.A.R.E. program, *International Journal of Environmental Research and Public Health*, 6(1), 267–77.
Parent, K.B., Wodrich, D.L. and Hasan, K.S. (2009) Type 1 diabetes mellitus and school: a comparison of patients and healthy siblings, *Pediatric Diabetes*, 10(8): 554–62.

Patel, V. et al. (2007) Mental health of young people: a global public-health challenge, *The Lancet*, 369(9569): 1302–13.

Payton, J. et al. (2008) *The positive impact of social and emotional learning for kindergarten to eighth-grade students: findings from three scientific reviews*. Chicago, IL: Collaboration for Academic, Social, and Emotional Learning (CASEL).

PHSE Association (2012) *Personal Social Health and Economic Education*. London: PSHE Association. http://www.pshe-association.org.uk [accessed 24 June 2013].

Pommier, J. et al. (2010) School health promotion: organization of services and roles of health professionals in seven European countries, *European Journal of Public Health*, 20(2): 182–8.

Portwood, M.M. (1999) *Developmental dyspraxia: identification and intervention: a manual for parents and professionals*, 2nd edn. London: David Fulton.

Prevention Action (2012) *What is the lifetime cost of a child maltreatment case?* http://www.preventionaction.org [accessed 26 June 2013].

Reading, R. et al. (2009) Promotion of children's rights and prevention of child maltreatment, *The Lancet*, 373(9660): 332–43.

Richardson-Todd, B. (2003) *Multi Agency Drop in at East Bergholt High*. Colchester: East Bergholt High School.

Ringwalt, C.L. et al. (2010) The effects of Project ALERT one year past curriculum completion, *Prevention Science*, 11(2): 172–84.

Sagan, A. et al. (2011) Poland health system review, *Health Systems in Transition*, 13(8): 1–193.

Sahota, P. (2003) Obesity: an intervention in the primary school setting, *Centre for Health Promotion Research Newsletter*, 28: 1.

Salonen, P. et al. (2004) How are Finnish schoolchildren? Findings from the broad health examination among 5th graders, *Duodecim*, 120: 563–9.

Save the Children (2011) *2010: a year in review. School Health and Nutrition Program Update, 7, 1*. Westport, CT: Save the Children.

Sawyer, S.M. et al. (2007) Adolescents with a chronic condition: challenges living, challenges treating, *The Lancet*, 369(9571): 1481–9.

Schonert Reichl, K.A. et al. (2012) Promoting children's prosocial behaviors in school: impact of the "Roots of Empathy" program on the social and emotional competence of school-aged children, *School Mental Health*, 4(1): 1–21.

SDQ. Information for researchers and professionals about theStrengths & Difficulties Questionnaires. http://www.sdqinfo.com/a0.html (28 June 2013).

Schuller, T. and Desjardins, R. (2007) Chapter 5: Health Outcomes of Learning. In: OECD (ed.) *Understanding the Social Outcomes of Learning*. Paris: Centre for Educational Research and Innovation, Organisation for Economic Co-operation and Development.

Sermier Dessemontet, R. and Bless, G. (2013) The impact of including children with intellectual disability in general education classrooms on the academic achievement of their low-, average-, and high-achieving peers, *Journal of Intellectual and Developmental Disability*, 38(1): 23–30.

Sigmund, E., El Ansari, W. and Sigmundová, D. (2012) Does school-based physical activity decrease overweight and obesity in children aged 6–9 years? A two-year non-randomized longitudinal intervention study in the Czech Republic, *BMC Public Health*, 12: 570.

Slingerland, M., Borghouts, L.B. and Hesselink, M.K. (2012) Physical activity energy expenditure in Dutch adolescents: contribution of active transport to school, physical education, and leisure time activities, *Journal of School Health*, 82(5): 225–32.

Snyder, F. J. et al. (2012) Improving elementary school quality through the use of a social-emotional and character development program: a matched-pair, cluster-randomized, controlled trial in Hawaii, *J Sch Health*, 82(1): 11–20.
South Leeds NHS Primary Care Trust and Leeds City Council (2003) Teenage Health Bus. Executive Summary. Leeds: South Leeds PCT.
St James-Roberts, I. and Samlal Singh, C. (2001) *Can mentors help primary school children with behaviour problems? Final report of the three-year evaluation of Project CHANCE carried out by the Thomas Coram Research Unit between March 1997 and 2000.Home Office Research Study 233*. London: Home Office.
Steptoe, A. et al. (2011) Educational attainment but not measures of current socioeconomic circumstances are associated with leukocyte telomere length in healthy older men and women, *Brain Behav Immun*, 25(7): 1292–8.
Stewart-Brown, S. (2006) *What is the evidence on school health promotion in improving health or preventing disease and, specifically, what is the effectiveness of the health promoting schools approach?* Copenhagen: WHO Regional Office for Europe (Health Evidence Network report).
Stewart, J. (1911) Medical inspection of schools: report to the Canadian medical association, *Canadian Medical Association Journal*, 1(5), 425–39.
Stickler, G.B. (2000) Are yearly physical examinations in adolescents necessary? *Journal of the American Board of Family Practice*, 13(3): 172–7.
Streng, I. (2009) Using therapeutic board games to promote child mental health, *Journal of Public Mental Health*, 7(4): 4–16.
Strid, O. (1996) From health examination to school health. A study of health examinations of 6th graders in Lappeenranta in 1996: (in Finnish) Aiheita 28/1996. Helsinki Stakes.
Thomson, K. et al. (2007) Health facilitation in primary care seen from practice and education, *British Journal of Nursing*, 16(18): 1156–60.
Torvik, F.A. et al. (2011) Parental alcohol use and adolescent school adjustment in the general population: results from the HUNT study, *BMC Public Health*, 11: 706.
Tylee, A. et al. (2007) Youth-friendly primary-care services: how are we doing and what more needs to be done? *The Lancet*, 369(9572): 1565–73.
United Nations World Food Programme (2010) *Global Mapping of Initiatives in School Health and Nutrition, with Emphasis on Health Education*. Rome: World Food Programme.
Wade, T.J. et al. (2008) Improvements in health-related quality of life among school-based health center users in elementary and middle school, *Ambulatory Pediatrics*, 8(4): 241–9.
Wadsworth, M.E. (1997) Health inequalities in the life course perspective, *Social Science and Medicine*, 44(6): 859–69.
Wang, L.Y. et al. (2003) Economic analysis of a school-based obesity prevention program, *Obesity Research*, 11(11): 1313–24.
Weare, K. and Nind, M. (2011) Mental health promotion and problem prevention in schools: what does the evidence say? *Health Promotion International*, 26(Suppl 1): i29–69.
Weichselbaum, E. and Buttriss, J. (2011) Nutrition, health and schoolchildren, *Nutrition Bulletin*, 36(3): 295–355.
West, S.L. and O'Neal, K.K. (2004) Project D.A.R.E. outcome effectiveness revisited, *American Journal of Public Health*, 94(6): 1027–9.
WHO (1997) *Promoting Health Through Schools*. Technical Report Series 870. Geneva: World Health Organization.
WHO (1998) *Global school health initiative. Health promoting school*. WHO/HPR/HEP/98.4. Geneva: World Health Organization.

WHO Regional Office for Europe (2008) *Inequalities in young people's health. HBSC international report from the 2005/2006 survey*. Copenhagen: WHO Regional Office for Europe.
WHO Regional Office for Europe (2010) *European Mortality Database*. Copenhagen: WHO Regional Office for Europe.
WHO (2011) *School and youth health. What is a health promoting school?* Geneva: World Health Organization. http://www.who.int/school_youth_health/gshi/hps/en/index.html [accessed 24 June 2013].
Wiegersma, P.A. (1999) *Long-term effects of preventive activities of youth health care for schoolchildren in The Netherlands*. Nijmegen: University of Nijmegen.
Wiegersma, P.A., Hofman, A. and Zielhuis, G.A. (1999) Prevention of suicide by youth health care, *Public Health*, 113(3): 125–30.
Wiegersma, P.A., Hofman, A. and Zielhuis, G.A. (2000) Prevention of unhealthy behaviour by youth health care in The Netherlands, *Journal of Public Health Medicine*, 22(3): 386–92.
Wiegersma, P.A., Hofman, A. and Zielhuis, G.A. (2001) Evaluation of community-wide interventions: the ecologic case-referent study design, *European Journal of Epidemiology*, 17(6): 551–7.
Wilson, J. and Jungner, G. (1968) *Principles and practice of screening for disease*. Geneva: World Health Organization.
Wiss, K. et al. (2007) Human resources of school health care in Finnish comprehensive schools, *Suomen Lääkärilehti*, 62: 53–9.
Yankenauer, A. and Lawrence, A. (1955) A study of periodic school medical examinations. I. Methodology and initial findings, *American Journal of Public Health*, 45(1): 71–8.
Zielhuis, G.A. (1985) *Preconditions for scientific research in school health care*. Nijmegen: University of Nijmegen.

chapter seven

Young people's health and health services

Rose Crowley, Jasmine Armour-Marshall, Ingrid Wolfe

"We cannot always build the future for our youth, but we can build our youth for the future."

Franklin D. Roosevelt

Introduction

Adolescent health has received comparatively little attention in the field of child health, which itself is a minority interest in population health and in health services research. This inequity is particularly striking because most indicators of health among Europe's adolescents have remained stable or worsened in recent decades, while most child health indicators have improved substantially. Adolescents have historically received few targeted health services and have risked getting lost in the gap between paediatric and adult-oriented provisions. There is growing recognition of the need to provide suitable services for the increasing number of children with chronic health conditions surviving into adolescence and making the transition to adulthood. See Chapters 3 and 4 for further discussion about chronic disease care and transition services. All young people also need access to services targeted to their specific health needs, including sexual and reproductive health and the promotion of mental well-being.

Adolescence is a key time in which adult health behaviours – including smoking, alcohol and drug use – can develop, but progress in optimizing health during this period has been hindered by an historical focus on single issues. The classic vertical systems approach ignores the connectedness of physical and mental health, and the interaction between education, health behaviours and environment. See also Chapter 6 for further information about school health services for young people. The epidemiological risk factors underpinning many issues of particular importance during adolescence – accidental injury, risk-taking behaviour, alcohol and substance use – are increasingly being recognized. However exploratory behaviours are part of normal behaviour in adolescence. Young people are too often subject to negative stereotypes and the perception that their health or social problems are self-inflicted or that it is 'just a stage' they are going through. By contrast, the life-course approach highlights the key importance of adolescent health as a determinant of, or window of opportunity for, building adult health (Sawyer et al., 2012).

Setting the context

Adolescence is a time of profound physical and emotional change. It is a time when young people are learning to exert an independent identity and to take responsibility for some of their own health needs. They may feel reluctant to engage with adult health services, but equally not feel catered for in settings designed for infants and children. Health promotion in adolescence is particularly important, because lifelong health behaviours, such as smoking, may be established in these years. Indeed, it has been estimated that up to 70% of premature deaths in adulthood are linked to behaviours started during adolescence (WHO, 2009). See Chapter 5 for more detailed discussion of risk factors for disease, and public health interventions. Health promotion can be challenging, given the important role of peer and social groups in young people's lives, who often prove more influential than health professionals. The communication skills needed to engage with adolescents, who are trying to make decisions about their health while their abstract reasoning skills are not yet fully developed, differ from those needed for communicating with younger children or with adults. Health professionals may feel ill-prepared to communicate with adolescents, as many will have had little exposure to adolescent medicine during paediatric or primary care training.

Although young people are often healthy, they have specific health needs that are distinct to those of younger children. They are more likely to engage in exploratory and risk-taking behaviour and suffer injuries; their emotional ell-being may be compromised by difficulties with family, peers or educational/vocational transitions; they are likely to initiate sexual relationships and experiment with drugs and alcohol. Disorders such as chronic fatigue syndrome and eating disorders increase greatly in prevalence during adolescence, and require specific expertise not usually incorporated in paediatric or primary care training. Carving out an independent identity means establishing more equal relationships with adults; in the health sector, this can bring unique challenges, for example, in the ethics of sexual and reproductive health and issues regarding consent and confidentiality. Furthermore, young people may give preference to enhancing well-being rather than avoiding risks and have a different understanding of the relative importance of short- and long-term gains. The risk-taking behaviours that many young people engage in reflect a distinct developmental stage, as they are developing abstract reasoning skills, testing boundaries and establishing their unique identity.

Adolescence poses a particular challenge for young people with chronic health conditions, due to the physical, social and psychological changes they are undergoing. For example, the physiological changes brought about by puberty may pose challenges for glycaemic control in those with diabetes mellitus or increase seizure frequency in those with epilepsy. Lifestyle factors – such as alcohol and drug use, irregular meals and sleeping patterns – may prove challenging for those with chronic health conditions, who may not wish to stand out from their peers by adhering to a rigid medication schedule. Conflicts between young people and their parents, or a wish to rebel against authority figures, may be played out as refusal to adhere to health regimes. Health services therefore need to be well attuned to the needs of young people, and to focus on making them feel listened-to, involved and respected (Hargreaves, 2011).

Assessing the challenges: needs and trends

Adolescence is often considered to be a time of good health and adolescent health has received comparatively little attention in comparison to that focused on younger children. It is increasingly recognized, however, that adolescents have benefited significantly less than younger children from improvements in health care over the past 50 years. Indeed, the global improvement in under-5 mortality rates has been such that mortality rates are 2 to 3 times higher in men aged 15–24 years than boys aged 1–4 years, while death rates for girls in both age groups are equal (Viner et al., 2011).

A significant quantity of information on morbidity and related socioeconomic factors amongst European adolescents is provided by the Health and Behaviour in School-aged Children (HBSC) study, conducted every 4 years across 43 regions of Europe and North America (HBSC, 2012). See also Chapter 5. The questionnaire is limited by the fact that it surveys only 11, 13 and 15-year-olds, and depends upon self-reported data. However, it provides useful information from a very large number of young people, using a questionnaire that is standardized between countries and indicators that have been mapped over time, giving data on Europe that is more comprehensive than for many other regions of the world (Patton et al., 2012). The report of the most recent study (2009/10) has again highlighted the importance of the social determinants of adolescent health; the relevance of family affluence; and the appropriateness of the life-course approach (Currie et al., 2012).

In addition to the management of long-term health conditions in adolescence and transition to adult care (see Chapter 4), and the importance of mental health and well-being (see Chapter 8), there are a number of particular issues affecting adolescents and their health services that warrant further discussion and are covered next in this chapter.

Obesity

Obesity is increasing in prevalence across Europe (International Obesity Task Force, 2004), and increasing numbers of adolescents and young adults are suffering from complications, such as the metabolic syndrome, hypertension and type 2 diabetes mellitus. Although many obese young people will have become overweight in childhood, adolescence can be a critical period for the development of health behaviours that contribute to obesity, including more sedentary behaviour and changes in diet (Alberga et al., 2012). Such health behaviours often persist into early adulthood and beyond, having a significant impact on adult health (Bertheke Post et al., 2001). The HELENA study (Healthy Lifestyle in Europe by Nutrition in Adolescence cross-sectional study) has involved thousands of adolescents across ten European countries, and recorded nutritional status, eating behaviour, physical activity, body composition and metabolic profile (Santaliestra-Pasias et al., 2012). Known socioeconomic gradients in lifestyle behaviours (including physical, diet, alcohol and smoking) that contribute to inequalities in health outcomes in adulthood, are likely to be reinforced during adolescence. A number of preventive programmes in Europe, involving interventions aimed at the general adolescent population using health education, environmental interventions or policies, are currently being evaluated in the TEENAGE project (van Lenthe et al., 2009). See Chapter 5 for more discussion on obesity.

Injuries

The significant contribution that injuries make to death and disability amongst young people worldwide is well established (Patton et al., 2009) and injuries are still the leading cause of death in the European Region for those aged 10 to 24 years. The majority of these are due to road traffic accidents, the risk of which is greatly increased in lower or middle-income countries (Morrison and Stone, 2000). Far from being random, unpredictable events, there are established risk factors for accidents, providing important opportunities for public health intervention (Gore et al., 2011). Poverty, poor housing, having a single parent, low maternal age or education, large family size and parental drug/alcohol abuse all increase the risk of sustaining a fatal injury (Sethi et al., 2006). See Chapter 5 for further detail on the scale of the problem and on strategies for reducing injury.

Alcohol use

Alcohol use amongst young people is increasing in many European countries, yet the risk and protective factors for this and associated behaviours (risk-taking and substance use) are not clearly established. The ongoing AAA-Prevent study is investigating the epidemiology of alcohol use across 26 European countries, including individual, social and country-level risk factors (Alcohol Abuse among Adolescents in Europe, 2012). HBSC data from 77,586 adolescents confirmed significant differences between eastern and western European countries in the longitudinal pattern of teenage drunkenness. Between 1997/8 and 2005/6, the mean frequency of drunkenness increased by 40% in all seven eastern European countries involved, while it decreased by an average of 25% in western European countries (Kuntsche et al., 2011). In the 2009/10 data, gender differences are still apparent, with boys more likely to report drunkenness and earlier age at initiation of drinking. See Chapter 5 for further information on the scale of the problems with alcohol and young people, and interventions to prevent and reduce alcohol misuse.

Sexual and reproductive health

Supporting sexual and reproductive health, providing access to contraception and the prevention of teenage pregnancy have become key aspects of adolescent health services in many European countries. Yet, enormous variations in access to sexual health services exist, as do levels of knowledge among young people. Comparing indicators of sexual and reproductive health (including age of first sexual activity, condom use, rates of teenage pregnancy and STIs) is complicated by the variation in age ranges and indicators between countries, and the large reliance on self-report surveys such as the HBSC (Avery and Lazdane, 2008).

However, certain patterns are clear from the available evidence. The age of first sexual intercourse has been declining for a number of decades, and the gap between genders has narrowed; by the age of 15 years old, 24% of girls and 30% of boys are sexually active (WHO Regional Office for Europe, 2008). Condoms are the most widely used contraceptive amongst young people in Europe, with oral contraceptive use being much greater amongst girls in western than eastern Europe. The rate of abortion varies substantially, with eastern Europe having much higher rates than any other area of Europe. This has been linked to lack of availability and the high cost of other contraceptive options (Sedgh et al., 2007). The most widely tracked STIs are Chlamydia, gonorrhoea, syphilis and HIV. Of these, Chlamydia has shown a significant increase in many countries (although this is partly attributable to increased detection), while gonorrhoea has shown a less significant increase, limited to only a few countries (European Centre for Disease Prevention and Control, 2011).

The rate of teenage pregnancy varies from approximately 12 per 1000 women aged 15–19 years in Italy to 64 per 1000 in the Russian Federation, with generally lower rates in western Europe, other than in the United Kingdom (Avery and Lazdane, 2008). The consequences of unwanted teenage pregnancy can be profound; having a child while still a teenager is associated with increased risk of disadvantage in later life, including a doubling of the risk of living in poverty, worsening of socioeconomic inequalities and increased risk of social exclusion (Paranjothy et al., 2009). Teenage mothers are less likely to complete education and training and, since teenage pregnancy is more common in lower socioeconomic groups, it may perpetuate an intergenerational cycle of poverty.

Youth-friendly services

Our increasing understanding of the distinct health needs of adolescents, and their unique developmental context, has resulted in attempts across many

European countries to design health services that are 'youth-friendly', in design, accessibility and delivery. This has been interpreted in a range of ways, but a key underlying principle is that young people are encouraged to become involved in shaping services, rather than services being imposed on them by others. Such an approach is underpinned by Article 12 of the United Nations 'Convention on the Rights of the Child', which states that 'the child who is capable of forming his or her own views' has the 'right to express those views freely' with 'the views of the child being given due weight'. It is clear that involving young people in decision-making improves engagement and health outcomes (de Winter, Baerveldt and Kooistra, 1999) and it is proposed that involving them in the development of the services they use will enhance this. There is also increasing use of patient satisfaction as a quality outcome in health services, although a recent United Kingdom review concluded that children and young people have only rarely been included in patient satisfaction surveys to date (Hargreaves and Viner, 2012).

WHO has identified five key attributes of adolescent responsive health services (WHO, 2013):

- **Accessible**: where and when services are provided should suit adolescents' needs. Opportunities to access them without parents, if preferred.
- **Acceptable**: adolescents should be assured that privacy and confidentiality will be maintained, and they should be offered choices and an open discussion.
- **Appropriate**: treatment should be suited to adolescents' needs, evidence-based and up-to-date.
- **Effective**: outcomes should be measured and make a positive contribution to adolescent health.
- **Equitable**: services should not be affected by ability to pay, ethnicity, sexuality or gender.

In the United Kingdom, the targets for adolescent-friendly services have been further developed into the 'You're Welcome' quality criteria, which provide standards for youth-friendly services across ten key areas:

- accessibility
- publicity
- confidentiality and consent
- environment
- staff training, skills, attitudes and values
- joined-up working
- young people's involvement in monitoring and evaluation of patient experience
- health issues for young people
- sexual and reproductive health services
- specialist child and adolescent mental health services (CAMHS).

The criteria have been formalized into a self-assessment toolkit that services can use to assess and improve how youth-friendly they are. Interpretation of the various facets has varied; for example, some regions of the United Kingdom have increased accessibility by offering 'no worries' appointments, in which the school can authorize a young person to miss school to attend a doctor's appointment, without parental knowledge. Clinics may open in the evening or at weekends, so young people do not need to miss school. Mobile 'drop-in' sexual health services, which provide services in a location convenient to them, have proved popular with many young people (Box 7.1).

Box 7.1 The 4YP sexual health outreach bus for young people

4YP is a sexual health outreach bus for young people in London, taking information, advice and contraception services to young people in accessible places in the community. Young people set the agenda, asking questions on all aspects of sexual health, from puberty and body changes to relationships, peer pressure, sex, contraception, STIs, and where to go for more help. They can access free condoms, most forms of contraception, pregnancy testing, Chlamydia screening and treatment.

'People are able to talk freely on the bus without embarrassment.'

Since the project was launched in 2001, in one area of London, it has been extremely popular with young people, particularly boys and young men. In its first year, the 4YP bus had 3142 visits from young people, 59% of whom were young men and 64% from black and minority ethnic groups. Boys and young men accounted for 76% of visits to the bus in 2009/10. Young men have traditionally been seen as 'hard to reach', although the experience of the 4YP bus has revealed a huge appetite amongst young men for a safe and trusted place where they can get unbiased information and advice without fear of judgement.

'This is good because it comes to the places that I hang out.'

Rather than seeing particular groups of young people as 'hard to reach', 4YP embraces the idea that it is often health services themselves that are hard to reach. 4YP targets those groups of young people who do not always access health services readily, such as young men, particularly young black men and those from minority ethnic groups, young offenders, looked-after young people and those leaving care.

'I prefer to come to the bus for advice as no one else knows your business here, because it's all out of school and that. It's all about you here.'

4YP is a branded identity that is recognized by young people locally as indicating a service that is confidential and will welcome them. The 4YP 'brand' is shared by a range of local sexual health services for young people, including young people's sexual health clinics, drop-ins and the 4YP pharmacy (emergency contraception in pharmacies) scheme.

'Here you can come and talk to someone that's not your parents and not your friends either as there are some things you don't even want to share with your friends.'

The approach of the staff on the 4YP bus is to make young people feel welcome and to encourage them to ask whatever questions they have without fear of judgement. When giving information, staff aim to give it in non-didactic ways, in language that the young people understand, and in ways that relate to their experiences.

'There's no way I could get this kind of advice at home. My parents would just say "don't", and at school the advice isn't this practical. I just don't want to get anyone pregnant.'

The emphasis is on encouraging young people to make informed choices by answering their questions, allowing them time to discuss their concerns and not by telling them what to do.

'[At 4YP] they tell you everything, if you are going to have sex then think about it, use protection. At school they just tell you all the bad stuff and that just becomes really boring so you just switch off and don't listen.'

Note: For further information, see www.shharingey.co.uk.
Source: Harriet Yudkin, personal communication.

Routine health services can be co-located with sexual health, drug and alcohol, mental health and employment services, to provide a 'one-stop shop' that encourages adolescents to access all the health and vocational services they need, and promote a holistic understanding of adolescents.

Young people have repeatedly cited the attitude of health professionals as being central to their satisfaction with health services, and there have been a number of attempts to improve training in adolescent health and communication skills. Curricula include the EuTEACH programme (EuTEACH, 2013) and an e-learning package developed by the RCPCH in the United Kingdom (e-learning for Healthcare, 2013). The HEADSS screening tool, which offers a standardized framework for communicating with adolescents, incorporates techniques for raising sensitive subjects and assessing risk (for example, of suicidality) (Cohen, Mackenzie and Yates, 1991).

Young people's health services: the European experience

A 2009 analysis of the provision of adolescent health care across Europe (Ercan et al., 2009) identified significant differences in practice, with regard to the upper age limit of paediatric care (from 14 to 17 years); the training provided (undergraduate or postgraduate, the latter being within paediatric or general practice training); and whether or not adolescent medicine was a recognized subspecialty. The questionnaire survey conducted for this book identified broadly similar themes, as well as significant diversity of opinion with regard to the provision of sexual health services, contraception, consent and confidentiality, and the development of specific adolescent inpatient or outpatient facilities. The varied role played by school health services in different countries, in both health promotion and routine health care, was also evident. It was notable that a number of respondents reported that mental health services had overtaken other services in the development of specific adolescent provision.

Training

Adolescent medicine is recognized as a subspecialty in its own right in Italy, while in most countries, particular training or a special interest is available for general paediatricians in this area (Austria, France, Israel, Netherlands, Norway, Poland, Scotland and Sweden). By contrast, adolescent psychiatry is a separate specialty mentioned by Finland, Poland and Scotland, the respondent for the latter commenting that 'mental health services are probably setting the pace in this direction'.

Adolescent inpatient facilities

A few countries have developed adolescent-only inpatient wards in some areas (e.g. Austria, England and France) but provision is very patchy. This finding is supported by a recent review of the development of adolescent wards in the United Kingdom and Australia (Payne et al., 2012), which highlighted a move towards the inclusion of adolescent wards in designing new-build hospitals, while only a minority of existing facilities have either dedicated wards or separate bays within paediatric wards. The respondents from Finland, Israel and Scotland reported there are more adolescent-only wards available in psychiatric services.

School health services

School health services play an important role in routine adolescent health care in Finland, Sweden, the Netherlands and parts of Norway. Elsewhere, adolescents receiving routine health care will attend paediatric clinics or be seen within primary care. Health promotion is an important component of school health services; a comparative analysis of seven European countries identified significant international differences in the way health promotion was provided (whether community-based, school-based or focused) and whether health professionals were permanently located in schools (Pommier et al., 2010). Many respondents cited schools as being of key importance in primary prevention of teenage pregnancies (Austria, Finland, Israel, Italy, Poland, Sweden and Scotland). Sex education is integrated within the school curricula in all countries, with a variable contribution by teachers, school nurses and doctors. None of the respondents mentioned preventive mental health programmes in schools or strategies to reduce bullying and promote emotional resilience, although these have been recommended in many countries (European Pact for Mental Health and Well-being, 2013). Chapter 6 covers school health services in greater detail, Chapter 5 discusses public health, and Chapter 8 provides detailed information about mental health in children and young people.

Sexual health services

Adolescent sexual health services were reported as being provided within routine adult genitourinary medicine (France, Italy, Isle of Man, Poland,

Scotland); as a separate adolescent service within adult services (Austria, Norway, Sweden); or within the school health services (Finland). In the Netherlands, a group separate from routine health services, but funded by the Ministry of Health, Welfare and Sports, provides adolescent-specific services.

Countries or regions vary in whether adolescents are charged fully for contraception (Italy), pay a reduced price (Israel, Sweden), or are not charged (France, Isle of Man, Scotland). In Finland, it is nationally recommended that contraception is free for the under-20s, although there is significant variation between municipalities. In Poland, natural family planning is reported to be the preferred method. The morning-after pill is available in Italy for those over 14 years of age. All countries that gave a clear response to the question answered that abortions are available to adolescents, and that illegal abortions are thought to be a rare occurrence.

Screening for STIs varies between entities, but no country reported a well-established adolescent-specific screening programme. In Italy, the adult screening programme is open to adolescents as well, while in Scotland and England there is screening available to under-25s for Chlamydia (including significant attempts to improve accessibility, such as a self-test kit that can be ordered online without attending a sexual health clinic) (National Health Service, 2013). Austria, France, Israel, the Isle of Man, Poland and Sweden reported no STI screening, while in Finland any adolescent who requests contraception should be screened for Chlamydia, and the Netherlands is also considering a Chlamydia screening programme. Our respondent from the Netherlands also described free vaccination of 12-year-olds against HPV to protect against cervical cancer. A 2009 report highlighted disparity in HPV vaccine provision, with only nine European countries offering it free, and three more requiring a co-payment (European Cervical Cancer Association, 2009). In the remainder of countries, it is available only in the private sector.

Confidentiality and consent

A key component of sexual health programmes for adolescents is confidentiality, which has repeatedly been cited by adolescents as an important issue when they access any health service. Policies vary widely: at one extreme, parents are automatically informed of an adolescent's attendance (Austria, Israel); at the other, it is guaranteed the consultation will remain confidential (Finland). In the United Kingdom and the Netherlands, the specific adolescent's age and ability to consent is assessed and a decision taken at an individual level, for example, using the Fraser guidelines (Great Britain Court of Appeal, 1985). The Israeli respondent highlighted the paradox that adolescents require parental consent to access contraceptives, yet can consent to an abortion without parental involvement.

Youth-friendly services

A number of respondents highlighted a lack of services targeted specifically towards adolescents, echoing the growing recognition of the importance of youth-friendly services across Europe. Our French respondent summarized this: 'We have a lot to do about adolescent medicine . . . There are few settings dedicated to adolescents, needs are growing.' The Scottish representative similarly reported that 'adolescents have access to the full range of NHS services but there are few specific services designed to meet their particular needs'.

Such responses marry with the report of a 2009 WHO meeting which compared approaches to youth-friendly services across Europe, highlighting individual examples of good practice but very patchy provision. Delegates described the challenges to providing youth-friendly services in geographically, economically and ethnically heterogeneous populations across nine European countries (Georgia, the Republic of Moldova, Portugal, the Russian Federation, Sweden, Switzerland, the former Yugoslav Republic of Macedonia, Ukraine and the United Kingdom) (WHO Regional Office for Europe, 2010).

Future challenges

Adolescent health services in Europe face significant financial challenges, with many having their budgets reduced at the same time as ever greater numbers of young people are being subjected to increasing economic disadvantage. The number of young people not in education, employment or training (NEET) has increased across Europe, with an estimated 7.5 million young people currently in that category (European Foundation for the Improvement of Working and Living Conditions, 2011). Such young people are likely to face multiple disadvantages, being more likely to have a disability, to be an immigrant and have a low education level. All of these factors combine with the socioeconomic and psychological consequences of unemployment to put them at significant risk of disenfranchisement, physical and mental ill health. A review of the impact of both structural and proximal determinants of health on adolescents highlighted the negative consequences of income inequality and unemployment on young people (although there are few comparative data available for the latter) (Viner et al., 2012). Employment and education policies must take into account the vulnerability of adolescent health to these broader influences.

Adolescents exist in a network of family, peer, community and structural influences. Understanding how risk factors for certain behaviours cluster together to create a subgroup of young people most likely to engage in risky behaviour or come into contact with mental health or criminal justice systems, can help us to target preventive health measures towards those who may benefit most. For example, a study of almost 70,000 women in the Nordic countries demonstrated an association between early initiation of smoking (<15 years), risk-taking sexual behaviours and adverse reproductive events (such as teenage pregnancy and STIs), suggesting a group that might benefit from targeted interventions (Hansen et al., 2010). Epidemiological data can also identify which protective factors may foster resilience in young people, strengthening family, school and community responses (WHO, 2002). The challenge now is to identify which interventions, in both childhood and adolescence, are effective (Catalano et al., 2012), and how they can be integrated into existing universal and targeted services to improve adolescent – and future adult – health.

Action at European regional level can do much to encourage efforts in strengthening research efforts and improving the quality of services for young people.

References

Alberga, A.S. et al. (2012) Overweight and obese teenagers: why is adolescence a critical period? *Pediatric Obesity*, 7(4): 261–73.

Alcohol Abuse among Adolescents in Europe (2012) *Effective Environmental Strategies for Prevention*. http://www.aaaprevent.eu [accessed 24 June 2013].

Avery, L. and Lazdane, G. (2008) What do we know about sexual and reproductive health of adolescents in Europe? *European Journal of Contraception and Reproductive Health Care*, 13(1): 58–70.

Bertheke Post, G. et al. (2001) Longitudinal trends in and tracking of energy and nutrient intake over 20 years in a Dutch cohort of men and women between 13 and 33 years of age: The Amsterdam growth and health longitudinal study, *British Journal of Nutrition*, 85(3): 375–85.

Catalano, R.F. et al. (2012) Worldwide application of prevention science in adolescent health, *The Lancet*, 379(9826): 1653–64.

Cohen, E., Mackenzie, R.G. and Yates, G.L. (1991) HEADSS, a psychosocial risk assessment instrument: implications for designing effective intervention programs for runaway youth, *Journal of Adolescent Health*, 12(7): 539–44.

Currie, C. et al. (eds) (2012) *Health Policy for Children and Adolescents, No 6. Social determinants of health and well-being among young people. Health Behaviour in School-aged Children (HBSC) study. International Report from the 2009–10 Survey*. Copenhagen: WHO Regional Office for Europe.

de Winter, M., Baerveldt, C. and Kooistra, J. (1999) Enabling children: participation as a new perspective on child-health promotion, *Child: Care, Health and Development*, 25(1): 15–23; discussion 23–5.

e-learning for Healthcare (2013) *Adolescent Health*. http://www.e-lfh.org.uk/projects/ah/index.html [accessed 24 June 2013].

Ercan, O. al. (2009) Demography of adolescent health care delivery and training in Europe, *European Journal of Pediatrics*, 168(4): 417–26.

European Centre for Disease Prevention and Control (2011) *Annual epidemiological report on communicable diseases in Europe*. Stockholm: European Centre for Disease Prevention and Control.

ECCA (2009) *HPV Vaccination Across Europe*. Brussels: European Cervical Cancer Association.

European Foundation for the Improvement of Working and Living Conditions (2011) *Young people and NEETs in Europe: first findings*. Dublin: European Foundation for the Improvement of Working and Living Conditions.

European Pact for Mental Health and Well-being (2013) http://ec-mental-health-process.net [accessed 24 June 2013].

EuTEACH (2013) *European training in effective adolescent care and health*. http://www.unil.ch/euteach [accessed 24 June 2013].

Gore, F.M. et al. (2011) Global burden of disease in young people aged 10–24 years: a systematic analysis, *The Lancet*, 377(9783): 2093–102.

Great Britain Court of Appeal (1985) *Re Gillick v West Norfolk and Wisbech Area Health Authority [1985] 3 All ER 402HL.*

Hansen, B.T. et al. (2010) Early smoking initiation, sexual behavior and reproductive health – a large population-based study of Nordic women, *Preventive Medicine*, 51(1): 68–72.

Hargreaves, D.S. (2011) Revised You're Welcome criteria and future developments in adolescent healthcare, *Journal of Clinical Research in Pediatric Endocrinology*, 3(2): 43–50.

Hargreaves, D.S. and Viner, R.M. (2012) Children's and young people's experience of the National Health Service in England: a review of national surveys 2001–2011, *Archives of Disease in Childhood*, 97(7): 661–6.

HBSC (2013) *Health Behaviour in School-Aged Children.* http://www.hbsc.org [accessed 24 June 2013].

IOTF (2004) *EU childhood obesity "out of control": Childhood Obesity Report.* London: International Obesity Task Force.

Kuntsche, E. et al. (2011) Cultural and gender convergence in adolescent drunkenness: evidence from 23 European and North American countries, *Archives of Pediatrics and Adolescent Medicine*, 165(2): 152–8.

Morrison, A. and Stone, D.H. (2000) Trends in injury mortality among young people in the European Union: a report from the EURORISC working group, *Journal of Adolescent Health*, 27(2): 130–5.

National Health Service (2013) *Checkurself.* https://www.checkurself.org.uk [accessed 24 June 2013].

Paranjothy, S. et al. (2009) Teenage pregnancy: who suffers? *Archives of Disease in Childhood*, 94(3): 239–45.

Patton, G.C. et al. (2012) Health of the world's adolescents: a synthesis of internationally comparable data, *The Lancet*, 379(9826): 1665–75.

Patton, G.C. et al. (2009) Global patterns of mortality in young people: a systematic analysis of population health data, *The Lancet*, 374(9693): 881–92.

Payne, D. et al. (2012) Developing and running an adolescent inpatient ward, *Archives of Disease in Childhood – Education and Practice*, 97(2): 42–7.

Pommier, J. et al. (2010) School health promotion: organization of services and roles of health professionals in seven European countries, *European Journal of Public Health*, 20(2): 182–8.

Santaliestra-Pasias, A.M. et al. (2012) Food consumption and screen-based sedentary behaviors in European adolescents: the HELENA study, *Archives of Pediatrics and Adolescent Medicine*, 166(11): 1010–20.

Sawyer, S.M. et al. (2012) Adolescence: a foundation for future health, *The Lancet*, 379(9826): 1630–40.

Sedgh, G. et al. (2007) Induced abortion: estimated rates and trends worldwide, *The Lancet*, 370(9595): 1338–45.

Sethi, D. et al. (2006) *Injuries and violence in Europe: why they matter and what can be done.* Copenhagen: WHO Regional Office for Europe.

van Lenthe, F.J. et al. (2009) Preventing socioeconomic inequalities in health behaviour in adolescents in Europe: background, design and methods of project TEENAGE, *BMC Public Health*, 9: 125.

Viner, R.M. et al. (2011) 50-year mortality trends in children and young people: a study of 50 low-income, middle-income, and high-income countries, *The Lancet*, 377(9772): 1162–74.

Viner, R.M. et al. (2012) Adolescence and the social determinants of health, *The Lancet*, 379(9826): 1641–52.

WHO (2002) *Broadening the horizon: balancing protection and risk for adolescents.* Geneva: World Health Organization.

WHO Regional Office for Europe (2008) *Inequalities in young people's health. HBSC international report from the 2005/2006 survey*. Copenhagen: WHO Regional Office for Europe.

WHO (2009) *Global health risks: mortality and burden of disease attributable to selected major risks*. Geneva: World Health Organization.

WHO Regional Office for Europe (2010) *Youth-friendly health policies and services in the European region: Sharing experiences*, Copenhagen: WHO Regional Office for Europe.

WHO (2013) *Maternal, newborn, child and adolescent health*. http://www.who.int/maternal_child_adolescent/topics/adolescence/health_services/en [accessed 24 June 2013].

chapter eight

Mental health and behavioural disorders

Rose Crowley, Rittakerttu Kaltia-Heino, Sebastian Kraemer

"What is a normal child like? Does he just eat and grow and smile sweetly? No, that is not what he is like. The normal child, if he has confidence in mother and father, pulls out all the stops. In the course of time, he tries out his power to disrupt, to destroy, to frighten, to wear down, to waffle, to wangle, and to appropriate . . . At the start he absolutely needs to live in a circle of love and strength (with consequent tolerance) if he is not to be too fearful of his own thoughts and of his imaginings to make progress in his emotional development."

DW Winnicot (1896–1971)
Paediatrician and psychoanalyst

Introduction

Mental health and behavioural conditions affect a large number of children and young people across Europe, providing a considerable challenge for paediatric, psychiatric and primary care services. Emotional or behavioural disorders affect one in five young people in Europe, while mental health conditions affect one in eight (Braddick et al., 2009). The range of conditions and health services that need to be addressed under the term 'mental health' is broad: from young children with emotional disorders to adolescents with psychosis or those who self-harm or misuse substances. The detection and management of such a variety of disorders requires the integration of paediatric and psychiatric input with education and welfare services, making this a particularly complex area of service provision.

The impact of child mental health disorders is profound, contributing a quarter of the DALYs associated with NCDs and disorders in western European children and young people (Lim et al., 2012). See Chapter 1 for further information about the burden of childhood disease and disability. Mental disorders directly impair quality of life and can threaten the acquisition of social, educational and vocational skills during crucial periods of childhood and adolescent development. This has lifelong consequences for individuals and, on a wider scale, threatens countries' economic productivity and social cohesion. The importance of child mental health in adulthood is profound: the majority of major adult mental health disorders have their onset during childhood and adolescence (Rutter, Kim-Cohen and Maughan, 2006), making detection and intervention during this period crucial; while adverse childhood conditions, particularly those involving maladaptive family functioning, account for almost 30% of adult mental health disorders worldwide (Kessler et al., 2010).

There is a persuasive economic argument for governments to increase funding for and awareness of child mental health services, in that effective programmes may drastically reduce the long-term costs to the state. These disorders have far-reaching consequences for individuals, families and wider society, and failure to address them results in significant costs to health, social and criminal justice systems in adult life, which could be avoided by effective prevention and treatment. One of the major difficulties in persuading governments to invest is that such savings may take many electoral terms to become apparent, and long-term follow-up is needed to determine which programmes are cost-effective. There is also a widespread view, not borne out by the facts, that children will 'get over it'. Moreover, most children with mental disorders look, and often are, physically healthy. The younger the child, the harder it is for busy policy-makers to contemplate and comprehend his or her mental pain.

This chapter will outline the existing data about the prevalence of mental health disorders across the European region, the difficulties in establishing these figures, and what evidence there is that mental disorders are increasing. The responses to the 'Child Health Services and Systems in Europe' survey conducted for this book will then be considered, focusing particularly on the interaction between paediatric and psychiatric services in both community and inpatient settings, and the fundamental role of the education sector in screening for and the promotion of positive mental health. The needs of adolescent patients are particularly challenging, as they often fall between the provision for children and that for adults, and risk being treated in facilities not suited to their stage of development. See Chapter 7 for further discussion about young people's health. Governments need to develop coherent policies that integrate health, welfare and education for the prevention and management of mental disorders in young people. The impact of changing family structures, immigration, inequality and social exclusion on such disorders also needs to be addressed in service provision across the region.

Overview of the issues

Before determining the issues that currently affect child mental health services in Europe, it is necessary to define what is meant by 'mental health'. Most simplistically, it could be considered as the absence of a mental illness, such as those with internationally agreed-upon classifications in the Diagnostic and Statistical Manual of Mental Disorders (DSM-V) or International Classification of Diseases (ICD-10). More holistically, however, WHO defines it as 'a state of well-being in which the individual realizes his or her own abilities, can cope with the normal stresses of life, can work productively and fruitfully, and is able to make a contribution to his or her community' (WHO, 2004). If the latter approach is used, it is more difficult to compare the provision for mental health services between countries, as health services *per se* account for only a small proportion of efforts to tackle broader societal forces (for example, poverty, social exclusion and vulnerable parents), which are known to increase the risk of children developing mental health disorders. A great deal of mental disorder in children and young people is concealed behind social problems and disorders, such as delinquency, crime, drug abuse, homelessness, poverty, domestic and peer-to-peer violence, self-harm, promiscuity, educational failure and bullying (either as perpetrator or victim). These phenomena are, in turn, strongly associated with early disruption or breakdown in attachments with parents and other significant caregivers. Of arguably greater importance, therefore, would be the numerous programmes within education and social services that tackle psychosocial risk factors for mental illness; target high-risk groups; and foster resilience during crucial periods of child and adolescent development.

This approach can be seen in recent policies aimed at improving child mental health across Europe, which embed mental health provision firmly within broader social policy and emphasize the importance of school health. These include the 2007 WHO Forum 'Social cohesion for mental well-being among adolescents' (WHO Regional Office for Europe, 2008), the 'Mental Health Action Plan for Europe' (WHO, 2005b) and the 'European Pact on Mental Health and Well-being' (2008) (European Commission, 2008), which focused on early intervention programmes in educational settings and combating social exclusion. The lack of existing comparative data in the region is being addressed by the Child and Adolescent Mental Health in the Expanded European Union (CAMHEE) project (Braddick et al., 2009), which is collating information on existing services, identifying examples of best practice, and establishing knowledge networks to allow examples of good practice to be shared. A preliminary report on the infrastructure and evidence base from 15 countries identified wide variation in data collection between countries, making any comparison of prevalence rates problematic (Braddick et al., 2009). The three key areas the CAMHEE project will now focus on clearly illustrate the intersectoral nature of services in this area: tackling destructive patterns of behaviour in schools; parent training; and community-based approaches as an alternative to institutionalization. The latter is of particular importance in the countries of the former Soviet Union, where the institutionalization of children with behavioural problems has often led to a 'vicious circle of stigma, social exclusion and helplessness' (Braddick et al., 2009).

Next, we will consider issues related to the workforce required in order to address the needs of children with mental health problems and their families, and ways to finance the necessary services.

Workforce

Two main workforce issues need to be considered in the provision of a comprehensive child mental health service: first, adequate numbers of suitably trained specialist providers (including child psychiatrists and psychologists); and secondly, sufficient knowledge of the disorders among those most likely to first detect them (such as paediatricians, primary care practitioners, teachers and social workers). A survey, answered by specialists in child mental health across 36 European countries, revealed key areas of variation in training and availability, and the provision of very limited training in child mental health for paediatricians and primary care physicians (Table 8.1) (Levav et al., 2004).

Paediatric liaison psychiatry has a crucial role to play in supporting the mental health of children and their families, and requires the close integration of psychiatric and paediatric services. Such services not only assess children thought to be at risk of mental distress or disorder, such as those presenting after self-harm or psychiatric crisis, but also arrange early medical attention to exclude physical causes in such situations. Other important, but often neglected, roles of mental health services located in paediatric departments include: the collaborative assessment of medically unexplained symptoms (including fabricated and induced illnesses) and of younger children with attachment, feeding, eating and sleeping ('regulatory') disorders (Schmid et al., 2010); children traumatized by accidents, burns or major surgical operations; children of parents in the same hospital who are seriously ill or have died (Dowdney et al., 1999); and the families of very premature babies (Jotzo and Poets, 2005). Joint care of chronic diseases, such as asthma, diabetes, epilepsy and cancers, in all of which higher levels of mental disorder can be seen, creates a major role for mental health liaison with paediatrics (Hysing et al., 2007). In general, paediatricians tend to overlook the majority of mental problems in

Table 8.1 Provision of child mental health services

Area of provision	*Responses*
Availability of child psychiatrists	• Minimum: 0.2 per 100,000 population (Bosnia Herzegovina, Turkey) • Maximum: 33 per 100,000 (Finland) • Overall negative correlation between the income level of a country and provision
Period of training in child mental health for paediatricians and GPs	• Range: 0 to 8 weeks • Median: 0 weeks
Coverage of child services	• Consensus: Worse than adult services
Quality of child services	• Consensus: Equal to or better than adult services

Source: Levav et al., 2004

their patients, hence the need for co-located mental health staff in wards and clinics (Glazebrook et al., 2003). Psychological distress may contribute to both the causes and consequences of illness for the whole family, yet the 2008 CAMHS review in the United Kingdom highlighted a 'tendency to overlook the impact of physical illness on mental health and vice-versa' as well as lack of expertise and appropriate coordination (CAMHS, 2008). Failure to address these shortcomings may adversely affect outcomes for paediatric patients and have important financial consequences (for example, on treatment, length of stay and readmission rates). For young people with asthma, demonstrable benefits were accrued from a family therapy intervention in terms of airway inflammation, patient's adjustment to asthma, and their parents' perception of asthma management efficacy (Ng et al., 2008). A systematic review concluded that glycaemic control in diabetes mellitus can be improved by psychological interventions, while mental distress is lessened (Winkley et al., 2006). The overall financial savings when psychological programmes are used successfully in the management of chronic disease can be significant (Barlow and Ellard, 2004). Indeed, a review in the United States of the impact of involving psychiatric teams more closely in care within children's hospitals concluded that 'fiscal success was associated with [. . .] better integration of the psychiatry program within the children's hospital' (Campo et al., 2000).

Finance

Comparing the budget available for child mental health services between countries is complicated by the wide variation in funding streams. Issues include: whether there is a ring-fenced budget for child and adolescent mental health services; whether it forms a variable percentage of mental health services decided at a local level; and what funding comes from child health services and/or from primary care or indeed from other governmental authorities. In many countries, mental health service budgets are decided independently at regional or federal level from their allocation for health care in general, with surprisingly little aggregate data available. Analysing spending within the health service will also fail to take into account the widely varying proportion of education and social care budgets that are spent on preventive programmes for child mental health in different countries. Significant numbers of projects are funded by NGOs and there is frequently little coordination between various government sectors and these programmes, plus there is often an emphasis on funding short-term projects rather than sustainable investment.

Despite these limitations in the economic information available, the worrying conclusion from the WHO ATLAS survey (2005) was that, globally, 'there is a universal absence of parity between adult and child mental health services' (WHO, 2005a). In the 25 countries from the WHO European Region that responded, only 77% had any specific programme for child mental health in place, and for 29% of countries, out-of-pocket payments were still the second most common means of financing mental health care (in all European countries, the most common method was taxation or social insurance schemes) (WHO, 2005a). The CAMHEE project identified a lack of transparency about funding for child mental health services and recommended earmarking of specific budgets for this population as they may become lost in the funding for adult services (Braddick et al., 2009). A need for greater coordination between different funding sources was also one of the key recommendations of the 2005 'Child and Adolescent Mental Health Services Review' in the United Kingdom, namely that 'The Government should clarify the extent to which all funding streams – direct and indirect – can be utilised to [. . .] improve [local and regional partners'] ability to pool and align funding' (Department for Children, 2008). An analysis of spending in the United Kingdom by the health think tank, the King's Fund, revealed that £143 million (€167 million), or 7.3% of the total mental health budget, was spent on child and adolescent services in 2007, and annual funding will need to increase to £237 million (€277 million) by 2026 (King's Fund, 2008). Well-meaning pronouncements from public bodies about the need for better mental health services for children tend to be overtaken by greater anxiety about – and fear of – adult mental disorders. As in most policy areas, except arguably education, children's voices and needs are minimized in the busy adult world of political negotiations and priority setting.

Assessing the challenges: needs and trends

A number of strategies have been used to compare the prevalence of psychiatric conditions or the state of mental well-being in children across Europe, each with its own limitations. At the severe end of the spectrum, data on deaths from suicide among young people are available for most European countries in the WHO mortality database, allowing direct comparisons to be made (WHO, 2010), and identifying suicide as the third leading cause of death worldwide among those aged 15 to 19 years old (Wasserman, Cheng and Jiang, 2005). Suicide is far more common among males, evidence of a gendered diffidence in asking for help (Kraemer, 2000). Adolescent girls more often harm themselves deliberately, yet also more often get help for their distress. Mortality rates need to take into account not only direct deaths from suicide, overdose or the physical consequences of anorexia nervosa, but the fact that mental health problems (particularly substance abuse) can increase the incidence of risk-taking behaviour and accidental injury, a leading cause of death among young people. Usage rates for child mental health services, while useful for service planning, will clearly underestimate the magnitude of the problem, as many problems will go unrecognized or untreated. See Chapters 5 and 11 for more detailed discussion around data and service planning. A large American survey, for example, found that almost 80% of children in need of mental health assessment were not receiving any care (Kataoka, Zhang and Wells, 2002). Undoubtedly, the stigma associated with mental health problems, particularly in childhood, coupled with gaps in service provision and inconsistent referral pathways, means that patterns of service use will provide a gross underestimate of the problem.

An alternative strategy has been the use of surveys, such as anonymous postal or school-based questionnaires, for young people or their carers or teachers. Such questionnaires can be used to assess the burden of probable 'hidden' mental illness, and can offer insights into patterns of disease prevalence within the community (e.g. differences between sexes and socioeconomic groups). For example, a large self-report survey to assess the prevalence of self-harming behaviour, the CASE (Child and Adolescent Self-harm in Europe) study (Scoliers et al., 2009), involved 30,000 young people completing anonymous questionnaires in six European countries and Australia. Over 30% of girls and 10% of boys said they had self-harmed, or thought about doing so, in the previous year, with the majority not telling anyone what they had done or seeking medical advice. Self-report surveys have demonstrated marked cultural (Hawton and James, 2005) and national (Grootenhuis et al., 1994) variations in the incidence of self-harm, its age distribution and risk factors. Self-report questionnaires can also incorporate standardized diagnostic tests, such as the Strengths and Difficulties Questionnaire, as has recently been used in a national survey in Germany (Box 8.1) (Holling et al., 2008; Ravens-Sieberer et al., 2008).

Using standardized questionnaires with children, parents and teachers, a comprehensive survey was conducted in the United Kingdom to determine the prevalence of emotional disorders, conduct disorders and hyperkinetic disorders among 5 to 15-year-olds; the prevalence was 3.7%, 5.8% and 1.5% of the population, respectively (Office for National Statistics, 2005). Higher rates were observed in those from a lone parent family, children with chronic illness (again reiterating the importance of psychiatric liaison services) and those with a lower socioeconomic status. Across Europe, the WHO HBSC, conducted every 4 years among 11, 13 and 15-year-olds, aims to assess both positive and negative indicators of health and well-being, as well as external factors affecting these (such as bullying, socioeconomic status, and peer and family support) (WHO Regional Office for Europe, 2012).

The question of whether mental health disorders in children and young people are increasing in prevalence is a complex one, and undoubtedly varies between

Box 8.1 Germany – The National Health Interview and Examination Survey

- Strengths and Difficulties Questionnaire administered to more than 14,000 3 to 17-year-olds across Germany
- 18.5% classified as 'borderline' or 'abnormal', suggesting they were at risk for psychopathology
- Higher rates among migrants and those of lower socioeconomic status
- Subset of 2863 children given specific standardized questionnaires to detect anxiety disorder, ADHD, conduct disorders and depressive disorders, and asked about substance abuse, self-harm and health-related quality of life
- 14.5% of children met the criteria for at least one diagnosable mental health problem; fewer than half were receiving treatment

Source: Hollings et al., 2008

types of mental disorder and age groups. Overall, a literature review concerning global prevalence cited figures for European countries, ranging from 8% in the Netherlands (13–18-year-olds) to 23% in Switzerland (1–15-year-olds) for any mental disorder (Patel et al., 2007). The authors concluded that 'evidence is mixed' about whether the rate of mental disorders has increased, and there is evidence that the trend has varied across different conditions and populations. In the United Kingdom, for example, the rate of suicide among young people fell 28% between 1997 and 2003 (Windfuhr et al., 2008) and rates of depression have not increased over the last 30 years (Costello, Foley and Angold, 2006), but rates of conduct disorder have significantly increased (Collishaw et al., 2004). A recent paper shows however, that there has been no decline in deaths in the United Kingdom due to self-harm or assault among older children, between 1980 and 2010 (Hardelid et al., 2013). There is also some evidence that trends in the prevalence of mental health problems may have differed across the age range covered by paediatrics, as well as across the spectrum of mental health disorders. The major disorders will now be considered in turn.

Affective and eating disorders

The prevalence of depressive disorders increases greatly from childhood to adolescence, and from adolescence they are about twice as common among girls than boys. In childhood, the prevalence of major depressive disorder is about 2%, from adolescence it is 4–8% (as in adulthood), and the cumulative incidence by age 18 is approximately 20% (Birmaher, Brent and Benson, 1998). Anxiety disorders similarly increase from childhood to adolescence, and they are also more common among girls; from adolescence their prevalence is 5–15% (Connolly and Bernstein, 2007). The prevalence of conduct disorders in adolescence is 2–5%, and these are more common among boys (AACAP, 1997). The prevalence of substance use disorders varies greatly across countries. Eating disorders are rare before puberty; while in adolescence their prevalence is 1–2%, and they are about 10-fold more common among girls than boys (Hsu, 1996).

There are great concerns about the possibility that, for example, depressive disorders and eating disorders might be increasing in prevalence among adolescents, and even also among children. Contacts to services due to these disorders are indeed increasing. However, epidemiologically valid studies do not confirm the assumed increase of eating disorders (Fombonne, 1996a, 1996b, 1998); indeed, a recent decline has been suggested in the incidence and prevalence of bulimia nervosa (Currin et al., 2005; Keel et al., 2006). Depressive symptoms may be increasing among children and adolescents, and their onset may be earlier, but there is no evidence that major depression has increased in prevalence (Birmaher et al., 1996; Birmaher, Brent and Benson, 1998; Sourander et al., 2008).

Psychoses

Psychoses, affecting about 1% of the population, often have their onset in adolescence. Productive psychotic symptoms are often preceded by a prodromal phase with varying and atypical symptoms, making diagnosis challenging in young people (Kumra et al., 1998; Frazier et al., 2007). Prodromal symptoms may mimic a variety of other mental disorders, and therefore the delay between the onset of a psychotic disorder and the beginning of appropriate treatment (duration of untreated psychosis, DUP) tends to be greater among minors than among adults (Ballageer et al., 2005). The incidence of psychoses is not increasing: on the contrary, schizophrenia may even be decreasing in younger age cohorts (Suvisaari et al., 1999; McGrath et al., 2008).

Developmental disorders: ADHD, autistic spectrum disorder

Developmental neuropsychiatric disorders, ADHD and autistic spectrum disorders (ASD) emerge in childhood. Based on a large systematic meta-analysis of epidemiological studies, the prevalence of ADHD in childhood is 6.48%, in adolescence it is 2.74% (Polanczyk and Rohde, 2007). ASD affect between 20 to 70 per 10,000 children and adolescents (Williams, Higgins and Brayne, 2006; Newschaffer et al., 2007; Fombonne, 2009). With the challenges of adolescent development, neuropsychiatric disorders of childhood often result in emotional and behavioural problems.

The disturbances in impulse control, attention and executive functions often result in poor development of social skills among children with ADHD and can also impair learning, resulting easily in academic failure and excessive negative feedback at school. In adolescence, peer relationships become of major developmental importance and, at this same time, academic demands usually increase. Adolescents with ADHD often experience a lot of frustration both in peer relationships and schoolwork, increasing the risk of antisocial development. The risk of conduct disorder and substance use disorders increases greatly in adolescence among subjects with ADHD (Galera et al., 2008). Critical epidemiological studies do not suggest any increase in the prevalence of ADHD, but increased interest, improved treatment options and assertive marketing of pharmacological treatments have resulted in an increase of treated ADHD in childhood and adolescence. Towards adulthood, ADHD symptoms often become milder and diagnostic criteria may no longer be fulfilled among children who have had ADHD.

The core difficulties for children and adolescents with ASD are in social interaction. Impaired social perception and communication frequently result in misunderstandings and conflicts. Impaired theory of mind and a lack of ability to understand that other people have their own thoughts and feelings are typical of ASD. In adolescence (when peer relationships become increasingly necessary developmentally and school poses all the greater challenges), those with mild ASD often display increased depressive and anxiety symptoms, aggression, and even psychotic symptoms, but ASD itself does not increase in prevalence. Indeed, ASD are not becoming more common in children and young people, even if this impression has been created by increased attention on the condition due to: expanding diagnostic criteria; changing classifications and epidemiological study methods; and increased service contacts enhanced by new treatment options (Fombonne, 2008, 2009).

The impact of socioeconomic factors on the development of mental health disorders is increasingly recognized and the consequences of these may vary for different age groups. For example, a Swedish study comparing figures of self-reported mental health problems from 1985/86 to those from 2005/06 reported an increased prevalence in adolescents but no change in younger children (Hagquist, 2010). The authors argue that the economic downturn during this period (and consequent high rates of unemployment) may have had a greater impact on adolescents than on younger children. The negative impact of income inequality on mental health, throughout the life-course, is increasingly recognized (Friedli, 2009), and may account for some of the variation between European countries in trends of incidence. For example, the United Kingdom saw a marked 'increase in non-aggressive conduct problems such as lying, stealing and disobedience rather than aggressive problems such as fighting' (Collishaw et al., 2004) during the period 1974 to 1999, which coincided with a massive increase in income inequality (Weeks, 2005). By contrast, the Netherlands, which experienced no significant change in income inequality, saw little change in adolescent problems (Verhulst, van der Ende and Rietbergen, 1997). With many European countries currently undergoing an economic recession, parental unemployment and income inequality may have a considerable impact on young people's mental well-being over the coming years. See Chapters 1 and 5 for more detailed discussion of social determinants of health.

Our understanding of the psychosocial risk factors for mental illness suggests that other circumstances that increase the probability of these conditions may also be increasing, due to changes in society, migration and family structure. A review of child and adolescent mental health services in England, for example, concluded that children from lone-parent families were twice as likely to develop mental health problems (Maughan, Vrock and Ladva, 2004) although, as noted in Chapter 1, this may be due to risks such as increased poverty. Very high rates of mental disorder (up to 37%) were found in looked-after children (those in the care of the State) in the United Kingdom (Meltzer et al., 2003), and they form one of the key vulnerable groups the CAMHS review identified. A systematic review of studies involving children who had been asylum-seekers in Denmark found an OR of 5.5 for the development of mental illness in those who had been detained in immigration centres for a year or more (Nielsen et al., 2008). Concerns about the long-term psychological impact of detention centres on children have been raised across Europe, with urgent calls for less damaging alternatives to be found (Hodes, 2010). See Chapter 1 for more discussion on children in detention, and other vulnerable groups of young people.

An assessment of the importance of mental health problems in childhood must also take into account their long-term effects, which may persist even if an initial recovery is made. For example, a longitudinal study in Sweden reported that at least one-third of those seen in child and adolescent psychiatry services would require later psychiatric input in adulthood (Engqvist and Rydelius, 2005). The impact of childhood conduct disorders on society is marked: analysis of a Canadian birth cohort revealed that 76% of boys who had a conduct disorder in childhood went on to have mental health problems (most commonly substance abuse) and/or a criminal record by the age of 30 years (Kratzer and

Hodgins, 1997). For females, the equivalent incidence was 30%, perhaps reflecting a greater tendency to seek and receive support. Similar figures were reported in Finland, with 62% of those who had a combination of conduct disorder and internalizing problems at age 8 years going on to have a criminal record, psychiatric disorder, or both, in adulthood (Sourander et al., 2008).

Child mental health care: the European experience

The 'Child Health Services and Systems in Europe' questionnaire addressed child mental health services, using a clinical scenario of a child presenting with symptoms of ADHD, and their pathway from initial presentation (whether to education, health or social services) to diagnosis and long-term management. Respondents were then asked to consider the provision for inpatient care for children and adolescents with mental illness, as well as how quality in this area was assured and improved. Elsewhere in the questionnaire, respondents were asked about programmes to prevent child abuse and neglect, but such programmes would also be included in a broader definition of services that promote child mental well-being, such as early intervention programmes and parenting support for vulnerable groups. In the context of adolescent medicine, they were asked to consider services for those abusing drugs or alcohol, or with eating disorders.

The country responses highlighted six key areas of variation in service provision, and some important examples of effective practice.

Professionals responsible for child mental health

A significant area of variation in services across Europe is who is primarily responsible for mental health care in children (Table 8.2).

Table 8.2 Professionals responsible for child mental health

Professionals mainly responsible for child mental health care	*Countries*	*Comments*
Psychiatrists	• Finland • Italy • Netherlands • Poland	
Paediatricians	• Austria • Sweden	
A combination of paediatricians and psychiatrists	• England • Scotland	
Psychologists, social workers	• Israel	Psychiatrists used for consultation; paediatricians 'unfortunately have minimal involvement'

Source: 'Child Health Services and Systems in Europe' questionnaire

Box 8.2 Child and adolescent psychiatry provision in Finland

- In Finland, child psychiatry and adolescent psychiatry are separate medical specialities.
- Each has a specialist training curriculum of 6 years.
- Child psychiatry covers psychiatric treatment until puberty, and adolescent psychiatric services are provided for adolescents aged 13 to 18 (or in some circumstances 21).
- In most hospital districts, adolescent psychiatric outpatient services provide treatment until the age of 20 to 21 years, when the contact has been initiated before the age of 18, but inpatient adolescent psychiatric services are, by law, defined as being for those under 18 years of age.
- Among adolescent psychiatrists in Finland, there is a clear belief that this is the direction other countries should follow, i.e. building a separate specialty and separate services for adolescents, because adolescence is a unique developmental phase that is very different from both childhood and adulthood.

In the United Kingdom, the condition involved partly determines this; for example, many behavioural disorders fall within the remit of community paediatricians, while affective or psychotic disorders would be managed by child and adolescent psychiatrists. More recently, a small number of posts have been developed for paediatricians subspecializing in child mental health, although these are not yet widely available and there is often a lack of understanding of the importance of psychiatric input in paediatric care, particularly in supporting those with chronic illness. In Finland, the age of the patient is a major determinant of who cares for them (Box 8.2).

Management of substance misuse

The range of professionals involved is more complex in the case of substance misuse, with adolescents being seen by a combination of child psychiatrists, adult psychiatrists who specialize in substance abuse, and paediatricians. Whereas in Italy, adolescent substance abuse is seen as a subset of adolescent medicine, in France and Finland, it is treated as a part of substance abuse in general, falling under the remit of adult services that also cover adolescents. In Austria, there is a combination of the two, while in Poland there is a clear age cut-off with a specific toxicology ward for adults while the under-16s are admitted to the children's ward. While adult psychiatrists specializing in substance misuse have particular expertise, it is not clear whether the overall health needs of adolescents, who may be at varying stages of development, will be best met by being seen wholly within adult services.

Provision of inpatient care

A particular challenge in caring for children and adolescents is the lack of suitable inpatient facilities. Undoubtedly, many young people are treated in less than ideal settings, for example, adolescents being admitted to adult psychiatric units, or children with eating disorders having prolonged admissions to acute general paediatric wards. Our respondents suggested the latter was often not due to a need for acute medical admission because of physical ill health, but rather due to a lack of more suitable alternatives. In France, for example, they reported there are four or five dedicated units for eating disorders, but 'adolescents are usually hospitalized in paediatric wards, because beds in specialized wards are difficult to find'. In Israel, similarly, 'in total there are 24 beds in psych hospitals for eating disorder patients – demand is great!! . . . Eating disorders are common.' The difficulty of finding suitable inpatient care for adolescents was highlighted by our respondent for the Isle of Man, who wrote that 'there is a protocol in place to have under-16s on the paediatric ward, which is less than ideal and, as a last resort, we have had to look to the adult mental health facility to help place children'. In Finland, 'according to the law, adolescents with mental illness are not to be treated in adult wards', while in France there are designated beds for adolescents in adult psychiatric wards. In Scotland, there has been a drive to strengthen existing inpatient adolescent facilities, in response to a 2004 report on psychiatric inpatient facilities (Child Health Support Group, 2004). Our respondent highlighted the fact that, in this respect, psychiatry had been earlier to recognize the importance of dedicated adolescent units than other paediatric specialties. In the United Kingdom, there is greater political pressure to keep under-18s out of adult psychiatric wards than there is to provide comprehensive mental health care in paediatric settings, where many young people in crisis are likely to be admitted.

Areas of difference: access to mental health services/referral pathways

The 'Child Health Services and Systems in Europe' questionnaire sought to capture differences in access to health care from the perspective of the patient or parent. The responses highlighted the range of means of referral to children's mental health services across the region, and the importance not only of primary care physicians but of education and social services as well in identifying these problems. Indeed, for behavioural problems such as ADHD, many respondents (Austria, England, Italy, Norway and Sweden) stated that teachers were the main source of referrals, after they or the parents noted the child was having difficulties.

Once a possible mental health problem has been noted, the speed with which a specialist assessment is offered varies, but many respondents highlighted the slow speed of referral as a weakness in their country's services, predominantly due to a lack of availability of specialist services. In Norway, the child is guaranteed to be seen within 10 days by a child and adolescent psychiatrist. If

Box 8.3 Referral pathways in Finland

- Legislation stipulates that: initial assessment must start within 3 weeks of referral; all the assessments to define required treatment have to be completed within 6 weeks; and the required treatment has to be initiated within 3 months from when the need was noted (health care law).
- National practice guidelines have been published for child and adolescent psychiatric disorders such as ADHD and eating disorders.
- The guidelines define the responsibilities of primary care and specialist level services in the treatment of a given disorder, and the indications to refer between service levels.
- In practice, however, great variation can be seen across the country, in the resources and service provision in primary and secondary care, and in cooperation between service levels.

a preliminary ICD-10 diagnosis is reached, there is a guarantee that treatment will be initiated within 90 days. In Finland, there are standardized criteria for determining access to specialized mental health care in a non-urgent situation, developed by consensus (Kaukonen et al., 2010), with priority rating tools to ensure equal access to specialist level child and adolescent psychiatric care across the country (Box 8.3).

In the United Kingdom, NICE has produced guidance on the referral and management of ADHD (National Institute for Health and Care Excellence, 2008) and depression (National Institute for Health and Care Excellence, 2005) in young people, and is currently developing guidelines for autistic spectrum and conduct disorders. A four-tier hierarchy, ranging from primary care to extremely specialized services, is used in the referral pathway.

Age range covered by child and adolescent mental health services

Most European countries use 16 or 18 years of age as the cut-off for adolescent services, and many countries highlighted the transition between paediatric and adult care as being particularly challenging for mental health conditions. For behavioural conditions, a major difficulty is the lack of appropriate adult services: for example, British studies have revealed concerns about the lack of services available for adults with ADHD (Brown et al., 2005), with only 22% of community paediatricians being aware of any adult services for ADHD in their area (Marcer, Finlay and Baverstock, 2008). In Norway, child mental health services, including the 10-day assessment target, are notable for covering adolescents and young adults up to the age of 23. It has been argued that an age range encompassing early adulthood (such as up to 24 years) more accurately reflects the psychological development of young people (Patel et al., 2007), as many will not make a significant transition to independent living at

16 or 18 years. While adult psychiatry services now tend to refuse to admit or assess under-18s, there remains a serious gap between them and CAMHS services, which often stop at 16 or 17 (see Chapter 4 for detailed discussion of transition services).

Early intervention services

Early intervention services to support vulnerable parents and prevent the development of mental health problems, vary in provision across Europe (see Chapters 5 and 6). Our respondent from Finland highlighted such services as one of the country's great strengths in child health: child and maternity health clinics are being modified to become 'family welfare clinics (preventive services [with increasing] emphasis on the welfare of the family, father's role, psychosocial factors in addition to pure physical health of the child)' in parallel with the focus of school health examinations being extended to have an 'emphasis on psychosocial wellbeing of the child in addition to pure physical health'. There is, however, fragmentation and variable provision between municipalities.

There is clear evidence that stress and the family environment have an impact on children's emotional well-being, even before birth, making a case for interventions to begin as early as possible. From conception onwards, the resilience of children is compromised by stress and insecurity in their parents (Kaufman and Charney, 2001), with an increased risk of behavioural problems in 2-year-olds whose mothers had greater levels of perceived stress during pregnancy (Gutteling et al., 2005). Both anxiety during pregnancy (O'Connor et al., 2005) and depression after it (Cooper and Murray, 1998; Poobalan et al., 2007) have serious effects on the health and development of the child, with the most socially deprived mothers being far more likely to have very premature births (Smith et al., 2007). This is damage that could be prevented with coordinated antenatal and postnatal care, with joint work between maternity, primary care and mental health workers. The physical and mental health of infants is powerfully determined by the quality of care they receive, which can be modified by evidence-based interventions (Barnes, 2003). Despite recommendations in the National Service Frameworks (NSF) in the United Kingdom, there is a woeful lack of services (and poor coordination of what does exist) for mothers and fathers between conception and the time of birth.

Future challenges

Referral for specialist child and adolescent mental health services needs to be combined with a universal recognition of the importance of promoting child mental health within general paediatrics, primary care, education and welfare services. The relative merits of different approaches in both arenas are being investigated, with a focus on establishing an evidence base of effective interventions, and the development of models to establish the long-term financial returns from services in this area. Of course, in addition to the paucity of high-quality RCTs in child and adolescent mental health, there is the difficulty of translating the evidence we do have into helping individual patients, who exist in a complex web of familial, social and cultural relationships, experiences and co-morbidities.

Of the many issues currently being considered, the relative efficacy of community services in comparison with inpatient services is a major focus, to determine whether the established usefulness of community treatment in adult mental health will be replicated in the paediatric population. A 2009 Cochrane review concluded that there is a scant evidence base for determining the relative efficacy of different strategies of outpatient care in an effort to reduce inpatient treatment rates (Shepperd et al., 2009). The authors recommend that, in the absence of RCT data (they could find only seven RCTs comparing inpatient and intensive outpatient treatment), prospective multicentre audits should be carried out.

It is clear that many approaches to community mental health care will involve sectors outside health care, and the crucial importance of education in prevention and outpatient treatment programmes is reflected in a major ongoing European study, the 'Saving and Empowering Young Lives in Europe' project (Box 8.4) (Wasserman et al., 2010).

School-based programmes are likely to prove of particular importance, reaching a far greater proportion of the population than any intervention based within child psychiatry and psychology (see Chapter 6). A recent systematic review in Australia, for example, identified 28 programmes based within schools that reduced depressive symptoms (effect sizes ranged from 0.21 to 1.4 in all identified studies) (Calear and Christensen, 2010). The most successful programmes were those which targeted children manifesting depressive symptoms and which used school-based CBT. Clearly, schools could play an important role in the delivery of mental health screening programmes, particularly in countries where there are regular mandatory school health examinations. It has been argued that child mental health disorders provide an attractive opportunity for screening, since the various disorders tend to manifest

Box 8.4 The Saving and Empowering Young Lives in Europe project

- A randomized controlled trial comparing three approaches to suicide prevention.
- Involves 11,000 young people across 11 European countries.
- Schools will be randomized to one of four groups:
  - gatekeeper training (training teachers to identify and refer those engaged in risky behaviours);
  - awareness training for adolescents on mental health promotion;
  - questionnaire-based screening for depression;
  - control group.

Source: Wasserman et al., 2010

within well-defined age ranges (e.g. attachment and autistic spectrum disorders in younger pre-school children; mood and conduct disorders in school-age children; and psychotic disorders, self-harm and substance misuse in young adulthood). The role of teachers and childminders, in addition to parents, in fostering emotional resilience in children must not be forgotten (Kraemer, 1999).

An evidence base is also being established to determine the success of parenting and early intervention programmes, which are increasingly recognized as having a crucial role in promoting mental well-being. A systematic review of preventive programmes from Canada, for example, supported the use of parent training and child social skills training to prevent conduct disorder; and universal school-based CBT programmes to reduce anxiety (Waddell et al., 2007). Identification of those parents most in need of support is required, with strengthened provision for specific high-risk groups, such as children of parents with mental illness and/or drug use. It is increasingly apparent that such interventions are key to tackling the pernicious effects socioeconomic inequality can have on child and subsequent adult mental health, and that they need to be started before birth. See also Chapter 5. Sir Michael Marmot's review of health inequalities in the United Kingdom prioritized early childhood interventions for reducing lifelong health inequalities; stressed the importance of pre- and postnatal interventions that reduce adverse outcomes in pregnancy and infancy; and recommended increasing the overall expenditure allocated to the early years, with this focused progressively across the social gradient (Marmot, 2010). The effect of policies in many sectors on child and adolescent mental well-being needs to be recognized. For example, the health benefits of providing paid parental leave in the first year of life for subsequent mental and physical health are clear: fully funded maternal leave is associated with lower child mortality, with 'a ten week extension in paid leave [. . .] predicted to decrease post neonatal mortality rates by 4.1%' (Tanaka, 2005). Social policy saves lives. However, deaths are merely the tip of an iceberg of physical, mental and developmental disorders afflicting children in the early years.

Economic evaluation of early intervention programmes is becoming more sophisticated, with economic analyses that take into account long-term savings not only to the health service, but to the criminal justice and welfare systems as well, reflecting the impact of early intervention across the life-course. The use of such social return on investment (SROI) analysis determines the benefits to the child, family and state, across all sectors, while recognizing that these benefits may take many years to accumulate. One early intervention scheme in Caerphilly, for example, is predicted to produce a return of £7.60 for each £1 invested, when savings across all sectors are taken into account (New Economics Foundation, 2009). Further work is needed to establish robust economic tools to evaluate mental health programmes, as they straddle the divide between health, education and social services. This will address the fact that their long-term benefits, as well as their delivery, will be intersectoral in nature, and reflects the complex role of social and economic deprivation, as both cause and consequence of mental ill health in the developing child.

References

AACAP (1997) Practice parameter for the assessment and treatment of children and adolescents with conduct disorders, *Journal of the American Academy of Child and Adolescent Psychiatry*, 36(10 Suppl): 122–39S.

Ballageer, T. et al. (2005) Is adolescent-onset first-episode psychosis different from adult onset? *Journal of the American Academy of Child and Adolescent Psychiatry*, 44(8): 782–9.

Barlow, J.H. and Ellard, D.R. (2004) Psycho-educational interventions for children with chronic disease, parents and siblings: an overview of the research evidence base, *Child: Care, Health and Development*, 30(6): 637–45.

Barnes, J. (2003) Interventions addressing infant mental health problems, *Children and Society*, 17(5): 386–95.

Birmaher, B., Brent, D.A. and Benson, R.S. (1998) Summary of the practice parameters for the assessment and treatment of children and adolescents with depressive disorders. American Academy of Child and Adolescent Psychiatry, *Journal of the American Academy of Child and Adolescent Psychiatry*, 37(11): 1234–8.

Birmaher, B. et al. (1996) Childhood and adolescent depression: a review of the past 10 years: Part I, *Journal of the American Academy of Child and Adolescent Psychiatry*, 35(11): 1427–39.

Braddick, F. et al. (2009) *Child and Adolescent Mental Health in Europe: Infrastructures, Policy and Programmes*. Luxembourg: European Communities.

Brown, R.T. et al. (2005) Treatment of attention-deficit/hyperactivity disorder: overview of the evidence, *Pediatrics*, 115(6): e749–57.

Calear, A.L. and Christensen, H. (2010) Systematic review of school-based prevention and early intervention programs for depression, *Journal of Adolescence*, 33(3): 429–38.

CAMHS (2008) *Children and Adolescent Mental Health Services Review*. London: Child and Adolescent Mental Health Services.

Campo, J.V. et al. (2000) Child and adolescent psychiatry in general children's hospitals. A survey of chairs of psychiatry, *Psychosomatics*, 41(12), 128–33.

Child Health Support Group (2004) *Inpatient working group – Psychiatric Inpatient Services for Children and Young People in Scotland: A way forward* (http://www.scotland.gov.uk/Resource/Doc/35596/0012563.pdf, accessed June 2013).

Collishaw, S. et al. (2004) Time trends in adolescent mental health, *Journal of Child Psychology and Psychiatry*, 45(8): 1350–62.

Connolly, S.D. and Bernstein, G.A. (2007) Practice parameter for the assessment and treatment of children and adolescents with anxiety disorders, *Journal of the American Academy of Child and Adolescent Psychiatry*, 46(2): 267–83.

Cooper, P.J. and Murray, L. (1998) Postnatal depression, *BMJ*, 316(7148): 1884–6.

Costello, E.J., Foley, D.L. and Angold, A. (2006) 10-year research update review: the epidemiology of child and adolescent psychiatric disorders: II. Developmental epidemiology, *Journal of the American Academy of Child and Adolescent Psychiatry*, 45(1): 8–25.

Currin, L. et al. (2005) Time trends in eating disorder incidence, *British Journal of Psychiatry*, 186: 132–5.

Dowdney, L. et al. (1999) Psychological disturbance and service provision in parentally bereaved children: prospective case-control study, *BMJ*, 319(7206): 354–7.

Engqvist, U. and Rydelius, P.-A. (2005) [Children and youth cared for by child and adolescent psychiatry – what is the outcome?] Barn och ungdomar inom BUP – hur går det för dem? *PsykiskHälsa*, 4: 39–44.

European Commission (2008) European Pact for Mental Health and Wellbeing, (http://ec.europa.eu/health/archive/ph_determinants/life_style/mental/docs/pact_en.pdf accessed June 2013).
Fombonne, E. (1996a) Anorexia nervosa: no evidence of increase, *British Journal of Psychiatry*, 168: 251–2.
Fombonne, E. (1996b) Is bulimia nervosa increasing in frequency? *International Journal of Eating Disorders*, 19(3): 287–96.
Fombonne, E. (1998) Increased rates of psychosocial disorders in youth, *European Archives of Psychiatry and Clinical Neuroscience*, 248(1): 14–21.
Fombonne, E. (2008) Is autism getting commoner? *British Journal of Psychiatry*, 193(1): 59.
Fombonne, E. (2009) Epidemiology of pervasive developmental disorders, *Pediatric Research*, 65(6): 591–8.
Frazier, J.A. et al. (2007) Treatment of early-onset schizophrenia spectrum disorders (TEOSS): demographic and clinical characteristics, *Journal of the American Academy of Child and Adolescent Psychiatry*, 46(8): 979–88.
Friedli, L. (2009) *Mental health, resilience and inequalities: how individuals and communities are affected*. Geneva: World Health Organization.
Galera, C. et al. (2008) Hyperactivity-inattention symptoms in childhood and substance use in adolescence: the youth gazel cohort, *Drug and Alcohol Dependence*, 94(1–3): 30–7.
Glazebrook, C. et al. (2003) Detecting emotional and behavioural problems in paediatric clinics, *Child: Care, Health and Development*, 29(2): 141–9.
Grootenhuis, M. et al. (1994) Attempted suicide in Oxford and Utrecht, *British Journal of Psychiatry*, 165(2): 73–8.
Gutteling, B.M. et al. (2005) The effects of prenatal stress on temperament and problem behavior of 27-month-old toddlers, *European Child and Adolescent Psychiatry*, 14(1): 41–51.
Hagquist, C. (2010) Discrepant trends in mental health complaints among younger and older adolescents in Sweden: an analysis of WHO data 1985–2005, *Journal of Adolescent Health*, 46(3): 258–64.
Hawton, K. and James, A. (2005) Suicide and deliberate self harm in young people, *BMJ*, 330(7496): 891–4.
Hodes, M. (2010) The mental health of detained asylum seeking children, *European Child and Adolescent Psychiatry*, 19(7): 621–3.
Holling, H. et al. (2008) Assessing psychopathological problems of children and adolescents from 3 to 17 years in a nationwide representative sample: results of the German health interview and examination survey for children and adolescents (KiGGS), *European Child and Adolescent Psychiatry*, 17(Suppl 1): 34–41.
Hsu, L. K. (1996) Epidemiology of the eating disorders, *Psychiatric Clinics of North America*, 19(4): 681–700.
Hysing, M. et al. (2007) Chronic physical illness and mental health in children. Results from a large-scale population study, *Journal of Child Psychology and Psychiatry*, 48(8): 785–92.
Jotzo, M. and Poets, C.F. (2005) Helping parents cope with the trauma of premature birth: an evaluation of a trauma-preventive psychological intervention, *Pediatrics*, 115(4): 915–19.
Kataoka, S.H., Zhang, L. and Wells, K.B. (2002) Unmet need for mental health care among U.S. children: variation by ethnicity and insurance status, *American Journal of Psychiatry*, 159(9): 1548–55.
Kaufman, J. and Charney, D. (2001) Effects of early stress on brain structure and function: implications for understanding the relationship between

child maltreatment and depression, *Development and Psychopathology*, 13(3): 451–71.
Kaukonen, P. et al. (2010) Child psychiatry in the Finnish health care reform: national criteria for treatment access, *Health Policy*, 96(1): 20–7.
Keel, P.K. et al. (2006) Point prevalence of bulimia nervosa in 1982, 1992, and 2002, *Psychological Medicine*, 36(1): 119–27.
Kessler, R.C. et al. (2010) Childhood adversities and adult psychopathology in the WHO World Mental Health Surveys, *British Journal of Psychiatry*, 197(5): 378–85.
King's Fund (2008) *Paying the price: the cost of mental health care in Britain to 2026.* London: King's Fund.
Kraemer, S. (1999) Promoting resilience: changing concepts of parenting and child care, *International Journal of Child and Family Welfare*, 3: 273–87.
Kraemer, S. (2000) The fragile male, *BMJ*, 321(7276): 1609–12.
Kratzer, L. and Hodgins, S. (1997) Adult outcomes of child conduct problems: a cohort study, *Journal of Abnormal Child Psychology*, 25(1): 65–81.
Kumra, S. et al. (1998) "Multidimensionally impaired disorder": is it a variant of very early-onset schizophrenia? *Journal of the American Academy of Child and Adolescent Psychiatry*, 37(1): 91–9.
Levav, I. et al. (2004) Psychiatric services and training for children and adolescents in Europe: results of a country survey, *European Child and Adolescent Psychiatry*, 13(6): 395–401.
Lim, S.S. et al. (2012) A comparative risk assessment of burden of disease and injury attributable to 67 risk factors and risk factor clusters in 21 regions, 1990–2010: a systematic analysis for the Global Burden of Disease Study 2010, *The Lancet*, 380(9859): 2224–60.
Marcer, H., Finlay, F. and Baverstock, A. (2008) ADHD and transition to adult services – the experience of community paediatricians, *Child: Care, Health and Development*, 34(5): 564–6.
Marmot, M. (2010) *Strategic Review of Health Inequalities in England Post-2010.* London: University College London.
Maughan, B., Vrock, A. and Ladva, G. (2004) Mental Health. In: Office of National Statistics (ed.) *The Health of Children and Young People*. London: Office of National Statistics.
McGrath, J. et al. (2008) Schizophrenia: a concise overview of incidence, prevalence, and mortality, *Epidemiologic Reviews*, 30: 67–76.
Meltzer, H. et al. (2003) *The mental health of young people looked after by local authorities.* London: Office of National Statistics.
National Institute for Health and Care Excellence (2005) Depression in children and young people: Identification and management in primary, community and secondary care, NICE clinical guideline 28 (http://www.nice.org.uk/nicemedia/live/10970/29856/29856.pdf accessed June 2013).
National Institute for Health and Care Excellence (2008) Attention Deficit Hyperactivity Disorder: Diagnosis and Management of ADHD in children, young people and adults, NICE clinical guideline 72 (http://www.nice.org.uk/nicemedia/live/12061/42059/42059.pdf accessed June 2013).
New Economics Foundation (2009) *The economic and social return of Action for Children's Early Intervention Team / 5+ project, Caerphilly.* London: New Economics Foundation.
Newschaffer, C.J. et al. (2007) The epidemiology of autism spectrum disorders. *Annual Review of Public Health,* 28: 235–58.
Ng, S.M. et al. (2008) Incorporating family therapy into asthma group intervention: a randomized waitlist-controlled trial, *Family Process*, 47(1): 115–30.

Nielsen, S.S. et al. (2008) Mental health among children seeking asylum in Denmark – the effect of length of stay and number of relocations: a cross-sectional study, *BMC Public Health*, 8: 293.
O'Connor, T.G. et al. (2005) Prenatal anxiety predicts individual differences in cortisol in pre-adolescent children, *Biological Psychiatry*, 58(3): 211–17.
Office for National Statistics (2005) *Mental Health of Children and Young People in Great Britain, 2004*. London: Stationery Office.
Patel, V. et al. (2007) Mental health of young people: a global public-health challenge, *The Lancet*, 369(9569), 1302–13.
Polanczyk, G. and Rohde, L.A. (2007) Epidemiology of attention-deficit/hyperactivity disorder across the lifespan, *Current Opinion in Psychiatry*, 20(4): 386–92.
Poobalan, A.S. et al. (2007) Effects of treating postnatal depression on mother–infant interaction and child development: systematic review, *British Journal of Psychiatry*, 191: 378–86.
Public Health Group (2005) *Victorian burden of disease study: mortality and morbidity in 2001*. Melbourne: Victorian Government Department of Human Services.
Ravens-Sieberer, U. et al. (2008) Prevalence of mental health problems among children and adolescents in Germany: results of the BELLA study within the National Health Interview and Examination Survey, *European Child and Adolescent Psychiatry*, 17(Suppl 1): 22–33.
Rutter, M., Kim-Cohen, J. and Maughan, B. (2006) Continuities and discontinuities in psychopathology between childhood and adult life, *Journal of Child Psychology and Psychiatry*, 47(3–4): 276–95.
Schmid, G. et al. (2010) A prospective study on the persistence of infant crying, sleeping and feeding problems and preschool behaviour, *Acta Paediatrica*, 99(2): 286–90.
Scoliers, G. et al. (2009) Reasons for adolescent deliberate self-harm: a cry of pain and/or a cry for help? Findings from the child and adolescent self-harm in Europe (CASE) study, *Social Psychiatry and Psychiatric Epidemiology*, 44(8): 601–7.
Shepperd, S. al. (2009) Alternatives to inpatient mental health care for children and young people, *Cochrane Database of Systematic Reviews*, CD006410.
Smith, L.K. et al. (2007) Socioeconomic inequalities in very preterm birth rates, *Archives of Disease in Childhood – Fetal and Neonatal Edition*, 92(1): F11–14.
Sourander, A. et al. (2008) Changes in psychiatric problems and service use among 8-year-old children: a 16-year population-based time-trend study, *Journal of the American Academy of Child and Adolescent Psychiatry*, 47(3): 317–27.
Suvisaari, J.M. et al. (1999) Decline in the incidence of schizophrenia in Finnish cohorts born from 1954 to 1965, *Archives of General Psychiatry*, 56(8): 733–40.
Tanaka, S. (2005) Parental leave and child health across OECD countries, *Economic Journal*, 115(501): F7–28.
Verhulst, F.C., van der Ende, J. and Rietbergen, A. (1997) Ten-year time trends of psychopathology in Dutch children and adolescents: no evidence for strong trends, *Acta Psychiatrica Scandinavica*, 96(1): 7–13.
Waddell, C. et al. (2007) Preventing mental disorders in children: a systematic review to inform policy-making, *Canadian Journal of Public Health*, 98(3): 166–73.
Wasserman, D. et al. (2010) Saving and empowering young lives in Europe (SEYLE): a randomized controlled trial, *BMC Public Health*, 10: 192.
Wasserman, D., Cheng, Q. and Jiang, G. (2005) Global suicide rates among young people aged 15–19, *World Psychiatry*, 4(2): 114–20.
Weeks, J. (2005) *Inequality Trends in Some Developed OECD Countries*. DESA Working Paper No.6. New York: United Nations.

Williams, J.G., Higgins, J.P. and Brayne, C.E. (2006) Systematic review of prevalence studies of autism spectrum disorders, *Archives of Disease in Childhood*, 91(1): 8–15.
Windfuhr, K. et al. (2008) Suicide in juveniles and adolescents in the United Kingdom, *Journal of Child Psychology and Psychiatry*, 49(11): 1155–65.
Winkley, K. et al. (2006) Psychological interventions to improve glycaemic control in patients with type 1 diabetes: systematic review and meta-analysis of randomised controlled trials, *BMJ*, 333(7558): 65.
WHO (2004) *Promoting Mental Health: Concepts, emerging evidence, practice*. Geneva: World Health Organization.
WHO (2005a) *Atlas: Child and Adolescent Mental Health Resources*. Geneva: World Health Organization.
WHO (2005b) *WHO European Ministerial Conference on Mental Health: Facing the Challenges, Building Solutions*. Helsinki: World Health Organization.
WHO (2010) *WHO Mortality Database*. http://www.who.int/healthinfo/morttables/en/index.html (accessed 12 August 2010).
WHO Regional Office for Europe (2008) *Social cohesion for mental well-being among adolescents*. Copenhagen: WHO Regional Office for Europe.
WHO Regional Office for Europe (2012) *Health behaviour in school aged children (HBSC) study: International report from the 2009/2010 survey*. Copenhagen: WHO Regional Office for Europe.

chapter nine

Services for vulnerable and maltreated children

June Thoburn

> "It always grieves me to contemplate the initiation of children into the ways of life when they are scarcely more than infants. It checks their confidence and simplicity, two of the best qualities that heaven gives them, and demands that they share their sorrows before they are capable of entering into our enjoyments."
>
> Charles Dickens
> *The Old Curiosity Shop*

Introduction

This chapter describes and analyses the different European approaches to the provision of preventive, therapeutic and out-of-home placement services for vulnerable children and their parents and carers (Box 9.1). In some countries, services are focused around investigating and responding to reports of maltreatment, especially by parents and other caregivers: in others, protection services are part of a broader child welfare approach to assisting families at times of stress, or coping with a range of adult and child difficulties that impact on the child's health and development. Although the volume of descriptive and research literature on child protection and out-of-home care is considerable, there are still many gaps in our knowledge about how best to identify and then provide appropriate and cost-effective services to combat the well-documented long-term negative impacts of maltreatment, separation and poor parenting in childhood. In the light of the differences in definitions, contexts and thresholds to services, caution is required when comparing statistics on prevalence and outcome across European nations.

Although the focus of this chapter is Europe, space is given to the contrasting child welfare model that predominates in the United States and some other Anglophone jurisdictions for two reasons. Firstly, the United Kingdom components (especially England, Northern Ireland, the Isle of Man and Channel Islands) have more similarities with these jurisdictions than do other European entities and, secondly, much of the English language literature that has an influence on United Kingdom practice (and to a lesser extent policy) originates in the United States, so it is important for European scholars and professionals to understand the differences in context and jurisdictions.

Overview of European policies and services

A recent article in *The Lancet* (Gilbert et al., 2009a) described two broad (though at times converging) approaches to identifying and assisting children who have been, or are at risk of being, abused or neglected. The authors define these approaches as 'child and family welfare' and 'child safety', the first being the dominant approach in Europe, Japan, New Zealand and a minority of provinces/states in Australia and Canada; and the second, dominant in Australia, Canada and the United States, being characterized as a 'child safety' or 'child protection' approach. In essence, in 'child safety' jurisdictions, the trigger for assessment and the provision of services is the 'report' or 'notification' that a child may have been maltreated or is at risk of maltreatment. The service starts with an 'investigation' of whether the report is 'substantiated', and intervention, often with a judicial component, focuses around the maltreatment. This 'targeted' approach means that these countries are able to provide robust statistics on the incidence of identified maltreatment, although much maltreatment remains unrecognized. Because of the volume of reports, coordinated supportive and therapeutic services are actually provided in only a minority of cases where maltreatment is substantiated. The maltreated child will be the focus, and any services provided to the family will be primarily directed to whatever has led to the maltreatment rather than on more general family stressors. Partly as a result of this approach, and also because of heavy reliance on insurance-based systems of care rather than on needs-based welfare systems, child protection agencies tend to commission specific 'programmes' or 'interventions', often from private or not-for-profit third-sector agencies, and assistance tends to be of time-limited (usually less than 12 months) duration. Where maltreatment is not substantiated, or substantiated maltreatment does not reach a threshold for provision of services, some families are provided with social support through referral to voluntary sector agencies, and a small (but growing) proportion are provided with services commissioned by the statutory agencies as a preventive measure. The out-of-home care service in these countries is viewed as an integral part of the child protection service: few placements are organized by agreement with parents and almost all are court sanctioned, often with the termination of parental rights after a comparatively short period in care. There is low usage of out-of-home care for reasons other than maltreatment, although in the United States health insurance-funded residential treatment for young people with challenging behaviour or mental health problems is provided within the health sector for families covered by insurance and, less frequently, the child protection services fund residential treatment provided by the health services (see also Chapter 8). Young offenders placed away from home are provided for separately within the criminal justice system.

In contrast, in most of western and much of central and eastern Europe, the emphasis is on 'referral' of a child or family experiencing psychosocial or relationship problems or serious environmental stresses, 'assessing' the problems and providing appropriate assistance to families (or specific children within families) that are experiencing difficulties, including those in which children are suffering or are likely to suffer 'impairment to their health or development' (the language of the England and Wales Children Act 1989) because of a range of psychosocial stresses. These stresses will include abuse or neglect but also a wide range of others that may or may not be attributable to parental fault. In most countries, the services to prevent and deal with the consequences of abuse and neglect are integrated within the generally available locality-based social services. In some (e.g. Italy, Scotland and Sweden), these include services for adults experiencing difficulties (including a range of physical, mental health and relationship problems and the elderly) and some neighbourhood-based community development services. They are likely to have specialist child and welfare sections, but in small communities, the service is provided by 'generic' social work teams. In some countries, child and family social services are separate from the other social services, for example England, where they are a part of the local authority education services and other countries, where they are part of the community health services. In some European jurisdictions, although child and family welfare is part of the locality social services, some more specialist aspects of the service are provided by other agencies, such as child and family mental health services or justice services. In France, for example, a separate agency closely linked with the health service is responsible for services for children with disabilities, and child protection and youth justice services are provided by a specialist section of the Justice Department, though working closely with the locality social services.

The legislation in most European jurisdictions has been reviewed in response to the United Nations 'Convention on the Rights of the Child' (United Nations, 1989), and there are many commonalities in the approach to assessment and service provision. The emphasis is on working collaboratively with parents and older children in order to ensure that children are only placed away from home if this is necessary to ensure their safety and development and/or they are likely to benefit from this provision. Self-referral is encouraged, often by the availability of social work in open-access neighbourhood settings such as family centres (for example, Sure Start Children's Centres in England).

Across Europe, most children and adolescents who enter out-of-home care do so on a voluntary basis; the service is viewed as a response to a range of child well-being issues, and since many of these children are difficult to parent because of emotional and behavioural difficulties, there is collaboration with mental health services in assessment and the provision of therapy. There is also a cross-over with criminal justice services, through criminal prosecutions of parents who maltreat their own or others' children and through youth justice services directed at young offenders. In some countries, for example, Scotland and Sweden, youth justice services are integrated within social services for all

Box 9.1 Child welfare approaches in a range of European jurisdictions

ENGLAND

Broad child and family welfare approach: Protection and out-of-home care services integrated with social work and family support to vulnerable families. There are specific guidelines for multiprofessional assessment and intervention when child maltreatment is suspected. Children's services keep a record of and coordinate multiprofessional work with children where a multiprofessional case conference concludes the child has suffered or is likely to suffer 'significant harm' and a formal child protection plan is necessary.

Main child protection agencies: Children's social services, but mechanisms for interprofessional collaboration. If evidence of a serious assault or acute/chronic neglect first becomes known to a health service professional, a paediatrician/trauma specialist is likely to join a specialist police officer and social worker as part of a 'strategy group' to decide on next steps. Health visitors/school nurses are usually key members, alongside a local authority allocated social worker, of the 'team around the child'/'core group' providing ongoing protective and support service.

Mandatory reporting of child abuse? No, but an agreed referral system, which professionals are expected to follow when maltreatment is suspected. Formal substantiation of maltreatment only recorded if formal child protection measures are needed or by the courts. No rate of 'substantiated' maltreatment available.

FINLAND

Broad child and family welfare approach: Family support, protection and out-of-home care services integrated. Municipal social services departments are mandated to assess cases of children referred because there may be a need for a social care service and to provide appropriate services to meet identified need. A client plan is drawn up for all children and families receiving a child welfare service.

Main child protection agencies: Municipality social work services. Links with paediatric clinic and hospital social workers and child psychiatrists/psychologists.

Mandatory reporting of child abuse? Yes, but this applies to a wide range of welfare needs/services including protection. Duty placed on a wide range of agencies to refer children who may be in need of services.

FRANCE

Broad child and family welfare approach: Local social work departments provide a range of social work/social care/socio-educative services (or commission from the voluntary sector). Collaborate with court services in providing services to children at risk of maltreatment or in need of out-of-home care.

Main child protection agencies: Family court services attached to the Justice department and coordinated by a 'juge d'enfants' for assessment and judicial decisions about more serious cases and some out-of-home care. Extensive use of health professionals (attached to the juge d'enfants service for assessment and therapy). Locality social work teams provide longer-term family work and placement services.

Mandatory reporting of child abuse? Yes, of suspected maltreatment, to children's courts. Substantiated maltreatment officially recorded and data available.

ISRAEL

Broad child and family welfare approach: Formal child protection services are an integral part of the services provided by local Departments of Social Services (DSS) and partner agencies. A range of services from home-based (i.e. family support) through community-based (i.e. day care) to out-of-home care.

Main child protection agencies: Local DSS. A multidisciplinary team in the DSS, together with the parent/s and child (when relevant), decide on the treatment plan. Courts if compulsion is necessary in serious abuse cases.

Mandatory reporting of child abuse? Yes. Since 1989, by law, every adult citizen who has a reasonable thought that a minor has been offended against by a guardian/s is required to report this to the police or to a child protection officer.

ITALY

Broad child and family welfare approach: Municipality social services departments provide family support and educative services and therapy to vulnerable children and their families, including those who have been maltreated and are in need of out-of-home care. Close links with health services.

Main child protection agencies: Municipality social services departments work with multiprofessional teams, including paediatrician, gynaecologist, children's neurospsychiatrist, social worker, psychologist, nurse, police officer.

Mandatory reporting of child abuse? No, but an agreed referral system which professionals are expected to follow when maltreatment is suspected.

NORWAY

Broad child and family welfare approach: Family support, child protection and out-of-home care policy is determined nationally. Integrated services are provided by municipalities.

Main child protection agencies: Municipality social work departments. Decisions about compulsory intervention (including care) are taken by the County Child Welfare Boards.

Mandatory reporting of child abuse? No. Policy requires all agencies to collaborate with child and family social care services, which have a duty to assess and provide services to vulnerable children and families and to use legislative protection provisions when necessary.

SCOTLAND

Broad child and family welfare approach: Family support, child protection, out-of-home care and youth justice services are provided as coordinated services by local authority social work departments, which also provide services for adults in need of social care services (including the probation service for adults found guilty of offences including child maltreatment). Strong emphasis on multidisciplinary policy and practice.

Main child protection agencies: Local authority social work departments provide (or commission from the voluntary sector) child protection and out-of-home care services. If elements of compulsion are needed, cases are referred to children's panels.

Mandatory reporting of child abuse? No, but an agreed referral system that professionals are expected to follow when maltreatment is suspected.

SWEDEN

Broad child and family welfare approach: Protection services integrated with social work and family support to vulnerable families.

Main child protection agencies: Locality social work departments providing or coordinating services to all age/disability/needs groups. Some provision of out-of-home care by NGOs and private for-profit sectors.

Mandatory reporting of child abuse? Yes, but this incudes all possibly in need of a social work service and not just child maltreatment. No mandatory decision about whether maltreatment has occurred unless a court order is needed in order to provide services. No accurate incidence data on substantiated maltreatment.

but very serious offenders, while in others (e.g. England and France), there are separate youth justice services and custodial establishments.

European jurisdictions require assistance to be provided to vulnerable families based on the assessment of need (irrespective, for most services, of the ability to pay, although in some countries based on a compulsory insurance system). Most countries have similar legislation to the England and Wales Children Act 1989 (section 17) which places a duty on local authorities to provide a service to children assessed as 'in need' of additional services beyond those 'universally' available, to ensure they achieve 'a reasonable standard' of well-being, or their health or development is not 'significantly impaired'. They also have provisions for compulsory intervention if it can be shown that, without a court order (the majority) or an administrative decision (e.g. Norway), the child is likely to suffer significant harm. State agencies are often required, as in United Kingdom jurisdictions, to show that they have provided appropriate assistance in order to demonstrate that placement in care against parental wishes, or compulsory supervision at home, is necessary. The requirement to provide services in response to assessed need and risk to well-being (in theory at least) for as long as needed, means that several services are usually provided both concurrently and sequentially, and 'universal' 'tier 1' health, education and neighbourhood services are integrated with 'specialist' and 'targeted' child welfare services. Something similar to the coordinated approach spelled out in the England guidance 'Every Child Matters' (Her Majesty's Government, 2003) is in place, although not always so well documented, monitored and reported on, in most European countries (ChildOnEurope, 2009).

There are, however, differences among European states in terms of which agencies actually provide the services. In some (e.g. Finland and Italy) most services are provided by professionals employed by national or local government departments, supplemented by the voluntary sector taking on specialized roles (e.g. Children's Villages in eastern Europe caring for separated children in both residential and family settings). In some, the statutory workers assess the referral and, once the shape of the service needed has been agreed, the voluntary sector becomes the main provider, with the state agency retaining a financing, monitoring and quality assurance role. In some countries, service provision is more mixed, although England is the only European country in which the private for-profit sector has a sizeable role (although at the moment this is almost entirely confined to providing out-of-home foster or residential placements). Differences can also be seen between countries in the settings in which the service is usually provided. In some countries, family members are most likely to attend a day centre or clinical setting, whereas in others the emphasis is on home visiting.

Professionals involved in the assessment of need and provision of services to vulnerable children

As indicated above, accountability for the coordination and provision of services to vulnerable children is, in most European jurisdictions, placed on social services departments, mainly staffed by professionally qualified social workers or para-professionals, variously referred to as 'family support workers', 'social care workers' or 'family aides'. Even when accountability is shared between government departments (e.g. health, justice, education), social workers tend to have a lead role as case managers and to take lead responsibility for ensuring that appropriate services and resources are provided. However, the importance of interagency and interprofessional practice is recognized, with some version of the United Kingdom 'team around the child' or 'team around the family' (Department for Children Schools and Families, 2010) approach being apparent in all jurisdictions. Depending on the country or the characteristics of the child, the lead professional may be a health professional, such as a hospital or community-based paediatrician or community nurse, or (as in France in child protection cases) a 'juge d'enfants'.

One important difference is the existence in mainland Europe but not, until very recently (and still in very small numbers) in the United Kingdom nations, of the profession of 'social pedagogue', 'éducateur spécialisé' or 'educatore sociale'. Although its roots date back further, this profession (which, despite its name, is regarded as a 'social' rather than a 'teaching/school-based' profession) expanded rapidly in numbers after 1945. In broad terms, the social pedagogue tends to be more 'hands on', working sometimes alongside children and parents in the family home (especially in France and Italy), but more often in residential settings, and more often than social workers in the voluntary/NGO sector. Although United Kingdom 'family support workers' often fulfil a similar role, the European social pedagogues are more highly qualified – usually having a 4-year degree-level qualification, although diploma-qualified para-professionals are beginning to appear to meet growing demand (Boddy et al., 2009a, 2009b).

Another difference is that in some countries (Belgium, France and Italy are examples), child psychiatrists and clinical or counselling psychologists play a more significant role as lead professionals and case managers than is the case elsewhere.

The role of the police also varies. In some countries this is confined to responding to emergency calls for help or reports of an offence against a child, or intimate partner violence, and prosecuting alleged offenders; in others, specialist police teams are integrated within the child protection structures, especially in cases of interparental violence or treatment programmes, such as anger management or sexual perpetrator programmes.

All professions have a duty of confidentiality to both children and parents, and to members of the public and professionals providing information, with data protection rules and ethical codes (which differ between professions and jurisdictions) setting out when confidentiality may be broken. Usually this is only when there is serious risk of harm to a child. In most cases, the consent of the person providing the information should be sought before disclosure, unless there is serious and imminent risk of harm to the child or serious danger to another person.

Administrative data and research studies from across Europe indicate that pressures on families are increasing, with: alcohol and substance addictions, mental ill health and cognitive and physical disabilities in parents; challenging behaviour in children; relationship difficulties; and inter-parent violence and parent–child conflict, all on the increase amongst those receiving services. Added to this are environmental and financial problems (such as increased homelessness, poor living conditions and debt) and inter-ethnic tensions all likely to increase as a result of the economic downturn and reduced funding for public services (Bradshaw, Hoelschire and Richardson, 2007; UNICEF, 2007). Looking specifically at the social work and child care workforce, increasing demand is putting pressure on social workers, resulting in a rapid turnover of professional staff in some countries, and with reports from some, such as the four parts of the United Kingdom, that many of those 'in the front line' (especially in child protection services) are inexperienced. There is an acute shortage of foster carers in most countries, resulting in greater use of kinship carers, and in England and Sweden, for example, in the growth of the private for-profit residential care sector.

Services for vulnerable children: the European experience

Broadly speaking, western European child welfare services were much influenced by a post-war consensus about the importance of family life. This was especially the case in countries which are traditionally Catholic, where there remains a resistance to state interference in family life and a strong emphasis on family preservation services and retaining family links when children enter care. In former Eastern Bloc countries, the strong influence of the church was, for a period, overlaid by powerful state controls and surveillance, but families also benefited from the provision of universal health and education services. Partly linked to a knowledge base influenced by academic and professional exchanges with academics and practitioners in the United States, there is a stronger emphasis on children's needs and rights, and a greater willingness to over-rule parental wishes, in Israel and the United Kingdom (seen especially with respect to services for children in care – see below). These positions are not fixed and at different times in their history (often in response to a high-profile case where things have gone wrong) societal attitudes will move along the 'kinship defender'/'state as parent' continuum (see Fox-Harding, 1991, for a discussion of these different positions towards the role of the state in family life). All endorse a children's rights perspective, but interpret this differently (Reading et al., 2009). Some, for example Scandinavian countries as exemplified in the work of a pan-Nordic NGO nobab (www.nobab.org), move closest to the position of giving children of a certain age the right to make key decisions, while others follow the United Nations Convention requirement by ensuring that children have a right to be heard and to influence key decisions.

There are many similarities between the different countries in Europe in the actual shape and content of service provision when children remain with their families, with services characterized by a combination of practical and emotional support, parenting education, relationship-based psychosocial casework, and a range of specific therapeutic interventions, which can be provided either for children, for parent/s, or for the whole family, sometimes on a one-to-one basis and sometimes in groups (see Thoburn, 2007 for a short account of child and family social work in the United Kingdom).

Services aimed at preventing or responding to child abuse and neglect

Information on child protection systems around the world is to be found in Gilbert et al. (1997) and Gilbert, Parton and Skivenes (2011). In the dominant European model of service provision, child protection services are an integral part of child and family welfare services.

Even where there is a separate agency to whom possible maltreatment is reported (as in France and the Netherlands), there is close liaison on the provision and funding of support and therapeutic services once the administrative or judicial processes have taken their course. Preventive services may be delivered in the family home, in community settings (such as neighbourhood family centres), in schools, or in clinical settings (such as family psychiatry or specialist child development centres). Usually a combination of practical help (to reduce poverty, improve housing or provide day care or practical help in the home); educative services (such as parenting groups, counselling, advice services); and a range of approaches to therapy for parents and children are provided. MacMillan et al. (2009) have surveyed the literature on services and specific interventions aimed at preventing and responding to maltreatment. They identify those 'model programmes' (mainly originating in the United States or Australia, but increasingly used in Europe) that have been found to be effective in improving parenting at early stages of the identification of difficulties, although actually linking these positive results to reduced levels of maltreatment is problematic. These authors conclude that, once serious maltreatment has occurred, there is as yet very little robust experimental-design research about 'what works' in preventing re-abuse or helping children to recover from the trauma of abuse or severe neglect.

All countries provide guidance and/or regulations on the detail of investigation, service provision and interprofessional collaboration, alongside legislation for securing the prosecution of offenders and the immediate safety of the children (although the English 'Working Together to Safeguard Children' guidance is probably the most comprehensive) (Her Majesty's Government, 2010). In all countries, the key agencies in the early investigation of serious physical assault, sexual assault and life-threatening neglect are specialist hospital and community doctors, social workers and the police.

One big difference between countries is whether there is legislation requiring specified professionals (or even in some cases, such as Israel, adult citizens) to report to the designated authorities all cases of possible child maltreatment. Penalties for not doing so; which professionals are included as 'designated professionals'; and the types of maltreatment to be reported vary from country to country. The advantages and disadvantages of 'mandatory reporting' are discussed in Gilbert et al. (2009a). Much depends on the legislation and on the responses to reports. The mandated duty in Finland and Sweden is to refer all cases in which a child may be suffering from a range of social and relationship adversities that may be relieved by the provision of a social welfare service. Referrals lead to a social work assessment to ascertain which services are appropriate and, since child protection services are integrated with other services, data are not collected specifically on 'substantiated' child maltreatment cases (as is the case in those jurisdictions in which the 'mandate' is specifically to report only those cases in which maltreatment is suspected). Thus, there are no specific incidence data on maltreated children (and, as an aside, it is therefore not possible to know whether legislation in Sweden and some other countries, where it is an offence to physically chastise children, impacts on the rate of substantiated maltreatment). In France, the mandate is to report cases of suspected abuse and data on substantiated cases of maltreatment are recorded. In some countries, data on known cases of abuse are available even without a system of mandatory reporting. In England, Norway and other countries that have not legislated for mandatory reporting, data on referrals of possible maltreatment are available, but there is no record of the total number of substantiated cases of maltreatment. In the nations of the United Kingdom, national-level data are only available on those cases where a multidisciplinary conference concludes that maltreatment has occurred or is likely to occur, and for which there is need for a formally agreed child protection plan (usually cases of more serious abuse, or where an element of (administrative or judicial) coercion to ensure parental compliance with protection plans has been considered necessary. Multidisciplinary and interagency child protection conferences are a feature of the child protection services of all jurisdictions but the degree of formality varies. The extent of involvement in decision-making of parents and older children varies, with some systems being more 'paternalistic' in their approach (professionals meeting away from family members) and others holding meetings such as family group conferences that include family members. The United Kingdom practice of routinely inviting parents to child protection conferences at which decisions are taken about whether formal intervention is needed is unusual. In part, this difference has opened up because of the greater potential consequences to family integrity of British legislation (see section below on care orders and adoption), and the stronger imperative to observe the principles of natural justice with such serious potential impact of the decisions taken at such meetings on the United Nations convention 'right to family life'.

Out-of-home care services

The differences between European countries are most marked when it comes to out-of-home placement services (Colton and Williams, 1997; Eurochild, 2009; Fernandez and Barth, 2010; Thoburn, 2010b). Legislation in all the European countries provides for short- or longer-term placement away from the family home as a family support measure, or for the provision of 'care and upbringing' for those children whose parents cannot, for whatever reason, meet their needs, even with the support of community-based services. In most countries, this is usually on a 'shared care' basis, even for a long period of time, with strong attempts made to preserve links with birth family members. Care is often provided in response to a request by the parent, or sometimes an older child. In broad terms, the nations of the United Kingdom (although Scotland less so) follow the other Anglophone nations in having a generally negative view about the ability of the care services to meet the needs of children, and there is an ethos of resisting taking children into care and of getting them back to their parents or on to alternative carers, as soon as possible. Italy and France are in some respects closer to the United Kingdom in that children are more likely to come into care via a court order. The result, as shown in Table 9.1, is wide discrepancies in the rate of children in care on a given date from close to 100 or more per 10,000 children under 18 in Finland, France and Poland, and below 50 per 10,000 in Italy and Israel.

The factors that contribute to these differences are complex (Thoburn, 2010b). Although the incidence of deprivation is important, countries with

Table 9.1 Comparative data on rates per 10,000 children in nine western European countries receiving services for vulnerable children (dates of data collection between 2005 and 2010)

Country	*Population 0–17 years old*	*Rate receiving a social care/ social work service because of identified child/family difficulties*	*Rate receiving a service primarily because of substantiated maltreatment*	*Rate in out-of-home care per 10,000*	*% in out-of-home care on a court order*
England	11,012,300	339	32*	58	69
Finland	1,088,456	618	N/A	151	20
France	13,426,557	**	187	97	87
Israel	2,447,258	1760	218	42	N/A
Italy	10,090,805	**	N/A	32	75
Norway	1,174,489	303	82	79	68
Scotland	1,049,100		24*	76	78
Sweden	1,910,967	294	N/A	63	34

* Only those maltreated children currently receiving a formal child protection service (currently on child protection register/with a formal protection plan)
** Only collected as aggregated data from individual localities
Source: Derived from Gilbert et al. (2009) and Thoburn (2010b)

similar relative deprivation (for example, Italy and France) have very different rates in care. Part of the explanation is historical and, in particular, relates to the use of institutional or group care (Browne et al., 2006). Although the use of institutional care for young children is being reduced in favour of foster family care, most countries in Europe retain confidence in the value of good-quality longer-duration residential care as a family support or therapeutic service for teenagers experiencing difficulties. This is apparent from the older age profile of children entering care in Denmark, Finland, France and Sweden. Denmark, France and Germany have rates of children in group care (all over 40 per 10,000 children aged 0–17 years) considerably higher than England (7 per 10,000). However, in this respect, the placement profile of Norway and Sweden is more similar to England (around 13 per 10,000 in group care). There are big differences across Europe in both rates of those in foster care and in the proportions of those in care who are in 'stranger' foster family care or formal kinship care. Italy and Spain have, for many years, made greater use of kinship care than France, the nations of the United Kingdom and Nordic countries, but the percentage in kinship care is growing across Europe. While in general terms the increased use of kinship care is a positive direction, since research indicates that kinship carers are on average more successful on a range of measures than 'stranger' foster parents, nevertheless in a minority of cases what can be a 'default' and ill-planned response exposes children to additional risks.

Another explanation for difference in length of stay, especially of young children, is differential use of adoption as a route out of care. The nations of the

United Kingdom are alone in Europe in making extensive use of adoption without parental consent when (mainly young) care entrants are not able to return safely to parents or relatives within a short space of time. Children who in the United Kingdom are likely to leave care via adoption will, in other European states, more likely grow up in foster family care, usually with some continuing birth family contact. England has a higher rate of entry into care in a given year (25 per 10,000) than Norway (13 per 10,000), but has the same rate in care since Norwegian children stay longer in care. This is despite the fact that Norwegian legislation has moved away from the rest of Europe in making it easier for children to be adopted from care without parental consent. This usually only happens when children have lived for some time with their foster families, as opposed to the British practice of placing young care entrants quickly with adopters not previously known to them. Another explanation for the difference is the extent of use of kinship care, either within the formal care system (as in Spain) or outside it (as is more common in the Nordic countries, which tend to provide support for most kinship carers via 'routine' family support services).

Assessing the challenges: needs and trends

Before moving on to discuss the challenges inherent in comparing and contrasting service delivery, and especially reported child health and welfare outcomes for vulnerable children across Europe, it is necessary to reflect on data collection conventions.

The different approaches to service provision for vulnerable children across Europe impact on the nature of the knowledge base. In part, they explain differences between the approach to 'evidence-based' child welfare practice and research methodologies in Europe and in the Anglophone nations other than the United Kingdom. There is very little use of the RCT research methodology in European child welfare research, with a preference for descriptive and quasi-experimental process, longitudinal and epidemiological methodologies. These tend to measure change over time for individuals with particular problems, rather than comparing those who receive a specified intervention with those who receive a 'service as usual'. They use statistical techniques to seek to identify variables about the children, their families and the services that appear to be associated with more or less successful outcomes, but can rarely claim that a particular intervention 'works' because there is no randomly allocated control group. In the United States the commissioning approach to service provision, and the narrower range of families provided with a child and family social service, result in 'programmes' or 'interventions' that have a clear beginning and end point. This makes it more feasible to randomly allocate children to different programmes or to a 'service as usual'/no service group and to identify whether a defined intervention or 'model programme' works. Although, increasingly, model programmes that have been evaluated using experimental methodologies and found to be effective in the United States are being incorporated into European child welfare practice, it is still difficult to know whether they, or other services likely to be provided at the same time, are contributing to any observed changes. 'Service as usual' is also very difficult to define or standardize in a needs-based welfare system, as was discovered in two recent European trials of multidimensional treatment foster care in England (Biehal, Ellison and Sinclair, 2011) and Sweden (Hansson and Olsson, 2012).

There are often robust cross-sectional administrative data on children in care, or for those receiving a child protection service at national or local level at a specific date each year, but only a minority of countries can provide longitudinal data on those who start to receive a service in a given year, which gives a more reliable guide to recent policies and trends. This is largely because it is still only a minority of countries that require social service agencies to report child-level rather than aggregated data to the national authorities. All jurisdictions recognize the need for national governments to monitor the care it gives to these children, a duty reinforced by the Resolution of the United Nations General Assembly of 15 June 2009 (Guidelines for the Alternative Care of Children GE.09–14213 (E) 160609) (United Nations, 2009). These guidelines build on the UN 'Convention on the Rights of the Child'. Para 68 of the United Nations resolution states:

> It is a responsibility of the State or appropriate level of government to ensure the development and implementation of coordinated policies regarding formal and informal care for all children who are without parental care. Such policies should be based on sound information and statistical data.

In furtherance of this General Assembly Resolution, UNICEF, via its Better Care Network Secretariat, published a 'Manual for the Measurement of Indicators for Children in Formal Care' (UNICEF Better Care Network, 2009). EuroChild (a network of child welfare organizations in 32 European countries supported by the European Commission and the Council of Europe) reported in 2010 on the generally poor level of data collection and analysis in a majority of European countries, and recommended that all EU States refer to the UNICEF Monitoring Guidelines when deciding on data collection systems. They particularly stress the importance of the individual child being the unit of return for data collection to allow for data analysis (Eurochild, 2010).

Epidemiological data on prevalence, incidence and outcomes

Gilbert et al. (2009b) review evidence (from high-income countries across continents), which indicates that many children who are being harmed in their own homes, or in unsupervised private arrangements, are either not known to professionals or not referred for appropriate services. Sweden and England are cited in the paper by Gilbert et al. (2009b:29) as examples of European jurisdictions (one with a mandatory reporting system and the other without) that provide national data on the incidence of referrals for investigation of possible maltreatment (62 per 10,000 children aged 0–17 for England, 177 for Sweden and 486 for the United States). With respect to substantiated maltreatment (Table 9.1) one can compare the rate of 146 per 10,000 substantiated cases in the United States in the Gilbert et al. paper with 177 for France and 82 for Norway. The rate of 32 per 10,000 on a protection plan in

England includes only those children for whom services were being provided and the coercive elements of a formal plan had been considered necessary. However, given the high thresholds for receipt of services in most countries, the rate of children allocated to a social worker's caseload can be considered as indicative of the rate actually or potentially suffering some degree of harm and for whom a service has been considered necessary. The article by Gilbert et al. (2009b) hypothesizes that children in those countries with a broadly 'child welfare' approach are more likely to be identified as vulnerable and provided with a service than those in countries with a narrower 'child safety' approach. Although there was a lower rate of referrals/notifications for service in England (499 per 10,000) and Sweden (424 per 10,000) than notifications of possible maltreatment in the United States (810 per 10,000), there was a higher rate of children actually receiving services in England (262 per 10,000) and Sweden (294 per 10,000) than in the United States (225 per 10,000) (Gilbert et al., 2009b:29). The more recent figures in Table 9.1 demonstrate that some European countries have more children receiving services, with Israel particularly interesting with a high rate for service provision but a comparatively low rate for children in care. These data suggest that the likelihood of children who may be at risk of maltreatment receiving a service is influenced less by protocols for responding to child protection referrals such as mandatory reporting but rather by the meaning ascribed to referral/notification by families, professionals making referrals and those responding to them. Thoburn (2010a discusses 'hard to reach' as well as 'hard to engage' families and supports the line taken by Gilbert et al. (2009a), in arguing that a non-stigmatizing approach to service delivery is more likely to encourage earlier referrals by professionals and also self-referral, and that this should contribute to services reaching those who need them most. There is some evidence from British research that GPs are particularly reluctant to refer families in the early stages of maltreatment because of what they often see as a non-consultative and overly coercive likely response (Tompsett et al., 2009). On the other hand, it has been argued that rigorous data collection systems that specifically record cases of substantiated maltreatment result in greater specificity of approach to intervention based on types of maltreatment.

Because of these different reporting conventions; different definitions of 'vulnerable' and 'maltreatment'; and different measures and time-frames used for reporting outcomes, comparing child well-being outcomes for maltreated children across jurisdictions is problematic. Service-level 'outputs', such as whether the child receives a particular service or has remained in the family home, tend to be used as 'proxies' for child well-being outcomes. As noted above, MacMillan et al. (2009) identify some model programmes that appear to be associated with improved parenting, both as preventive measures and as post-maltreatment interventions. However, once abuse has occurred, given the complexities of families and the number of factors involved, it becomes problematic to identify a causal link between a particular programme or intervention and a positive well-being outcome. This is even more the case in Europe when a range of services and specific interventions tend to be provided concurrently and sequentially.

Detailed analyses of serious case reviews conducted in England consider associations between services provided (or not) and child deaths and serious injuries (Brandon et al., 2009). These researchers concur with the conclusion of Gilbert et al. (2009a) that a proportion of even these most serious cases remain unrecognized by any of the services until a critical incident, or even death, occur. Using WHO statistics, Gilbert et al. (2009a) report that child murder rates have changed very little despite the development of child protection services. They also note that child murder rates are lower in the broadly 'child welfare' based countries, such as Sweden, than in those with less well-developed universal health and welfare services. A more recent analysis of WHO data by Pritchard and Williams (2010) concludes that child abuse related deaths fell in most European countries between 1974–76 and 2004–06, and that the decline was steeper in England and Wales than in comparable 'rich' countries. This more positive finding can be read alongside findings from the most recent prevalence study from the United Kingdom (self-report of victimization during childhood) of a decrease over the past 30 years in the proportions of young adults reporting that they were seriously maltreated by a parent or carer during their childhood, with the largest decrease in physical assault (including chastisement inflicting an injury) (Radford et al., 2012). Set against this encouraging trend is the increase in victimization (especially of children past infancy) at the hands of peers and unrelated adults.

As noted above, out-of-home care is used differently across Europe as a child protection intervention, and the resultant differences in the characteristics of in-care populations can be expected to have an impact on reported outcomes. Outcome data for children with different characteristics, and for different placement options, are only beginning to be available (Sinclair et al., 2007; Thoburn, 2010b; Thoburn and Courtney, 2011). A 2010 book on foster care, edited by Fernandez and Barth, is a particularly useful source, with chapters from Denmark, England, Ireland, the Netherlands, Scotland, Spain and Sweden, plus comparisons with Australia, Canada, and the United States (Fernandez and Barth, 2010). These newly available sources concur with earlier reports that the generally negative view of the value of out-of-home care, especially for children who have suffered neglect, is not supported by the evidence. Most maltreated children do better in care than would be the case if they had remained at home, unless high-quality and sustained services are provided (and the evidence is not encouraging that such services are likely to be provided). The broad conclusion (Bullock et al., 2006; MacMillan et al., 2009) is that the younger children enter care and the longer they remain there, the better their well-being on reaching adulthood. The important caveat is that they must be provided with stable, good-quality parenting and, where necessary, their needs for therapy should be met and their carers supported. Most want, and will benefit from, continuing contact with some, although not necessarily all, their birth family members. An understanding of these findings is leading all countries to seek ways of improving the stability of placements for children in care, including the introduction of more permanent legal guardianship that stops short of adoption, especially for kinship carers and some long-term foster carers. The United Kingdom is also following the lead of France, Germany and the Scandinavian countries in encouraging young people to remain in their care placements until they are in their early 20s.

Lessons learned

In all European countries, children's rights to be protected from trauma, assaults, neglectful parenting and the consequences of a range or adversities are recognized, and services and specialist programmes have been developed to identify and then provide appropriate remedial assistance. The public health impact of failing to identify children at risk of maltreatment, and then failing to provide effective preventive and remedial services and targeted interventions, is also recognized and there has been an increase in collaborative research and the sharing of practice approaches across national boundaries. However, within these shared aims, countries have reached differing conclusions about their detailed responses. As an example, the Nordic countries were the first to ban the physical disciplining of children. Despite pressure from health and social care professionals, successive United Kingdom governments have not gone down that route, but have sought to discourage physical chastisement by public health campaigns and by increasing resources to support and encourage vulnerable parents to find alternative parenting strategies. Some countries have been more ready to use coercive routes to service provision than others and some have been more confident about the value of out-of-home care or adoption as a response to family stresses and maltreatment. All recognize that the response to childhood vulnerability requires collaboration between professionals: some have developed elaborate procedures to attempt to improve interprofessional and interagency working, while others rely on professional competence and confidence. With something as multifaceted as child maltreatment, touching on cultural norms, historical contexts and views about the respective roles of parents and the State, the diversity of detailed service approaches is to be anticipated. Understanding and respecting cultural and contextual differences is an essential part of learning from each other, and indeed presents researchers with opportunities for 'natural experiments'.

There is evidence, from scoping the research, policy and practice literature, that this learning, both between professionals and across national boundaries, is gathering speed. The United Kingdom government is interested in what the social pedagogue approach might have to offer, especially to troubled young people in residential care, and British professionals have learned from European colleagues, and from young people themselves, that remaining in stable family care until early adulthood is essential for some young people who have been severely traumatized by maltreatment. Those in other European countries are learning from British child placement workers and from research that some young people in care need to be guaranteed a sense of permanence and stability so that they can put down roots in a foster or adoptive family rather than constantly wondering if and when they will be sent home.

The future

If countries across Europe are to learn from each other, a first step is the collection and analysis of more robust data. As evidenced by the Eurochild

(2010) survey and conclusions, this will require agreements about definitions for the coding of baseline and outcome data on children and families, and on aspects of service provision, so that the impact of services for children with similar characteristics can be compared. As well as continuing to introduce and rigorously evaluate promising interventions for different groups of vulnerable children, more work is needed on describing and providing agreed codes for capturing 'service as usual' practice of the different professional members of what is increasingly being referred to as the multidisciplinary 'team around the child' or 'team around the family'. Finally, going back to the evidence about the extent of unrecognized suffering amongst children and young people, a particular focus for cross-national learning must be on how best to encourage primary health care professionals and others such as teachers to recognize vulnerability and seek appropriate and timely specialist services.

References

Biehal, H., Ellison, S. and Sinclair, I. (2011) Intensive fostering: An independent evaluation of MTFC in an English setting, *Children and Youth Services Review*, 33(10): 2043–9.

Boddy, J. et al. (2009a) *Working at the 'edges' of care? European models of support for young people and families*. London: Thomas Coram Research Unit.

Boddy, J. et al. (2009b) *International perspectives on parenting support: non-English language sources*. London: Thomas Coram Research Unit.

Bradshaw, J., Hoelschire, P. and Richardson, D. (2007) An index of child wellbeing in the European Union, *Social Indicators Research*, 80(1): 133–77.

Brandon, M. et al. (2009) *Understanding Serious Case Reviews and their Impact*. London: Department for Children, Schools and Families.

Browne, K. et al. (2006) Overuse of institutional care for children in Europe, *BMJ*, 332(7539): 485–7.

Bullock, R. et al. (2006) Can the corporate state parent? *Children and Youth Services Review* (reprinted in *Adoption and Fostering* (2006), 30: 6–19).

ChildOnEurope (2009) *Guidelines on Data Collection and Monitoring Systems on Child Abuse*. Florence: Instituto degli Innocenti.

Colton, M. and Williams, M. (eds) (1997) *The World of Foster Care: An International Sourcebook on Foster Family Care Systems*. Aldershot: Arena.

Department for Children, Schools and Families (2010) *Support for All: The Families and Relationships Green Paper*. London: The Stationery Office.

EuroChild (2010) *Children in Alternative Care: National Surveys*. Brussels: Eurochild.

Fernandez, E. and Barth, R.P. (eds) (2010) *How does foster care work? International evidence on outcomes*. London: Jessica Kingsley.

Fox-Harding, L. (1991) *Perspectives in Child Care Policy*. London: Longman.

Gilbert, N. (ed.) (1997) *Combating Child Abuse: Comparative Perspectives on Reporting Systems and Placement Trends*. New York: Oxford University Press.

Gilbert, N., Parton, N. and Skivenes, M. (2011) *Child Protection Systems: International Trends and Orientations*. New York: Oxford University Press.

Gilbert, R. et al. (2009) Burden and consequences of child maltreatment in high-income countries, *The Lancet*, 393(9657): 68–81.

Gilbert, R. et al. (2009a) Recognising and responding to child maltreatment, *The Lancet*, 373(9658): 167–80.

Hansson, K. and Olsson, M. (2012) Effects of multidimensional treatment foster care (MTFC): Results from a RCT study in Sweden, *Children and Youth Services Review*, 34(9): 1929–36.
Her Majesty's Government (2003) *Every Child Matters*. London: The Stationery Office.
Her Majesty's Government (2010) *Working Together to Safeguard Children*. London: The Stationery Office.
MacMillan, H. et al. (2009) Interventions to prevent maltreatment and associated impairment, *The Lancet*, 373(9659): 250–66.
Pritchard, C. and Williams, R. (2010) Comparing Possible 'Child-Abuse-Related-Deaths' in England and Wales with the Major Developed Countries 1974–2006: Signs of Progress? *British Journal of Social Work*, 40(6): 1700–18.
Radford, L. et al. (2012) *Child abuse and neglect in the UK today*. London: National Society for the Prevention of Cruelty to Children.
Reading, R. et al. (2009) Promotion of children's rights and prevention of child maltreatment, *The Lancet*, 373(9660): 332–43.
Sinclair, I. et al. (2007) *The pursuit of permanence: A study of the English care system*. London: Jessica Kingsley.
Thoburn, J. (2007) Social Work with Children and Families. In Davies, M. (ed.) *The Blackwell Companion to Social Work* (chapter fully revised for 3rd edn). Oxford: Blackwell.
Thoburn, J. (2010a) Towards knowledge-based practice in complex child protection cases: a research-based experts' briefing, *Journal of Children's Services*, 5(1): 9–24.
Thoburn, J. (2010b) Achieving safety, stability and belonging for children in out-of-home care. The search for 'what works' across national boundaries, *International Journal of Child and Family Welfare*, 12(1–2): 34–48.
Thoburn, J. and Courtney, M. (2012) A guide through the knowledge base on children in out-of-home care, *Journal of Children's Services*, 6(4): 210–27.
Tompsett, H., Ashworth, M., Atkins, C., Bell, L., Gallagher, A., Morgan, M. and Wainwright, P. (2009) The Child, the Family and the GP: Tensions and Conflicts of Interest in Safeguarding Children, *DCSF Research Brief* RBX- 09–05.
United Nations (1989) *The United Nations Convention on the Rights of the Child*. New York: United Nations.
United Nations (2009) *Guidelines for the Alternative Care of Children*. GE.09–14213 (E) 160609. New York: United Nations.
UNICEF Better Care Network (2009) *Manual for the Measurement of Indicators for Children in Formal Care*. New York: UNICEF.
UNICEF (2007) *Child poverty in perspective: An overview of child well-being in rich countries*. Florence: Instituto degli Innocenti.

chapter ten

Prescribing for children in Europe

Martin McKee

"There are anomalies and diseases which are met within the infant and child only . . . Therapeutics of infancy and childhood are by no means so similar to those of the adult that the rules of the latter can simply be adopted to the former by reducing doses. The differences are many."

Abraham Jacobi
1830–1919
Paediatrician and founder of the first children's clinic in New York

Children are not just small adults

Children are not just small adults. Yet, for decades they were treated this way, as medicines tested on adults were administered to them without any additional evaluation. Even though they comprise about 20% of the population in European countries, the particular needs of children have largely been ignored in the process of drug discovery and development. Studies from many countries have suggested that up to 75% of medicines administered to children had not been evaluated adequately in this population (Turner et al., 1998; Conroy et al., 2000; Cuzzolin, Zaccron and Fanos, 2003; Pandolfini and Bonati, 2005), a phenomenon referred to as 'off-label' prescribing. The percentages are even higher for children treated for cancer (Paolucci et al., 2008), now one of the most common causes of death in children in Europe, and for neonates this situation persisted for many years (Turner et al., 1996), despite the fact that some of the worst disasters associated with drug use, such as thalidomide, have affected children. Adverse drug reactions have been reported to be more common with off-label prescribing (Turner et al., 1999). However, a study in Germany, found no difference in the number of adverse drug reactions associated with on- and off-licence medicines, but did find that patients treated with the latter had a greater risk of adverse reactions, suggesting that the latter may have been more vulnerable for other reasons, such as impaired metabolism

(Neubert et al., 2004). It is more difficult to ascertain efficacy. While one study using a primary care database in the United Kingdom found that children with asthma prescribed off-label preparations had worse control, once again the direction of causation could not be established (McCowan, Hoskins and Neville, 2007).

Frequently, the prescriber will adapt the dose to the characteristics of the child. This usually involves reducing dosage in line with body weight or, perhaps, surface area. In some cases, the adjustment may simply be based on age. Yet, such adjustments are entirely arbitrary. There are many other factors that may need to be taken into account. Pharmacokinetics may be quite different in children, sometimes in ways that are unexpected (Ginsberg et al., 2002). Some drugs have quite different pharmacological effects in children and adults, in some cases because of delayed maturation of certain receptors. Diazepam may cause agitation in children even though it is widely used as a sedative in adults. Age divisions are also arbitrary, conventionally divided into neonates (up to 28 days), infants (one to 23 months), children (2 to 11 years) and young people (12 to 18 years) (International Conference on Harmonisation, 2000). Yet, the liver, which plays a crucial role in drug metabolism, continues to mature up until about 4 years of age. This can have profound implications. Thus, the immaturity of enzymes in the liver in neonates means that chloramphenicol is not metabolized, leading to the cyanosis and hypotension that characterize 'gray baby syndrome' (Craft et al., 1974; McIntyre and Choonara, 2004). Medicines may also have specific effects arising because of the stage of development of the child, such as the way that tetracyclines stain developing teeth. Steroids will affect growth in children. Suplhonamides given to neonates compete with bilirubin for binding sites on albumin, displacing the latter, which crosses the immature blood–brain barrier causing severe neurological damage. Adolescents seem especially at risk of avacular necrosis of bone when given dexamethasone (Mattano et al., 2000). Unfortunately, the scale of the problem is inadequately understood as there is known to be significant under-recording of adverse effects (Horen, Montastruc and Lapeyre-Mestre, 2002). It can be especially difficult to identify under-dosing.

A key issue is the way that drugs are formulated and administered (Nahata, 1999). The obvious challenges of using inhalers with very young children has led to the development of spacers, recommended in the under-5s (De Benedictis and Selvaggio, 2003). However, a more common, and less easily resolved issue arises where medicines are formulated as tablets that cannot be swallowed by young children. This can give rise to a wide variety of ad-hoc solutions. Captopril is a drug used in heart failure among children, yet there is considerable uncertainty about the optimal dosage (Shaddy, 2001) and its bioavailability is sensitive to the way it is formulated (Reiffel, 2004). A survey of 26 cardiac surgery centres and their referral hospitals in the United Kingdom found widespread variations in the products used (Mulla et al., 2007). Four simply crushed tablets and dissolved them in water before use, while the others used nine different liquid formulations, mostly prepared in the hospitals. Only one, imported from Australia, had any data on stability. Continuity of care was especially problematic; only three of the 13 cardiac surgery centres used the same preparations as their referral hospitals and, in some hospitals, parents were given prescriptions for different formulations for use after discharge. The formulation of medicines for children in hospital pharmacies is widespread across Europe (Brion, Nunn and Rieutord, 2003).

Paediatricians are therefore faced with a dilemma. Do they make these arbitrary decisions, based on untested assumptions and rules of thumb, so that the children for whom they care will receive treatment, even if this involves a risk of under- or over dosage? Or do they simply decide that the risks – medical, ethical and potentially medico-legal – counteract the potential benefits to the child? A survey in Scotland confirmed the widespread use of off-label prescribing by paediatricians but also found that 70% had concerns about safety, although many fewer (47%) were concerned about the efficacy of the drugs used (McLay et al., 2006). There was, however, widespread acceptance that such prescribing was inevitable, with 69% believing it unnecessary to advise parents that they were prescribing off-label and 67% did not inform the child's GP. Nor was there overwhelming acceptance of the need for trials of many of the medicines currently in use, reflecting in part the view that data on efficacy in adults can be extrapolated to children as well as concern about obtaining informed consent in children (see later). A survey of GPs in Northern Ireland obtained similar results, also noting that most prescribers gained their knowledge from personal experience rather than any more robust source of evidence (Mukattash et al., 2011a). Northern Ireland is also the setting for the only study that could be identified for this chapter in which children (aged 10 to 16 years) were asked their views. They felt that older children and parents should be informed when medicines were prescribed off-licence (Mukattash et al., 2011b).

Another Scottish study described the pattern of off-label prescribing in primary care, with the most common form being reduced dosage (40–50% of all off-label prescribing), mostly involving antibiotics and antihistamines, and higher than recommended dose (35%), mostly involving anti-asthmatics, topical corticosteroids and laxatives (Ekins-Daukes et al., 2004). Off-label prescribing according to age was less common and mainly involved children under 2 years of age, while that in respect of formulation was least common.

The pattern of off-licence prescribing is, of course, likely to be different from that in hospitals, given the different spectrum of disease. However, those studies conducted in secondary care settings have also reported high levels of use of off-label and unlicensed medicines (Di Paolo et al., 2006; Dell'Aera et al., 2007; Lindell-Osuagwu et al., 2009).

The barriers to evaluating medicines in children

The barriers to evaluating medicines in children are considerable (Rocchi et al., 2010). Beyond the common childhood ailments, the number of children requiring medication is small, and among those that do, there are very many rare disorders. Consequently, the market for paediatric medicines is small. This has implications for trial design, as it may be necessary to recruit from a very large number of centres to obtain sufficient eligible subjects and controls. Ethical approval may be difficult to obtain (see next section). Dosages and schedules evaluated are arbitrary, chosen by scaling down the regimes used in adults. Trials on children are usually a lower priority than adults for manufacturers. Consequently, they are likely to start much later so that, by the time any results are available, the product may be approaching patent expiry.

It is important to recognize that evaluation is a necessary but not sufficient requirement for licensing. In some specialities, and especially oncology, trials may be conducted by academic researchers independent of manufacturers. The manufacturer must then decide whether, on the basis of a business case, to seek approval (Conroy, Newman and Gudka, 2003).

Ethical considerations

For many years there was a widespread view that the perceived inability of children to give informed consent meant that clinical trials involving them would be unethical. However, there is now much greater recognition that the situation in which the only treatment for children is with unevaluated medicines is in itself unethical, a view encouraged by extensive evidence of the benefits to patients from participating in trials, regardless of the arm they are in (Chalmers and Lindley, 2001).

Saint Raymond and Brasseur (2005) reviewed in detail the ethical considerations relevant to trials in children. They highlight a number of contradictions and inconsistencies. Thus, while the European 'Clinical Trials Directive' (European Parliament and Council of the European Union, 2001) specifies that participants must give informed consent, and that participation by children 'must represent the minor's presumed will', they note that the Directive respects varying national provisions on parental consent. The situation is complicated further by the use of the concept of 'assent' to treatment, which can be given by a non-competent child under various European and international conventions, but is not mentioned in the Clinical Trials Directive. They note evidence that ability to understand the concepts necessary to give informed consent is not present until children reach the age 7 to 9 years old (Rossi, Reynolds and Nelson, 2003).

These uncertainties led to the development of a set of European guidelines addressing: trial design and methods; assessment of risks and benefits; safety monitoring; and the needs of specific populations (Sammons, 2009).

Contrary to what is sometimes assumed, parents are often very willing to give consent for their children to participate in trials once the nature of the trial has been explained and where there is a trusting relationship with the health professionals involved (Harth and Thong, 1995). In many other respects, such as the use of placebos, the same principles apply as in adults, such as the need for equipoise.

Towards a solution

By the 1990s, it was clear that the existing system of drug development was failing children. In 1990, the European Parliament had called upon the

European Commission to bring forward measures to address their needs. However, progress came first in the United States, where the Food and Drug Administration (FDA) introduced a provision for 'pediatric exclusivity' in its 1997 Modernization Act. This enabled the FDA to request manufacturers to conduct additional studies to evaluate the application of their products to children, both prior to approval for adults and subsequently. In return, the manufacturers would be given a 6-month patent extension. From the beginning this was viewed as a success. The FDA claimed it had 'done more to generate clinical studies and useful prescribing information for the pediatric population than any other regulatory or legislative process to date' (Food and Drug Administration, 2001), a view endorsed by subsequent independent research (Roberts et al., 2003).

This success led to the passage of the 2002 Best Pharmaceuticals for Children Act (BPCA) and the 2003 Pediatric Research Equity Act (PREA). The BPCA extended the pediatric exclusivity provision, which had originally been scheduled to run for only 5 years, and extended it to drugs whose patents had expired. The PREA converted the original scheme from a voluntary to a compulsory one, permitting the FDA to require manufacturers to undertake studies on the application of their products to children.

A European response

Progress was somewhat slower in Europe. In 1997, the European Medicines Agency (EMA) had issued a guidance note on clinical investigation of medical products in children. However, this was viewed widely as being inadequate, especially in the light of achievements in the United States. The National Institute for Health Research in England established the Medicines for Children Research Network in 2005, specifically to improve research on medicines for children and adolescents (http://www.mcrn.org.uk). However it was only a decade after the EMA guidance, in 2007, that a European Union Regulation with similar features to the earlier American legislation came into force (Commission of the European Communities, 2006).

The new Regulation invited manufacturers to apply for a paediatric investigation plan (PIP) for new products undergoing approval (Permanand, Mossialos and McKee, 2007). The PIP, submitted at the end of phase I or II studies, is assessed by a newly created Paediatric Committee (PDCO) of the EMA, comprising experts in child health and representatives of professional associations and patients' organizations from across Europe. As with the American legislation, there is a strong incentive to apply. If the PIP is accepted, the manufacturer gains an additional 6 months' market exclusivity (on top of the combined maximum 15 years granted by patent protection and the supplementary protection certificate (a measure that extends exclusivity of medicines and related products in recognition of the length of time taken to achieve authorization). This extra market exclusivity that comes with a PIP is awarded not on completion of the study, but on signifying the intention to do this. The incentives in respect of orphan drugs are more generous (defined in the EU as a product for the diagnosis, prevention or treatment of a life-threatening or chronically debilitating condition affecting no more than 5 in 10,000 people in the EU at the time of submission, or for a life-threatening, seriously debilitating or serious and chronic condition, where it would be unlikely without incentives that the revenue after marketing of the medicinal product would cover the investment in its development). In such cases, the acceptance of a PIP gives an additional 2 years on top of the 10 years' market exclusivity.

The PDCO can respond to a PIP in four ways:

1. It can reject it entirely as inadequate, which is unusual.
2. It can approve the PIP, in which case the manufacturer agrees to undertake additional work to establish the parameters (dosage, formulation, frequency etc.) in children of different ages or with other specific characteristics.
3. It can defer a decision until additional information is available, recognizing that the approval process begins early in the testing of a new medicine.
4. It can issue a waiver, signifying that evaluation in children is not required. This may be because the condition for which it is intended does not occur in children, or because there is no significant difference from existing treatments.

Given the importance of avoiding unnecessary investigations on children, the entire process is coordinated closely with the FDA to avoid duplication of research and, especially, trials.

The Regulation also makes provision for the EMA to provide free scientific advice on questions related to medicines in children. This can take the form of scientific advice or protocol assistance (where the medicines are for orphan diseases). This is designed to help companies design and conduct trials needed to demonstrate the quality, safety and efficacy of medicines in the paediatric population. The advice is provided by the Scientific Advice Working Party of the Committee for Medicinal Products for Human Use (CHMP), with active involvement by members of the PDCO. In addition, the EMA has produced a number of highly influential documents on issues such as paediatric formulations and organ maturity (Breitkreutz, 2008).

These provisions relate to new products being submitted for approval. However, there are many existing medicines, most of which are now off-patent, that offer considerable potential benefits to children but have never been evaluated for use in them. Consequently, the Regulation has established a second mechanism, called Paediatric Use Marketing Authorisation (PUMA). This only applies to medicines intended solely for children. Recognizing that there is little scope for commercial benefit, the Regulation includes provisions for funding the necessary evaluations. An initial draft of the Regulation provided for a specific Medicines Investigation for the Children of Europe (MICE) fund but this did not make it into the final version (Permanand, Mossialos and McKee, 2007). Instead, funding has been made available within the European Commission's Research Framework programmes, with priorities for research established by the PDCO.

The Regulation has also encouraged research by means of the establishment of a European Network of Paediatric Research (Enpr-EMA), which brings together centres of excellence in ways that maximize the opportunities for collaborative research, shared protocols and patient recruitment, while avoiding possible duplication of effort. Enpr-EMA came into being in 2011. At the time of writing, 33 networks have applied for membership and been allocated to one of three categories: Category 1 (18 networks and centres now full members); Category 2 (networks and centres still being evaluated); and Category 3 (networks and centres not currently qualifying for membership). However, all are informed of relevant information and invited to annual Enpr-EMA workshops.

The Regulation also promotes the inclusion of experts in paediatrics on ethical committees. The need for such measures to build capacity are apparent from a 2005 survey, which could identify only 18 paediatric clinical pharmacologists in Europe (Bonati et al., 2006).

The final strand in the Regulation relates to transparency. Details of all progress in trials on children should be included in the publicly accessible European Clinical Trials database (EudraCT), while information on decisions regarding PIPs is included on the EMA's website.

There are a number of other provisions, although not all have been implemented. For example, Article 32 of the Regulation envisaged the development of a symbol that could be used throughout the EU to designate medicines that were approved for use in children. However, it was not possible to agree what such a symbol would look like and the quest for consensus was abandoned in 2008.

Achievements

As the preceding sections show, much progress has been made in improving the regulatory framework for paediatric medicines in Europe. But how much difference has it made? It seems that progress has been mixed.

A first question is whether the formulation of medicines labelled as appropriate for children changes prescribing. This was evaluated in a Finnish study of the use of triptans, a treatment for migraine, between 1994 and 2007 (Lindkvist et al., 2011). A nasal formulation of sumatriptan was authorized for young people (age 12 years and over) in 2003. Sumatriptan was the market leader, contributing 64% of all triptans prescribed to children. Although on-label prescribing increased substantially, so did off-label prescribing. By 2007, 72% of paediatric prescriptions were still off-label.

A second is the extent to which the new Regulation has increased the availability of medicines for children. A recent paper has quantified progress in the first 3 years of the new regime, drawing on a detailed analysis of applications for PIPs; scientific opinions by the PDCO; and paediatric clinical trials registered on EudraCT (Olski et al., 2011). The largest number of PIPs was for endocrinological disorders (13.4%), followed by oncology (11%), infectious (10.8%) and cardiovascular diseases (7.1%). Of the PIPs, 23% involved the development of age-appropriate formulations, while 26% included studies on dosing, efficacy and safety in specific age groups, in particular neonates. However, the PDCO requested major modifications in 38% of PIPs submitted, in most cases to strengthen the methodology. There was less progress in boosting the proportion of trials undertaken on children, which increased only from 8.2% to 9.4% of all trials registered on EudraCT. The authors, who are from the EMA, concluded that the goal of increasing access to age-appropriate medicines will be achieved (albeit with considerable input from the PDCO) but that progress in increasing trials has been much more limited.

The task of increasing trials of paediatric medicines has been complicated by the challenges inherent in implementing the Clinical Trials Directive. This is widely viewed as having failed in its goal of promoting trials as it has led to a marked increase in bureaucracy and in the costs of complying with regulatory requirements, including a doubling of insurance costs. It has been cited as a major factor in slowing the growth of paediatric trials in Europe (Cannell, 2007; Welzing et al., 2007), as well as reductions in the numbers of subjects enrolled.

There has also been less progress than some hoped for in making off-patent drugs available through the PUMA process.

There has, however, been progress in the development of networks of researchers and practitioners, such as the Task-force in Europe for Drug Development for the Young (TEDDY) network (Ceci et al., 2009). This acts as a platform for researchers, regulators and practitioners, working to increase understanding of the changing regulatory environment, developing shared approaches to common problems, including common research tools, and strengthening links between the different stakeholders.

In summary, the regulatory situation with regard to prescribing for children has long lagged behind that of adults. This has, at last, changed in Europe with the passage of the paediatric medicines Directive and, while significant progress has been made in some areas, there is still an unfinished agenda.

Acknowledgement

We are grateful to Sir Alasdair Breckenridge, Chairman, Medicines and Healthcare products Regulation Authority, United Kingdom, for helpful comments.

References

Bonati, M. et al. (2006) Paediatric clinical pharmacology in Europe, *Paediatric and Perinatal Drug Therapy*, 7: 134–7.

Breitkreutz, J. (2008) European perspectives on pediatric formulations, *Clinical Therapeutics*, 30(11): 2146–54.

Brion, F., Nunn, A.J. and Rieutord, A. (2003) Extemporaneous (magistral) preparation of oral medicines for children in European hospitals, *Acta Paediatrica*, 92(4): 486–90.

Cannell, E. (2007) Clinical Trials Directive slows registration of paediatric studies, *The Lancet Oncology*, 8(1): 10.

Ceci, A. et al. (2009) The Task-force in Europe for Drug Development for the Young (TEDDY) Network of Excellence, *Paediatric Drugs*, 11(1): 18–21.

Chalmers, I. and Lindley, R.I. (2001) Double standards on informed consent to treatment. In: Doyal, L. and Tobias, J.S. (eds) *Informed consent in medical research.* London: BMJ Books.

Commission of the European Communities (2006) Regulation (EC) No 1901/2006 on medicinal products for paediatric use and amending Regulation (EC) No 1768/92, Directive 2001/20/EC, Directive 2001/83/EC and Regulation (EC) No 726/2004, *Official Journal of the European Communities,* L378 27/12/, 1–19.

Conroy, S. et al. (2000) Survey of unlicensed and off label drug use in paediatric wards in European countries. European Network for Drug Investigation in Children, *BMJ,* 320(7227): 79–82.

Conroy, S., Newman, C. and Gudka, S. (2003) Unlicensed and off label drug use in acute lymphoblastic leukaemia and other malignancies in children, *Annals of Oncology,* 14(1): 42–7.

Craft, A.W., Brocklebank, J.T., Itey, E.N., and Jackson, R.H. (1974). The "grey-toddler". Chloramphenicol toxicity. *Arch. Dis. Child.,* 49, 235–7.

Cuzzolin, L., Zaccaron, A. and Fanos, V. (2003) Unlicensed and off-label uses of drugs in paediatrics: a review of the literature, *Fundamental and Clinical Pharmacology,* 17(1): 125–31.

De Benedictis, F.M. and Selvaggio, D. (2003) Use of inhaler devices in pediatric asthma, *Paediatric Drugs,* 5(9): 629–38.

Dell'Aera, M. et al. (2007) Unlicensed and off-label use of medicines at a neonatology clinic in Italy, *Pharmacy World and Science,* 29(4): 361–7.

Di Paolo, E.R. et al. (2006) Unlicensed and off-label drug use in a Swiss paediatric university hospital, *Swiss Medical Weekly,* 136(13–14): 218–22.

Ekins-Daukes, S. et al. (2004) Off-label prescribing to children in primary care: retrospective observational study, *European Journal of Clinical Pharmacology,* 60(5): 349–53.

European Parliament and Council of the European Union (2001) Directive 2001/20/EC Of The European Parliament and of The Council of 4 April 2001 on the approximation of the laws, regulations and administrative provisions of the Member States relating to the implementation of good clinical practice in the conduct of clinical trials on medicinal products for human use, *Official Journal of the European Communities,* L121: 34–44.

FDA (2001) *The pediatric exclusivity provision: January 2001 status report to Congress.* Washington, DC: Food and Drug Administration, Department of Health and Human Services.

Ginsberg, G. et al. (2002) Evaluation of child/adult pharmacokinetic differences from a database derived from the therapeutic drug literature, *Toxicological Sciences,* 66(2): 185–200.

Harth, S.C. and Thong, Y.H. (1995) Parental perceptions and attitudes about informed consent in clinical research involving children, *Social Science and Medicine,* 40: 1573–7.

Horen, B., Montastruc, J.L. and Lapeyre-Mestre, M. (2002) Adverse drug reactions and off-label drug use in paediatric outpatients, *British Journal of Clinical Pharmacology,* 54(6): 665–70.

International Conference on Harmonisation (2000) *Clinical investigation of medicinal products in the pediatric population.* Geneva: International Conference on Harmonisation.

Lindell-Osuagwu, L. et al. (2009) Off-label and unlicensed drug prescribing in three paediatric wards in Finland and review of the international literature, *Journal of Clinical Pharmacy and Therapeutics,* 34(3): 277–87.

Lindkvist, J. et al. (2011) Evolution of paediatric off-label use after new significant medicines become available for adults: a study on triptans in Finnish children 1994–2007, *British Journal of Clinical Pharmacology*, 71(6): 929–35.

Mattano, L.A., Jr et al. (2000) Osteonecrosis as a complication of treating acute lymphoblastic leukemia in children: a report from the Children's Cancer Group, *Journal of Clinical Oncology*, 18(18): 3262–72.

McCowan, C., Hoskins, G. and Neville, R.G. (2007) Clinical symptoms and 'off-label' prescribing in children with asthma, *British Journal of General Practice*, 57(536): 220–2.

McIntyre, J. and Choonara, I. (2004) Drug toxicity in the neonate, *Biology of the Neonate*, 86(4): 218–21.

McLay, J.S. et al. (2006) A prospective questionnaire assessment of attitudes and experiences of off label prescribing among hospital based paediatricians, *Archives of Disease in Childhood*, 91(7): 584–7.

Mukattash, T. et al. (2011a) Healthcare professional experiences and attitudes on unlicensed/off-label paediatric prescribing and paediatric clinical trials, *European Journal of Clinical Pharmacology*, 67(5): 449–61.

Mukattash, T. et al. (2011b) Children's views on unlicensed/off-label paediatric prescribing and paediatric clinical trials, *European Journal of Clinical Pharmacology*, 68(2): 141–8.

Mulla, H. et al. (2007) Variations in captopril formulations used to treat children with heart failure: a survey in the United Kingdom, *Archives of Disease in Childhood*, 92(5): 409–11.

Nahata, M.C. (1999) Pediatric drug formulations: challenges and potential solutions, *Annals of Pharmacotherapy*, 33(2): 247–9.

Neubert, A. et al. (2004) The impact of unlicensed and off-label drug use on adverse drug reactions in paediatric patients, *Drug Safety*, 27(13): 1059–67.

Olski, T.M. et al. (2011) Three years of paediatric regulation in the European Union, *European Journal of Clinical Pharmacology*, 67(3): 245–52.

Pandolfini, C. and Bonati, M. (2005) A literature review on off-label drug use in children, *European Journal of Pediatrics*, 164(9): 552–8.

Paolucci, P. et al. (2008) Challenges in prescribing drugs for children with cancer, *The Lancet Oncology*, 9920: 176–83.

Permanand, G., Mossialos, E. and McKee, M. (2007) The EU's new paediatric medicines legislation: serving children's needs? *Archives of Disease in Childhood*, 92(9): 808–11.

Reiffel, J.A. (2004) Formulation substitution: a frequently overlooked variable in cardiovascular drug management, *Progress in Cardiovascular Diseases*, 47(1): 3–10.

Roberts, R. et al. (2003) Pediatric drug labeling: improving the safety and efficacy of pediatric therapies, *JAMA*, 290(7): 905–11.

Rocchi, F. et al. (2010) The European paediatric legislation: benefits and perspectives, *Italian Journal of Pediatrics*, 36: 56.

Rossi, W.C., Reynolds, W. and Nelson, R.M. (2003) Child assent and parental permission in pediatric research, *Theoretical Medicine and Bioethics*, 24(2): 131–48.

Saint Raymond, A. and Brasseur, D. (2005) Development of medicines for children in Europe: ethical implications, *Paediatric Respiratory Reviews*, 6(1): 45–51.

Sammons, H. (2009) Ethical issues of clinical trials in children: a European perspective, *Archives of Disease in Childhood*, 94(6): 474–7.

Shaddy, R.E. (2001) Optimizing treatment for chronic congestive heart failure in children, *Critical Care Medicine*, 29(10 Suppl): S237–40.

Turner, S. et al. (1996) Use of "off-label" and unlicensed drugs in paediatric intensive care unit, *The Lancet*, 347(9000): 549–50.

Turner, S. et al. (1998) Unlicensed and off label drug use in paediatric wards: prospective study, *BMJ*, 316(7128): 343–5.
Turner, S. et al. (1999) Adverse drug reactions to unlicensed and off-label drugs on paediatric wards: a prospective study, *Acta Paediatrica*, 88(9): 965–8.
Welzing, L. et al. (2007) Consequences of Directive 2001/20/EC for investigator-initiated trials in the paediatric population – a field report, *European Journal of Pediatrics*, 166(11): 1169–76.

chapter eleven

Comprehensive strategies for improving child health services in Europe

Ingrid Wolfe, Giorgio Tamburlini, Matthew Thompson, Peter Gill, Martin McKee

It is justice, not charity that is wanting in the world.

Mary Wollstonecraft, 1792

Introduction

Europe is undergoing a process of rapid change, affecting the economy, welfare policies, demography, and social and cultural norms. All these factors greatly influence child health and development and, together with advances in science and technology, contribute to shaping the current and future lives of Europe's children. The health problems affecting children are changing as the diseases and disabilities they face evolve from predominantly acute and infectious illnesses towards chronic diseases and long-term conditions. Children's lives are changing too; for example, family structures and the social settings in which children live and grow up are being reshaped by technological advances. Together, these pose tremendous challenges to health systems throughout Europe, which will have to be met in order to ensure a healthy and thriving future for children.

There have been great successes in European child health in recent decades but, in many regards, the responses of health systems to advances in knowledge and to changing health and social needs, have been inadequate. There is increasing understanding that the roots of physical health, cognitive development, and social and emotional well-being are established early in life, but there has been a systematic failure fully to translate this knowledge into policy and practice. Furthermore, there has been a failure to anticipate the changes in children's health needs and in parental expectations of care, and too often a failure to respond adequately and appropriately to evolving needs and demands. The *World Health Report 2008* describes health systems' responses as 'too little, too late, or too much in the wrong place' and argues that a whole-system solution, rather than temporary and piecemeal remedies is required, involving society beyond the health sector (WHO, 2008). This certainly applies to children's health systems in Europe. National policies for children's health have too often focused on individual short-term issues, engendering needless competition for scarce resources and further fragmenting services, while paying inadequate attention to the underlying problems and preventing meaningful change. We believe that a system-wide transformation will be required to secure the health of Europe's children.

The purposes of this book have been to: examine European countries' approaches to children's health services and systems; identify common experiences; point out notable differences; and learn lessons from each other. The aim is to inform a strategy for improving child health services and systems, and ultimately the health and well-being of children.

Main findings

The findings of this book can be considered under three main themes. First, there is a mismatch between children's health needs and the services and systems that should be ready to meet those needs, and a failure to respond to progress in understanding child development. The consequences include suboptimal health outcomes; unnecessary variation in quality of care; inefficient, inconvenient services; and ultimately failure to realize children's full potential health and development. Secondly, there are missed opportunities to maximize children's health gain and well-being through a focus on population health and social equity. The consequences include: high rates of preventable NCDs; pervasive unmet needs among vulnerable children; and widening gaps between rich and poor. Thirdly, there is a failure to realize the rights-based approach to child health that underpins the United Nations 'Convention on the Rights of the Child', to which each European country has agreed. These three themes capture the variety of problems facing European child health services and systems. The next section sets out why these problems may have arisen, with a view to informing the section on strategy which will follow.

Mismatch between health needs, services and systems

There are many reasons why outcomes of health care among children are not as good, or consistently good, as they could be. We will consider three main categories: the shifting burden of disease; the organization of health care delivery systems; and advances in paediatric medicine.

The epidemiological shift away from infectious illnesses and towards chronic diseases, including conditions affecting mental health, mandates a change in approach to health services. Children with chronic diseases, long-term conditions, mental ill health and disabilities need different models of care from the traditional episodic reactive health service of the past. Currently, services for children with long-term conditions are fragmented and often of poor quality, inconvenient and sometimes unsafe. One of the reasons for this is that health services are still largely hospital-centric, and the multidisciplinary team-based planned care for children with chronic conditions is left to fit in around the needs of an urgent care-driven health model (Wolfe et al., 2011, 2013).

Second, and related, are suboptimally organized child health care delivery systems. Health services are too often driven by the needs of professionals and systems, and attempts to improve services are limited by inadequate data about health needs and insufficient knowledge about what works better and how to achieve it (Wolfe et al., 2011, 2013). Services should be organized to meet health needs, able to deliver equitable, accessible, high-quality, safe care. Irrespective of the type of health system and funding model, there needs to be a mechanism in place to ensure that children with needs, who would otherwise not be recognized, will be identified and cared for. This includes children from marginalized communities, such as the Roma, and other transient communities.

Finally, medicine advances exponentially and in some ways fails to deliver on its promises. The growing complexity and cost of technological medicine is one reason. Advances in medicine are outpacing our abilities to pay for, and deliver, care optimally. Furthermore, resources for research and development are often highly focused on problems that affect the adult population, and too often directed towards rare diseases at the cost of common problems where the majority of the disease burden lies (Modi et al., 2013). For example, while gene technology and telemedicine hold great promise and capture headlines, there are apparently insufficient funds to ensure social care for disabled children.

Missed opportunities to maximize health and well-being

Child health is about more than preventing illness and treating it when it occurs. It is about fostering good health and maximizing child development. Most child health services and systems in Europe remain focused on the former, while paying insufficient attention to the latter. Different interventions are needed at different life-stages; if an optimal balance is achieved, a healthy child will develop to reach their full potential. This reflects the life-course approach, illustrated in Figure 11.1. Understanding developmental trajectories gives an indication of the balanced approach to planning and providing services, which is needed in order to deliver maximal health gain for children.

Failure to translate the rhetoric of child rights to reality

Many European child health strategies, such as the English National Service Framework (Department of Health, 2004), are predicated, in part, on the United Nations 'Convention on the Rights of the Child'. Health strategies for the whole population, such as 'Health for All', WHO's global strategy aiming to achieve its goals by 2000, took the same laudable approach (WHO, 1981), for example. It is a gross social injustice that children and adolescents with

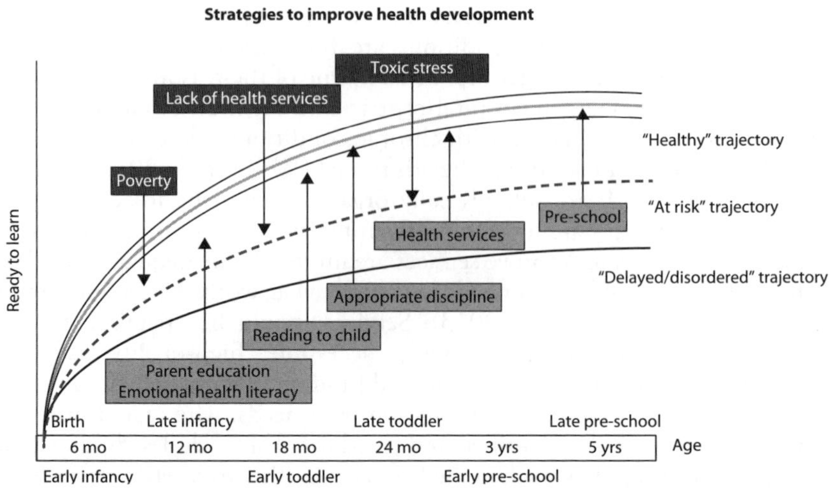

Figure 11.1 A life-course approach to child health and development

Source: Neal Halfon

mental health needs do not receive care commensurate with their problems, and equally so that the general health needs of adolescents remain inadequately addressed. Finally, child poverty and social inequalities persist in many countries, although in some very much more so than in others. Most of these problems are amenable to policy, and the failure of many countries to act is striking. Underlying many of these problems is the finding that countries lack mechanisms for the translation of high-level goals into meaningful deliverable policies, with effective accountability structures to ensure delivery.

A strategy for European child health

The three themes described in the preceding section derive from the various issues and challenges described in the chapters of this book. Every chapter has demonstrated that the problems confronting child health services and systems are complicated, meaning that solutions will inevitably be complex too.
Systems thinking acknowledges the huge complexity of the problems facing health systems, and the responses that will be required to meet health needs. For example, understanding, anticipating and reacting to the effects of an intervention on other parts of the system will be crucial if attempts to improve chronic care systems are to be successful (de Savigny and Adam, 2009). A whole-systems approach is needed to deliver the scale and scope of changes that will be needed to strengthen child health systems adequately to meet the current and evolving health needs of Europe's children. Action is needed in three broad and interdependent categories: practice, plans and policy (Figure 11.2).

Practice:

- Primary and first contact care
- A comprehensive chronic care model
- Public health
- Integrating services
- Workforce

Plan:

- Health services, systems and policy research
- Child health indicators
- Preparing for the future

Policy:

- Health in all policies
- Evidence and policy
- Accountability
- Commitment

A comprehensive strategy for child health relies on strengthening the capacity of European health systems to drive improvements in health and equity. This demands that health systems become more responsive. Responsiveness is a fairly new concept in the study of health systems; it recognizes that health systems should meet the legitimate expectations of the public, in particular, for quality of care and patient satisfaction. It also recognizes that health systems are one component of social systems, there to serve the public in meeting common goals (see Figure 1.1). Several international surveys have examined the responsiveness of national health systems, the two largest being the *World Health Survey 2002* (WHO, 2002) and the *WHO Multi-Country Survey Study*

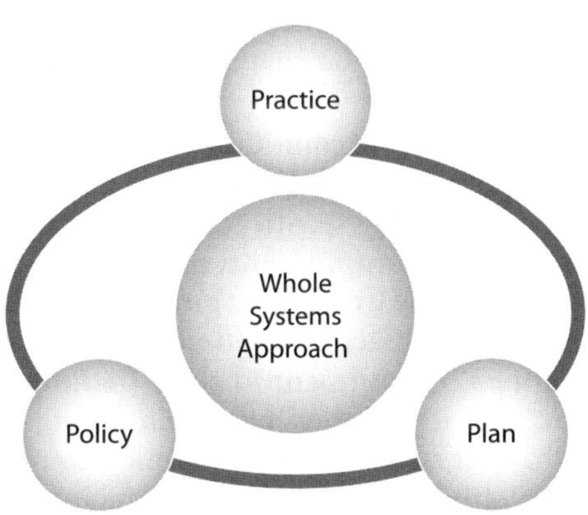

Figure 11.2 A whole-systems approach to strategy for European child health

Source: Adapted from Wolfe et al., 2013

2000/01 (Murray and Evans, 2003). Yet, while these included questions on children's health care, there is little published literature on responsiveness with respect to the child or young person per se. A preliminary survey by the Council of Europe in 22 of its Member States found that children are acutely aware of how they are treated by health care professionals and that they take a keen interest in the respect with which they are treated and in their need for information (Kilkelly, 2011). By establishing the values that define child health systems, we can strengthen our ability to translate a strategy into persuasive arguments for implementation and for holding those responsible for delivery to account for the results. A rights-based approach to child health services (Box 11.1) helps in articulating the values we should aspire to, because it allows health to be contextualized within the social and environmental conditions in which children live and grow up. The crucial point of the United Nations 'Convention on the Rights of the Child' is that it is about children in their own right, not as 'adults-to-be', whereby the period of childhood is seen merely as preparatory for adulthood. Thus, clinicians, health service managers and policy-makers should strive to meet the promises of the 'Convention on the Rights of the Child' by ensuring that child rights feature in every element of policy and practice.

Box 11.1 A rights-based approach to child health services

Clinicians and policy-makers should strive to realize children's rights to:

- A high standard of health care.
- Have special needs attended to.
- Have their best interests considered.
- Not suffer discrimination.
- Have their privacy and confidentiality respected.
- Receive direct and appropriate information about their health.
- Be able to participate in discussions and decisions.

Source: Adapted from Wolfe et al., 2013.

The Council of Europe adopted a resolution in 2011 to promote child-friendly health care, the provisions of which are summarized in Box 11.2. If the concepts articulated in the child-friendly health care resolution are implemented comprehensively, many of the commitments of the 'Convention on the Rights of the Child' would be realized (Council of Europe, 2011).

To deliver a rights-based approach to children's health services, as articulated by the Council of Europe's commitment to child-friendly health care, changes in practice are needed. This is where we begin our description of a strategy for European child health. Our strategy is not intended to provide a 'one size fits all' approach to child health; we acknowledge the regional and local variations in need and solutions, for example, the unique challenges of providing services in remote and rural settings. Our strategy is intended to provide a framework for adapting and refining according to local circumstances. Furthermore, as

Box 11.2 Child-friendly health care

The 47 Member States of the Council of Europe, in 2011, adopted guidelines on child-friendly health care, predicated on a rights-based approach to health care and key principles of the United Nations 'Convention on the Rights of the Child'.

- Children's rights guiding the planning, delivery and monitoring of health care services for children.
- Equitable access to quality health care services for all children.
- Appropriate integrated services for children with special needs.
- Eliminating discrimination against any child on any ground, such as sex, race, colour, language, religion, political or other opinion, national or social origin, association with a national minority, property, birth or other status.
- Facilitating the implementation of the principle in Article 6 of the Oviedo Convention with regard to the child's participation in medical decisions.
- Founding all decisions regarding children's health on their best interests, in a process involving the children themselves and their families.
- Evidence-based interventions by professionals with appropriate competences, dedication and knowledge of child-specific physical and well-being needs, as well as their psychosocial situation.
- Parents or carers being allowed, encouraged and helped to stay with the child receiving health care, unless this goes against the child's best interest.
- Health care institutions making the necessary arrangements to facilitate parents or carers staying with the child receiving health care.
- Working with ministries and other relevant stakeholders to effectively address the biopsychosocial development of every child and the social determinants of health.
- Improving health education to empower children to make informed choices about healthy lifestyles.
- Consulting and involving children and, where appropriate, their families, in the planning, assessment and improvement of health care services.
- Improving the infant mortality rates according to national goals, in order to achieve the United Nations Millennium Development Goal No 4 by 2015.
- Identifying and sharing good professional practices, research, policies and strategies focused on children's health and well-being, in partnership with other relevant stakeholders.
- Facilitating the development of appropriate practical tools for health practitioners to implement the child-friendly health care approach.

Source: Dr Simon Lenton (Council of Europe, 2011; http://www.cfhiuk.org).

illustrated in Figure 11.2 practice is contingent on service planning and policy, and all interact and depend upon each other.

Practice

Primary and first-contact care

The philosophy of primary care inherently suits children and families, and the ease of access is helpful too. However, there are difficulties in ensuring that there are sufficiently expert professional skills available at the first point of contact, while maintaining the family and person-centred approach of primary care. The tensions between generalism and specialism, and between access and expertise, have been referred to many times throughout this book. There is no simple 'one size fits all' solution to these problems. The debate about the best first-contact care model could start by asking the question: which services really need to be delivered in a hospital, and which do not? Hospitals are needed to provide safe care for children who are seriously ill, and for whom medical technology (such as ventilators) may be needed. Children with very rare diseases may also need hospital clinic appointments because providing community-based access to services for very few children may not be sustainable economically or enable maintenance of specialized clinical skills. However, hospitals are not needed to provide care for children with minor or common conditions, where sophisticated technology is not required, and where local access is an advantage.

Primary care is at the core of children's health care. A renewed focus on primary care and designing a team of professionals that achieves an optimal balance between access and expertise for medical, mental health, social care, and other specialties, should enable the majority of children's health needs to be managed in primary care settings.

The chronic care model

A comprehensive chronic care model is crucial to improving prevention and care of chronic conditions in children and young people. Such a model should incorporate the elements of medical, psychological, nursing, social, educational and other aspects of care for children with NCDs, together with wider policy actions to reduce risk and enhance resilience and quality of life. This sort of holistic comprehensive chronic care model is described by the philosophy of primary care, and of course, developing an effective chronic care model and improving first-contact care for children are closely related. Problems in one area worsen those in the other; for example, if acute services are excessively and inappropriately taken up with minor illness, there is inadequate resource available for chronic care services. And, because first-contact care often functions as gatekeeper to the rest of the health care system, a bottleneck results. Solving problems in first-contact care and gatekeeping will allow more time and resource for planned team-based care. Other services, such as mental health and transitioning to adult care, benefit in similar ways. A great deal of progress in child health care hinges on resolving the problems in everyday paediatric practice. There are immediate steps necessary to address the deficiencies we have described in this book, involving service reconfiguration and workforce, information technology and payment systems. Moreover, there are more distal policy actions that would enable these changes to occur.

Public health

The upstream determinants of health have a direct effect on downstream health services. Thus, the traditional dichotomy separating health services for the individual child from the population-focused child public health service is increasingly outdated. After all, a population is a group of individuals. Health care and public health are part of a continuum and each is necessary for the other to produce and promote health in individuals and in populations. Public health policies and services can work, for example, to promote health through education and action on social determinants. Clinicians provide health services in response to established disease, but they also deliver primary prevention, such as screening; secondary prevention by treating complications; and tertiary prevention, for example, by maximizing quality of life in palliative care. Health services are an important determinant of health in children and young people. The health care part of public health, where it exists, can help improve the effectiveness of health care through planning, procuring and evaluating services. Health care public health (HCPH) is about assessing children's needs, and ensuring services are in place to meet those requirement, and to help improve quality and equity of care. Children's HCPH is an underdeveloped field, yet has much to offer in a comprehensive strategy to improve children's health and health services.

Integrating services

Service integration is a key policy driver in some European countries. Integration takes two broad forms, each relevant to the problems described in child health services. Vertical integration combines services that traditionally operate in a hierarchical model, for example, by integrating primary and secondary care to achieve a better balance between access and expertise. Horizontal integration across sectors, such as health and social care, is a particularly important goal for population groups with specific needs. These include: children with long-term conditions; children with mental health problems; vulnerable groups such as children who are neglected or abused; school-age children; adolescents and young adults. Integration is also needed at the transition between children's and adults' health services representing a longitudinal dimension to integration. Continuity of care and consistency of communication are especially important to children with chronic conditions and, by ensuring these aspects of care, integrated services can help to empower families and provide a more responsive service.

Although effective integration is a common goal, all countries have struggled to achieve progress. Notable examples were discussed in Chapter 3, and a review of barriers and possible solutions is presented here in Table 11.1.

Table 11.1 Barriers and potential solutions to achieving service integration

Barriers to successful integration of health care systems, and how these might manifest in practice	• Professional self-interest: 'It's my turf.' • Organizational culture, competing values: 'Acute care takes precedence.' • Lack of trust: 'You want to take over my service?' • Fragmented services: 'I work here and you work there; our clinics are on different days, and I can't email you from this system.' • Lack of clarity about professional roles: 'It's not my job.' • Inadequate information available to plan services appropriately: 'Wrong solution for wrong problem.' • Separate, often competing, funding mechanisms for different services, such as hospital community, primary care: 'Preventing admissions prevents me earning money.'
Potential solutions	• Strong leadership to articulate shared vision. • Opportunities, resources and rewards for learning and working together. • Bringing together organizations and services into a system through merger or contract to ensure professionals work together in the common interest of patients. • Organizational structures that are more responsive to patients' needs, for example, 'flatter' structures rather than traditional hierarchical arrangements, to use the skills and insights of staff at all levels. • Financial incentives to improve recruitment, retention and quality of working life for staff entering new integrated systems. • Co-location. • Disease management programmes. • Use of electronic information systems to facilitate rapid communication between team members. • Frequent team meetings. • Invest in data collection and analysis and harmonizing information systems. • Stable defined population denominators for reliable needs assessments and service planning. • Mechanisms for pooling funds or aligning financing across services and sectors.

Source: Wolfe et al., 2013

Workforce

To achieve many of the changes necessary in order to refocus children's health services and systems better to meet current and evolving needs and expectations, a comprehensive re-examination of the child health workforce is required. At present, there is a lack of comparable data on child health care professionals in Europe, and available data are of limited value, for example, because the nuances of category definition make interpretation challenging. There is neither reliable evidence nor guidance on safe numbers of staff for a given population size or need and, in many instances, training programmes lack evidence to substantiate their systems. Moreover, in some services, such as child and adolescent mental health care, there is enormous variability between countries regarding which professionals are responsible, and in what ways, suggesting a lack of evidence or agreement about competency standards. In financially challenging times, country paediatric, general practice, and family medicine associations may need to justify why a longer training programme is better than a shorter one, or whether service requirements while training are a justifiable use of workforce.

An international commission on education of health professionals recommended that comprehensive educational reforms are needed to drive improvements in health systems. In order to provide universal access to high-quality comprehensive health care for children and to work towards equity in health, health professionals need to go beyond the acquisition of skills and knowledge and develop the ability to mobilize knowledge, reason critically and participate as members of teams that are fully engaged in health systems (Frenk et al., 2010).

Plans

Health services are planned in different ways in each health system, which in turn are shaped by historical and cultural influences. However, no country plans children's health services in rational ways that are based on a comprehensive assessment of population health needs. One reason is the lack of public health resources. The current way of planning services creates a mismatch between need and provision that was discussed in a previous section. But there are other unintended consequences. Children and their parents frequently fail to use services as intended by those who designed them. For example, perceived difficulties in accessing urgent services, together with expectations of rapid access to specialist expertise, have led parents in many countries to seek care directly from emergency departments. Yet, too many emergency departments still do not have facilities appropriate for the needs of children and young people, and inexperienced junior staff may admit too many children to inpatient wards. The situation is made worse by shortages in the children's nursing workforce in many countries, which impairs early hospital discharge and ambulatory management of children with long-term conditions near to their homes. These problems arise partly because, in many countries, there is a gap in skills, confidence and capacity between primary (generalist) and secondary (specialist) paediatric (including mental health) services, which leads to children with urgent care needs being referred between services, often without having their needs met satisfactorily by either. This problem is known as failure demand, when parents seek health care for children and, after failing to find what they are looking for, repeat the process until the desired outcome is reached.

Poorly planned services also affect families of children with chronic disease or complex conditions; they may report unsatisfactory care experiences, for example, with multiple appointments in different locations on different days, inadequate communication between professionals, and inadequate transition to adult care.

There are complex reasons underlying the continuing rise in health service demand, including changing social expectations and increasing parental anxiety, but one important reason is the way in which health services are planned and commissioned. There are consequences beyond the inefficient use of services and frustrating experience for families. As comparative health systems performance analysis has developed, quality of care has become one of the most prominent drivers of health system reform. Two seminal publications moved the quality improvement goal forward: the WHO *World Health Report 2000*, which ranked country performance (WHO, 2000), and *Crossing the Quality Chasm*, published by the US Institute of Medicine in 2001 (Institute of Medicine, 2001).

For all these reasons, it is clear that health services and public health are interdependent. A public health service with a geographically defined population should be able to: provide population-level data; determine health and health service needs; know how many vulnerable children are in the area and where they are from; anticipate trends in health and needs; and shape services along the entire spectrum from prevention to palliation, thereby meeting children's health needs and contributing directly to improving their health.

Health services, health systems and policy research

Basic science, preclinical research and clinical trials help us to develop better medicines and procedures. What we lack is detailed understanding about how to deliver those interventions to optimal effect. Applied health services research for children is a relatively new field. There is growing recognition that we need a deeper understanding of the conditions within which a health system operates, defining the factors that promote improvement in child health, and understanding how to drive improvements in quality of care and health outcomes.

Health systems and policy research (HSPR) is a transdisciplinary research field defining new methods and standards for evaluating evidence and producing recommendations that are useful for policy-makers and practitioners. Existing recommendations are often based 'on the best available knowledge' (Ghaffar et al., 2013). Yet, if it is a relatively new field in adult health care, it has barely begun for children's health services. And, just as in other areas of medicine, learning from adult medicine does not always apply to children.

Children's medicine traditionally was a subset of adult health care, when children were thought of as little more than small adults, and beds and drug doses alike were decreased proportionately to their size. Then aspirin, widely used in adults, was found to be associated with Reye's syndrome in children. And chloramphenicol, safe in adults, was found to be dangerous for babies who could not metabolize it. High concentrations of oxygen, used in adults with acute respiratory failure, caused blindness in premature babies. There are numerous examples where a failure to appreciate that children have different physiology from adults has led to harm. For example, the evidence base for child-specific treatment is still lacking in many areas, for example, in medicines prescribing (see Chapter 10).

In the decade since the 2000 *World Health Report* ranked country performance, interest has grown in comparative health systems analysis. Rankings of countries can be powerful political tools for change. The essential question is: what is the scope for health care to improve health for children? Comparative health systems performance, although criticized as simplistic (particularly by countries that perform poorly), can be helpful, showing not just who is better and who is worse, but what may be possible. It can point towards where the problems may lie, and it gives us an idea of what we can aspire to achieve.

One tool for comparing performance is avoidable mortality, defined as deaths that should not occur in the presence of effective and timely health care (Rutstein et al., 1976). Deaths from these conditions can be used as sentinel events, or markers of the quality of care. There are, of course, many contributing factors influencing health outcomes, but for these carefully selected conditions, medical care is central. Take, for example, a child with asthma who dies from an acute exacerbation. Medical care is responsible for secondary prevention (such as a written asthma treatment plan, use of steroid inhalers and trigger avoidance) and for treatment of the acute episode. But who is responsible for the parents who smoke; for particulate air pollution in the neighbourhood; for vehicle emissions surrounding the school? The answers are complex, and include tobacco manufacturers and advertisers, national and European legislation on tobacco control, air quality regulations, vehicle emissions legislation, local authority planning regulations, and so on. The common outcome is a child with asthma, the responsibility of a medical team, who can take a leadership role in advocating change in the distal determinants of this child's problems. There is strong policy interest across Europe now in avoidable mortality (Nolte and McKee, 2004), and attention is beginning to shift towards children's services.

Avoidable mortality can indicate the existence of a possible problem, but further research is usually required to understand it and what the solutions might be. Hansen et al. (2011) describe priority areas for research on health care organizations and service delivery:

- intra- and interorganizational, such as developing and testing integrated care models;
- supraorganizational, such as describing the inequalities in distribution of services;

- patient relations, for example, how to better balance needs and demands for care; and
- governance and accountability: how to assess and improve quality, and how to balance efficiency and quality.

Indicators of health and health service performance

Europe offers a remarkable natural laboratory, given the diverse policies pursued in each country, and even within countries. However, this can only be exploited with comparable data on morbidity, mortality, and a comprehensive set of indicators for measuring the effects of policy and multiple dimensions of health care quality, including structural or systems measures, process and outcome measures. Comprehensive and reliable comparable Europe-wide child health indicators would significantly enhance research capability and progress in European child health.

Currently, however, the best available comparative data are limited to mortality, a crude and incomplete measure of health, and selected measures of preventive services. Although some indicators are widely available, such as immunization coverage, which is included in the OECD's 'Healthcare Quality Indicator Project' (Arah et al., 2006) and WHO's European 'Health for All' database (WHO Regional Office for Europe, 2012), even this is fraught with problems of comparability, with many countries extracting the data from systems designed to manage immunization programmes, thus tracking uptake in real time, but others, such as Germany, only collecting data at school entry.

There are, however, a few exceptions to the generally dismal coverage of child health data in Europe, such as in the Nordic countries, which have created comprehensive registers with unique personal identifiers allowing linkage across sectors. This has enabled them to remain at the forefront of child health research and policy across Europe. The Nordic model could be replicated elsewhere if there were the political will to do so. However, attempts are often impeded by over-zealous interpretation of European data protection legislation which, although harmonized in a European Union Directive designed to enable cross-border data sharing, is often interpreted more narrowly, even though this means the services that can be provided for children will be suboptimal, with adverse consequences for their health and well-being.

There are a number of European initiatives designed to address these weaknesses. Thus, the European Collaboration for Healthcare Optimization (ECHO) project seeks to facilitate health system comparisons using hospital databases but, of course, this only captures a fraction of the care received by children (ECHO, 2012). There are also some discrete research projects, such as CHILD, which has identified key child health indicators covering the life-course as well as aspects of primary, secondary and tertiary prevention and policy (Rigby et al., 2003). The European Community Health Indicators (ECHI) project includes some indicators that are relevant to child health (European Commission, 2013) but again is constrained by what is collected nationally, using definitions that are not always comparable. There are also a number of Europe-wide surveys relevant to child health. These include the

HBSC surveys and PERISTAT reports on perinatal outcomes (Europeristat, 2013; HBSC, 2013). Finally, the EU has agreed a selection of structural indicators, including access to care for vulnerable children such as asylum-seekers, and indicators for the protection and promotion of child rights (European Union Agency for Fundamental Rights, 2010). However, despite all this activity, there is still remarkably little comparable information on health services for children, and particularly primary and secondary care. Progress has been made at country level, such as developing measures designed to monitor quality in primary care; for example, in Italy, frequency and choice of antibiotic use has been used as an indicator of quality of paediatric care and professional continuing education (Marchetti et al., 2005). Other examples of primary care quality indicators are discussed in Chapter 2.

A compendium of child health measures and indicators makes a good start (RICHE, 2012); however, establishing a comprehensive set of child health indicators across Europe, based on comparable national information systems, would allow comparison of the quality of health services for children across Europe. This would greatly facilitate efforts to improve services.

Future challenges include devising indicators of positive conditions of child health – salutogenesis, rather than health deficits – and developing indicators for the management of complex conditions, such as neurodisability, which must take into account, for instance, the fact that children with such conditions require interventions of many types from many different professions and organizations. The challenges of developing measures that are sufficiently sophisticated to reflect all these contributions are formidable. Other challenges relate to measures of quality of services provided to vulnerable children and young people, such as those who have been maltreated, have mental illness or disabilities, or live in the care of the State.

Preparing for the future

The development of child health strategies should be based on understanding the past and foreseeing the future. Describing trends in health needs is crucial for developing effective policies, including prioritizing investments. While research can provide accurate information on current health status and risk factors (Murray et al., 2012; Vos et al., 2012), projections into the future are much more difficult, due to complex multifactorial causal pathways. Child health experts should work with experts in other disciplines in building future scenarios of child health to enable far-sighted policy-making. Credible exercises to develop scenarios in health should take into account: temporal trends in health status; new knowledge about causality; technological developments relevant to health; trends in the most important determinants of health; and, last but not least, policy developments in health, and across all sectors, at both national and multinational levels.

Current trends show increases in risk conditions (such as premature birth, low birth weight, obesity and unhealthy lifestyles) and in chronic conditions (such as mental health disorders, cancer and NCDs) (Cattaneo et al., 2012). Preventing NCDs has already been identified as a major goal of all health systems, but there is still insufficient awareness of the most recent research on early onset of NCDs and gene–environment interactions. There is great, and as yet unexploited, potential for early prevention from conception to the first years of life and such a prevention approach should become a more prominent feature of European health policies and strategies as technological advances like genomic medicine are unlikely to be sufficient on their own to address the many lifestyle-related chronic illnesses in children, such as obesity, hypertension and dyslipidaemia. Similarly, very expensive new biological drugs are likely to be available to only part of the population. Developments in communications and technology, and access to social networks, will play a greater role in influencing lifestyles, but may also be the cause of new psychosocial threats.

Finally, the continuing economic crisis means that the proportion of children living in poor families is likely to increase (Tamburlini, 2011), with poverty especially great among children from migrant families. Increasing use of alcohol and drugs, and unhealthy lifestyles, will also be likely as a consequence of continuing uncertainty about the future. Increasingly restrictive migration and welfare policies will pose further challenges, while failing to address unmet gender and civil rights issues in many countries.

For these reasons, it cannot be assumed that European children will continue to improve their health status, and current inequities may become deeper. New investments and specific targeted measures are needed to protect children's health and to ensure the future health and security of the whole population. Exercises to explore future scenarios that go well beyond the child health arena should be conducted. The establishment of a European regional mechanism to facilitate access to current databases and surveys, and to promote more uniform data collection methods, would provide invaluable input to health-related policies in the future.

Policy

Despite technological advances that allow improved preventive, diagnostic and curative care for parents and children, the outlook for child health in Europe is uncertain. Further progress may be hampered by policy gaps in addressing key social determinants. Devising policy for improving child health in Europe will require a multidimensional approach, as illustrated in Figure 11.3.

Health in all policies

Within public policies, health systems have a unique, although not exclusive, role in preventing exposure to health risks, and ensuring effective and equitable care. Exposure to risk factors can be modified by public policies, interventions, and in most cases by individual actions. Child health is determined by a balance of risk and protective factors, as illustrated in Figure 5.1, and the likelihood of exposure to risk factors depends on the conditions in which children are

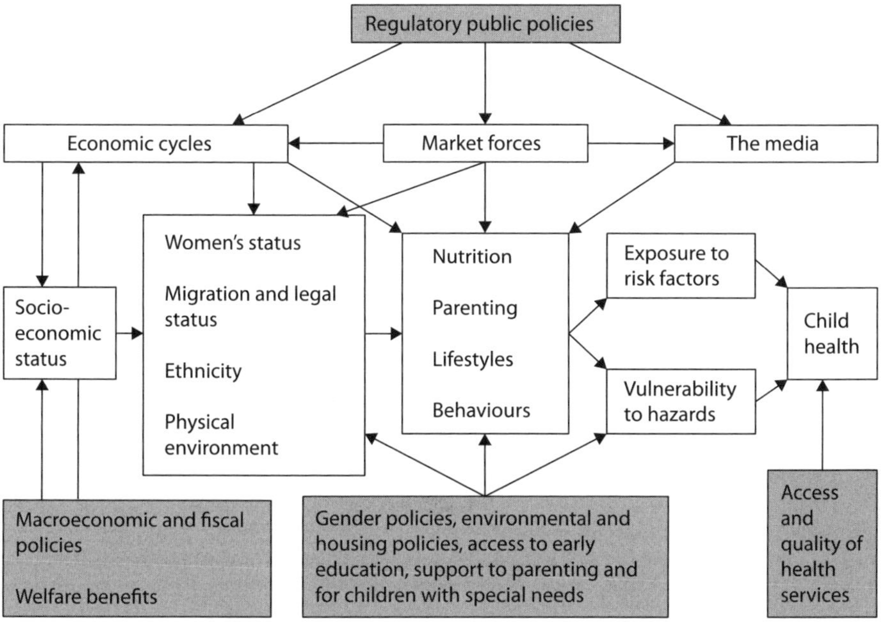

Figure 11.3 A comprehensive approach to addressing determinants of child health through policy

Source: authors' own (GT)

conceived, and in which they grow and live, as well as on a wide range of material, psychosocial, environmental and behavioural underlying factors. Risk factors and the social determinants that underlie them can only be addressed with a comprehensive, integrated and sustained policy response. In most cases, it will also require commitment from government in collaboration with civil society, local communities, the private sector and international institutions and agencies.

Evidence-based policy

Enhancing the knowledge base around child health policy would be enormously facilitated by a mechanism for improving European regional and country-level child health information. A concerted effort is needed to develop a research capacity in child health services, systems and policy research. Knowledge-brokering is especially lacking in child health policy and is urgently needed. There are numerous examples of research not being translated to policy and of policy-makers not having the evidence they require. Experiences of knowledge-brokering in the adult policy world should extend to child health.

Accountability

Accountability should ensure that the voices of children are heard effectively and that policy-makers fulfil their commitments. However, accountability is frequently promised but rarely delivered. Accountability can be realized through a framework of monitoring, reviewing and remedying processes. Oversight mechanisms for child health services should be put into place, and when problems are detected, action plans should be devised that address them. Countries could identify indicators for child health services that are contextually appropriate, and create a monitoring organization with responsibility for collecting and analysing data. A child health oversight committee could report either to the executive (ministers) or the legislature (parliament) and make recommendations for remedial action.

Commitment

A great deal is known about what could, and should, be done to improve children's health. What is lacking is sustained political will. Policy-makers must be prepared to translate into policies the increasing evidence that effective interventions early in life help build the foundations of lifelong health. Policy-making should reflect our commitments to the United Nations 'Convention on the Rights of the Child'. National and European governing bodies must demonstrate their obligation to improving child health in order to provide a secure future for us all.

Putting it all together

We have described a framework for a child health strategy in Europe, and the underlying social values of such a strategy. There is sufficient detailed knowledge about effective policies for improving health and reducing social inequalities to prompt the question: why has more progress not been made? Why do we, as a society, as child health professionals and policy-makers, and as parents, tolerate the poverty, deprivation and neglect of children that exist in otherwise relatively prosperous and thriving countries? We know that early investment is key to shaping the life chances of children, yet most health systems invest disproportionately in reactive services rather than preventive care; in medicine rather than health promotion; and in youth offender services rather than in building social resilience. Although there are many research questions in child health that need to be addressed, the immediate problem is the failure to translate the available evidence into policy, and then into measurable health gain.

The monumental scale of the task at hand will require effective advocacy. Abraham Jacobi, acknowledged as the founder of paediatrics in the United States, argued for improving the living conditions and medical care of children as a matter of social justice. Dr Jacobi's argument remains valid today.

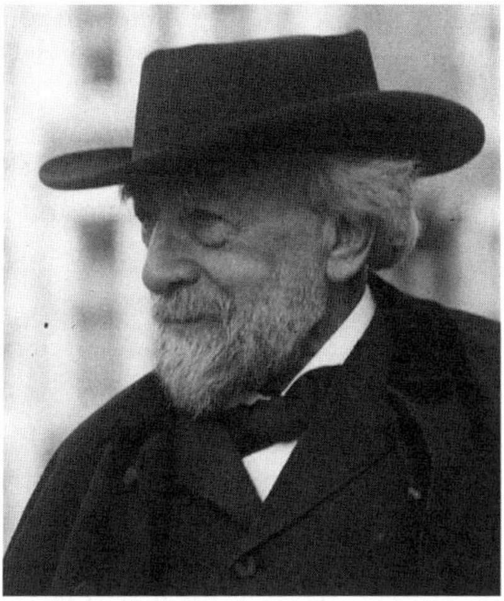

Dr Abraham Jacobi 1830–1919

A 'respectable rebel'. Founder of paediatrics in the United States as a medical specialty and academic discipline. He set up the first children's outpatients clinic in 1874, and the first hospital department of paediatrics; opened the first free clinic for children; and introduced bedside teaching and clinical teaching rounds. He was Clinical Professor of Diseases of Children at New York University in 1865 and Professor of Clinical Pediatrics at Columbia University in 1870.

Conclusions

European health systems are beginning to engage in attempts to adapt health services to meet the evolving health needs of their populations more effectively and efficiently. However, currently they tend to focus more on elderly people than the young, despite increasing evidence that the foundation of health over the life-course is built in the first years of life, from conception through adolescence. Although great gains have been made in improving child health and, on average, European children are enjoying unprecedentedly high standards of health and health care, the remaining challenges, in terms of both emerging health needs and risk factors, and of equitable distribution of the benefits to all children, are significant. Complex solutions will be needed for increasingly complicated problems in the health and lives of children. However, the present crisis of confidence and of financial means may contain the seeds of change and innovative solutions (Holland and Stewart, 1998). The current debate about child health and child health services indicates that there are reasons to be hopeful that child health services and societal policies will improve their ability to meet children's needs.

Child health is about early interventions, health promotion and prevention; and about social justice and protecting the vulnerable. It is also about fostering our futures. Providing universal opportunities for health and development, or universal health access,that goes beyond the goals of universal health coverage to address the social determinants of health, means adopting a more equity-based focus for improving child health. Such an approach should be underpinned by coherent intersectoral policies in order to be maximally effective in meeting children's evolving health and development needs. This will require political will at the highest levels.

The challenge for child health in the 21st century is to develop health systems and cross-cutting health policies that are more responsive to child and family health needs. This will be crucial to shape, promote and protect this generation and the next.

Acknowledgement

We are grateful to Professor Neal Halfon (Director Professor, David Geffen School of Medicine UCLA, Department of Paediatrics, Professor, UCLA Fielding School of Public Health, Department of Health Services and Luskin School of Public Affairs, Department of Public Policy, for comment and advice, and to Dr Simon Lenton for providing information on child-friendly health care, and Professor Staffan Janson for education on civil rights.

References

Arah, O.A. et al. (2006) A conceptual framework for the OECD Health Care Quality Indicators Project, *International Journal for Quality in Health Care*, 18(Suppl 1): 5–13.

Cattaneo, A. et al. (2012) *Child Health in the European Union*. Luxembourg: European Commission.

Council of Europe (2011) *Guidelines on child-friendly health care*. https://wcd.coe.int/ViewDoc.jsp?id=1836421andSite=COE (accessed 9 March 2013).

de Savigny, D. and Adam, T. (eds) (2009) *Systems thinking for health systems strengthening*. Geneva: Alliance for Health Policy and Systems Research.

Department of Health (2004) *National Service Framework for Children, Young People, and Maternity Services*. London: Department of Health.

ECHO (2012) *What is the ECHO project?* http://www.echo-health.eu [accessed 24 June 2013].

European Commission (2013) *European Community health indicators (ECHI)*. http://ec.europa.eu/health/indicators/echi/index_en.htm [accessed 24 June 2013].

European Union Agency for Fundamental Rights (2010) *Developing indicators for the protection, respect and promotion of the rights of the child in the European Union*. http://fra.europa.eu/en/publication/2012/developing-indicators-protection-respect-and-promotion-rights-child-european-union [accessed 24 June 2013].

Europeristat (2013) http://www.europeristat.com [accessed 24 June 2013].

Frenk, J. et al. (2010) Health professionals for a new century: transforming education to strengthen health systems in an interdependent world, *The Lancet*, 376(9756): 1923–58.

Ghaffar A, et al. (2013) Changing mindsets in health policy and systems research. *Lancet*, 381: 436–7.

Hansen, J. et al. (2011) European priorities for research on health care organizations and service delivery, *Journal of Health Services Research and Policy*, 16(Suppl 2): 16–26.

HBSC (2013) *Health Behaviour in School-Aged Children*. http://www.hbsc.org [accessed 24 June 2013].

Holland, W.W. and Stewart, S. (1998) *Public health: the vision and the challenge.* London: Nuffield Trust.
Institute of Medicine (2001) *Crossing the quality chasm: a new health system for the 21st century*. Washington, DC: National Academy Press.
Kilkelly, U. (2011) *Child-friendly health care: the views and experience of children and young people in Council of Europe member States*. Strasbourg: Council Of Europe.
Marchetti, F. et al. (2005) Delayed prescription may reduce the use of antibiotics for acute otitis media: a prospective observational study in primary care, *Archives of Pediatrics and Adolescent Medicine*, 159(7): 679–84.
Modi, N. et al. (2013) A healthy nation: strengthening child health research in the UK, *The Lancet*, 381(9860): 73–87.
Murray, C.J. et al. (2012) Disability-adjusted life years (DALYs) for 291 diseases and injuries in 21 regions, 1990–2010: a systematic analysis for the Global Burden of Disease Study 2010, *The Lancet*, 380(9859): 2197–223.
Murray, C.J.L. and Evans, D.B. (2003) *Health systems performance assessment: Debates, methods and empiricism*. Geneva: World Health Organization.
Nolte, E. and McKee, M. (2004) *Does health care save lives? Avoidable mortality revisited.* London: Nuffield Trust.
RICHE (2012) *Research Inventory for Child Health in Europe*. http://www.childhealthresearch.eu [accessed 24 June 2013].
Rigby, M.J. et al. (2003) Child health indicators for Europe: a priority for a caring society, *European Journal of Public Health*, 13: 38–46.
Rutstein, D.D. et al. (1976) Measuring the quality of medical care. A clinical method, *New England Journal of Medicine*, 294(11): 582–8.
Tamburlini, G. (2011) Economic crisis and child health, *Medico and Bambino*, 30.
Vos, T. et al. (2012) Years lived with disability (YLDs) for 1160 sequelae of 289 diseases and injuries 1990–2010: a systematic analysis for the Global Burden of Disease Study 2010, *The Lancet*, 380(9859): 2163–96.
WHO (1981) *Global strategy for health for all by the year 2000*. Geneva: World Health Organization.
WHO (2000) *World Health Report 2000: Health systems: improving performance.* Geneva: World Health Organization.
WHO (2002) *World Health Survey 2002, WHO Evidence and Information for Policy*. http://www.who.int/healthinfo/survey/whslongindividuala.pdf [accessed 24 June 2013].
WHO (2008) *World Health Report 2008. Primary health care: now more than ever.* Geneva: World Health Organization.
WHO Regional Office for Europe (2012) *European Health for All Database (HFA-DB)*. http://www.euro.who.int/en/what-we-do/data-and-evidence/databases/european-health-for-all-database-hfa-db2 [accessed 23 June 2013].
Wolfe, I. et al. (2011) Improving child health services in the UK: insights from Europe and their implications for the NHS reforms, *BMJ*, 342: d1277.
Wolfe, I. et al. (2013) Health services for children in western Europe, *The Lancet*, 381(9873): 1224–34.

Index